Interpreting Signs of Illness

Approaches to Semiotics
72

Mouton de Gruyter
Berlin · New York · Amsterdam

Interpreting Signs of Illness

A Case Study in Medical Semiotics

Kathryn Vance Staiano

Mouton de Gruyter
Berlin · New York · Amsterdam

Mouton de Gruyter (formerly Mouton, The Hague)
is a Division of Walter de Gruyter & Co., Berlin.

Library of Congress Cataloging in Publication Data

Staiano, Kathryn Vance, 1940–
Interpreting signs of illness.
(Approaches to semiotics ; 72)
Bibliography: p.
Includes index.
1. Black Carib Indians–Medicine. 2. Indians of Central America–Belize–Medicine. 3. Medical anthropology–Case studies. 4. Semiotics. I. Title. II. Series. [DNLM: 1. Attitude to Health. 2. Ethnopsychology. 3. Medicine, Traditional–Central America. 4. Symbolism (Psychology).
W1 AP535 v.72 / WB 50 DA3 S71]
F1505.2.C3S73 1986 306'.46 85-29337
ISBN 0-89925-155-2 (alk. paper)

CIP-Kurztitelaufnahme der Deutschen Bibliothek

Staiano, Kathryn Vance:
Interpreting signs of illness: a case study in medical semiotics / Kathryn Vance Staiano. – Berlin ; New York ; Amsterdam : Mouton de Gruyter, 1986.
(Approaches to semiotics ; 72)
ISBN 3-11-010361-3
NE: GT

Printed on acid free paper.

Typesetting: Asian Research Service, Hong Kong. – Printing: Druckerei Gerike GmbH, Berlin. – Binding: Dieter Mikolai, Berlin. Printed in Germany.

Dedicated to the memory of my mother
Ann Marie Hammer Smith

Contents

Acknowledgements

Part of the research for this book was funded by a doctoral fellowship from the Social Science Research Council. I am much indebted to the guidance of John Janzen who served as my advisor at the University of Kansas and Thomas Sebeok who has provided me with much advice and support over a period of many years. I would also like to thank Charles Gullick, Christian Guksch, and Allan Hanson who reviewed and commented on portions of the manuscript, and Marilyn Wells, Joseph Palacio, and Jon Schacht, who provided me with additional information on the Garinagu and Maya. I would also like to offer my appreciation to Liess Vantine for his assistance with phonetic transcriptions of certain Garifuna terms.

I owe my greatest debt to the people of Punta Gorda who made this book possible. In particular, I would like to thank Mr. John Zuniga, Mr. Justin Benguche, Mrs. Nunez, and Mr. Alceito Reyes, without whom this could never have been, Mr. Peter Benguche, who was kind, helpful, and always a good friend, Viola and Domingo who 'adopted' me as their mother, Elswith and Jim Porter, who accepted me as I am and always had a cold beer ready, Mr. Vincent Martinez and his wife who tried very hard to teach me Garifuna, Boniface Martinez, who is always cheerful in the face of adversity, Mrs. Catrina Lino and her children who saw to it I was well fed, Mrs. Presciliana Ordonez and her family who were friends and helpers, Mrs. Frances Gonzalez, Mr. Joseph Claro Villafranco, and Mr. Sam Vernon, who were always patient with my questions, Mr. Alex Chee and his family who provided me with shelter and friendship, Lottie Evans, who was always a help when I was working and when I wasn't, Gene West, who was a great neighbor, the staff of the hospital, who seemed not to mind that I was always in the way, and all the others who made me feel then and now that Punta Gorda is my home.

Finally, I would like to express my appreciation to and respect for Eugen Baer who has helped me find my way along this strange path called semiotics.

Preface

This is a book about the medical beliefs and practices of a people known variously as the Black Caribs, Caribs, Garif, Garifuna, or Garinagu. The Garinagu, as they prefer to be known, are scattered along the Caribbean coast of Central America from Belize to Nicaragua. The data offered here are derived from fieldwork conducted among the Garinagu of Punta Gorda in the country of Belize. Generalizations to other Garinagu in other communities must be undertaken with caution, for the Garinagu are an independent and clever people who have always exhibited the wisdom and ingenuity to alter the contours of critical cultural paradigms in the face of changing environments and new opportunities.

This study is also an exploration into the processes of communication, interpretation, and negotiation. It is, as well, an examination of the manner in which signs of health and illness serve as metaphors, functioning to represent an object, event, or relationship whose association to the sign itself is never obvious, or as metonyms, acting to 'stand for' some greater whole. The Garinagu do not live in isolation from other ethnic groups, nor have they been exempt from the transformations brought by the introduction of Western or bio-medicine. This study, therefore, describes conflict and competition among biomedical, ethnomedical, and sacred medical paradigms, but a story of co-existence, co-optation, and, in limited ways, cooperation emerges as well.

The analytic framework employed is semiotic. Semiotic, or, more commonly, semiotics, which differs from the traditions of semiology or semeiology, is derived from the work of the American philosopher, Charles Sanders Peirce (1839-1914). Semiotics is most frequently defined as the study or science of signs (or signs systems or sign functions). Despite the fact that the concept of interpretation of signs of illness (*semeiotike*) is at least as ancient as Greek medicine, the characteristics and boundaries of a semiotic have never been fully defined. Semiotics has been described as a theory (Eco 1976, Singer 1984), a model (Bouissac 1976), a system of significations (Greimas and Courtés 1982), a doctrine (Sebeok 1976, Deely, 1982), an approach (implying a methodology; see Baer 1975; Staiano 1979b), a body of ideas and techniques (MacCannell and MacCannell 1982), a discipline, a dimension, an endeavor, a perspective, a mode of reasoning, and so on. Whenever individuals and institutions deal with interpretive processes and undertake to examine the physiological, genetic, cultural, technological, and other codes which govern interpretive processes, they function as semioticians, whatever they call their enterprise or however they define it.

It is not my intention here to attempt to sort out these various descriptors and their possible significations, nor to delineate the present position of semiotics within all the sciences and humanities. My purpose is rather a more modest one: to describe the possible form and content of an explicitly medical semiotics (see also Sebeok 1983, Von Uexküll 1982, Baer 1982MS, Kahn 1978, Staiano 1979a, 1982). To this end, I have attempted to apply certain semiotic assumptions or perspectives to ethnographic data, to examine the relationship of interpretive activities to other experiential domains within a single ethnic collectivity, to evaluate the effects of access to alternative therapeutic resources on health-seeking behaviors, and to take up the subject of control over medical resources as a product of a broader system of social, spiritual, political, and economic relationships. In order to begin this task, it is necessary to describe those assumptions about culture, reality, and signs which are inherent to the semiotic enterprise.

1. Life is ordered by signs; that is, we structure and interpret our experiences according to pre-existing sets of signs or notions about the relations among signs.
2. Reciprocally, signs are ordered by life, that is, experience of the 'real world' contributes to the creation or production and ordering of signs.
3. We manipulate through signs and are, in turn, manipulated by them.
4. We communicate through signs and only through signs is communication accomplished.
5. The notion of communication is extended here to include that dialogue which one carries on with oneself, often referred to as 'inner speech." It includes as well the transmission and transformation of neural or physiological information.
6. To explain *culture* means to describe how signs are linked to their significations, how they are related syntagmatically and paradigmatically to one another, and the manner in which they are employed by social beings in specific social contexts.
7. We think with signs and every thought is itself as *interpretant* which is itself another signs. That is, no sign is ever completed, except through reference to another sign, or, in other words, no sign can be completed. This refers as well to signs generated at the physiological or biological level.

Guiraud (1975) describes the continuous unification of sign and signification:

At the beginning of Madame Bovary, Flaubert describes his hero's monstrous cap; he does so by means of words, and these words could be transcribed by an illustrator into a picture made of lines and colors. Words and picture are signs the meaning of which is this cap. But the cap in turn has a meaning; it is the sign of Charles' clumsiness, his lack of taste, his gaucheness in his relation with his friends.

The cap is thus both the signified meaning and the signifying sign. But the meaning does not stop there: Charles' clumsiness is the sign of his relations with Emma; his relations with Emma are the sign of a certain form of marriage; which in turn is the sign of a cultural situation, etc.

The meaning is a relation, and this relation envelops each meaning in a new meaning.

> Thus if semiology is to be the science of signs it encompasses all knowledge and all experience, for everything is a sign. everything is signified and everything is signifier (40).

This study is an exploration into this continuous union of sign and that for which it stands, or in Peircian terms, into the construction of the sign through the unity of object, representamen, and interpretant, and the ramifications of this semiosic process in relation to that event called illness.

What is the value of a semiotic framework in the analysis of illness epiodes? Deely (1982) argues that semiotics provides for the restoration of unity in traditions of thought; it offers a perspective which crosses the usual academic boundaries "simply by virture of the universal role of signs as the vehicle of communication within and between specialities...." (xiv). A semiotic anthropology is necessarily a pragmatic anthropology, for "It contains a theory of how systems of signs are related to their meanings, as well as to the objects designated, and to the experience and behavior of the sign users" (Singer 1984: 50). Semiotics allows us to examine the phenomena of communication and transformation without the use of an altogether new language to discuss these events at the physiological, ideological, and behavioral levels. This subject is taken up again in Chapter One.

The sign, from the Peircian perspective, is not static, an object with assigned or inherent significance, but a dynamic process referred to as semiosis. The unification of the thing or event or idea for which the sign stands (its object), the sign itself (or representamen in Peirce's schema, or signifier or signifying object) and the interpretant, which is variously defined as an interpretation, a thought or idea, an impression, a reaction or response, a signification, and so on, is an event without beginning and end. Man himself is seen by Peirce as a sign, or rather a continuous sign process. The tripartite sign of the Peircian tradition is conceptually more complex, but analytically more productive from my perspective than the bi-facial sign of the semiological tradition which treats the sign as composed of a signifying object or sound and the object or idea or event for which it stands.

Following Morris (1971), I have divided semiotic into three branches: syntactics, semantics, and pragmatics. Because of the obvious implications for a medical semiotic, those concepts are introduced here.

Syntactics is defined, for our purposes, as the relationship among signs and combinations of signs. In a medical semiotic, syntactics describes the expression of physical signs, their order of appearance, and the assumed relationships existing among several signs. The inclusion or exclusion of signs within a specific case or 'text' varies according to the needs of the various actors and the medical model(s) which constrain them. In general, the biomedical model of illness or disease evaluates only signs produced by or about the body, whereas ethnomedical models tend to include signs produced externally which are the product of social relationships and which are referrable to the body only under conditions imposed or allowed by the specific ethnomedical paradigm under which they were generated. Thus it is apparent that no single medical model can be used to examine the 'illnesses' which are produced by another. This is a significant problem for ethnomedical or biomedical studies which seek to make cross-cultural comparisions.

Since syntactics involves the relationship between signs, it must also deal with the ability of signs to substitute or 'stand in' for other signs. To use a simple example, a physician may determine by touch that a patient has a fever. The reading of a thermometer will offer the same information. The two signs are not identical, but can be substituted for one another. Since this quality of 'standing for' another sign is related to the signification, meaning, or semantic aspect of signs, syntactics and semantics can never be treated altogether separately.

In the medical semiotic proposed here, the relation of signs to diagnostic or symptom labels is a semantic relation. That is, these labels are assumed to have meaning or significance or to provoke a response or responses. The semantic dimension explores the relationship between individual signs or syndromes and the explanatory models which are employed to make sense of misfortune. But semantics deals with more than the labeling or categorizing of signs, for through the production, interpretation, and treatment of the signs of illness, seemingly disparate areas of experience are connected. For example, in Chapter VII, the illness histories of five Garifuna individuals are offered. These case histories serve as minor 'culture texts', which, when read together, document dominant themes of Garifuna culture – that past, present, and future generations are irrevocably linked, that death is but one transition in a series of transitions which does not remove individuals from participation in the activities of the living, and that respect for one's fellow men, both those living and those deceased, is an essential attribute if one is to live long and well.

Pragmatics examines the contexts in which signs occur and are interpreted and the manner in which signs are exploited by individuals and institutions to some end. The goal may be the reversal of a disease process or a change in an existing personal relationship or an alteration in social status. The action may be intentional as when an individual fails to report a sign in order to avoid certain moral judgments about behavior which is assumed to have led to the illness episode, or it may be unintentional, as when a diagnosis is rendered according to a conventional model of interpretation through which alternative cause-effect explanations have been eliminated.

There are four activities in which all healers engage, regardless of the medical model employed. They identify causative factors in general and specific instances of illness (etiology), they distinguish one illness from another and label specific cases according to existing classes of illness (diagnosis), they forecast the likely outcome of an illness episode (prognosis), and they intervene in the patient's production of signs (therapy). The relation between syntactics, etiology, and prognosis should be apparent. Etiology examines the production of signs by the body and by the social collectivity synchronically and diachronically. Prognosis implies the ordering of future signs yet to be produced. Prognosis is determined by the medical paradigm, and actual outcomes, though often not in conformity with the proffered prognosis, tend always to reinforce culturally important assumptions about illness, its cause and treatment. The process of imposing a diagnostic label and prescribing a therapy involves an interaction between patient and healer, the afflicted individual and his family or social group, the healer and other healers or other professionals who are responsbile for carrying out the prescribed therapy, and so on. Though each case can be assumed to be partially idiosyncratic, communicative patterns emerge which can be described in syntactic terms and which distinguish patient-healer interactions under the control of different medical paradigms.

Every diagnosis is derived from basic assumptions about cause and effect relationships which are part of the healer's and/or patient's medical paradigm. Cultural 'rules' or models of and models for behavior are thoroughly embedded in the medical paradigm. This is as true for biomedicine as it is for ethnomedical systems. Thus the process of diagnosis generates meaning through application of a label which carries important information regarding prognosis and therapies; but diagnoses are also meaningful in the additional sense that they are linked to critical cultural paradigms as well. Thus etiology, diagnosis, prognosis, and therapy clearly have semantic values at several levels of analysis.

This is the reason the patient, despite a thorough explanation of disease organism-host organism interactions, may continue to ask "How could this have happened to me?" and to search for meaning beyond the simple diagnostic label. The current emphasis in the United States on stress and its relation to illness, as well as research into environmentally caused illnesses and disorders (cancer, for example, now fits into both categories), indicates an attempt to expand responsibility for poor health to 'significant others', to specific industries, and to governments in general. I am not attempting to comment on the appropriateness of this shift, but merely to point out that, while diagnostic labels may remain essentially the same, the significance of the illness changes with modifications in broader cultural paradigms.

The inclusion or exclusion of certain signs within that chain of events which precedes or is part of the illness episode cannot be isolated from what I shall refer to as the politics of medicine, for the imposition of one medical model or one alternative cause-effect relationship from among several in a single paradigm represents the struggle for control over information and resources – illness being but one sort of resource exploitable by healers. The ability to successfully impose a particular medical model usually indicates the relative social and political status of the several actors. This, too, is the subject matter of the semantics of illness.

While illnesses may exist apart from their actual manifestations in human beings (that is, as theoretical cause-effect relationships), the more interesting aspects of a medical paradigm emerge in an actual examination of the 'practice' of medicine and the manner in which the potential range of explanations available is exploited. Every explanantory paradigm is capable of manipulation and when several explanatory models are available, the potential for producing satisfying and still culturally appropriate cause-effect relationships is dramatically increased. For example, the wide range of practitioners and numerous theories of illness causation available to the 'afflicted' in the United States makes possible an almost endless search for cause and for effective therapy in cases which do not yield to initial diagnosis and treatment.

The production and observation of signs diachronically or synchronically is dependent upon both the medical model employed and the techniques, materials, and facilities available to generate and classify signs. Ethnomedical systems tend to be 'complete', that is, they tend to have at their disposal the necessary materials and techniques to produce, arrange, and interpret signs which will yield culturally appropriate and satisfying diagnoses. Biomedicine, on the other hand, incorporates many theories about illness causation which cannot be effectively tested in third-world settings where the required materials, such as x-ray equipment, microscopes, centrifuges, refrigerated units, and so on, are not always available.

Diagnoses are obviously dependent on the total range of diagnostic and symptomatic labels available, and, less obviously but equally important, on the particular end sought by the various actors involved. Prognosis and outcome are based on several factors: the therapeutic resources available, the skill of the practitioner, the interaction between healer and patient, and interactions between the patient and his social group of which the healer may know little or nothing. All this is the focus of a medical pragmatics.

In summary, the syntactic, semantic, and pragmatic elements of illness events are closely interwoven and the story of a disease tells something of the history of a culture and much about the relation among individuals and the social networks in which they are embedded.

Notes on Research and Language

Research for this book was partially funded by a Doctoral Dissertation Fellowship from Social Science Research Council. Fieldwork was conducted from January of 1979 to May of 1980 and in March and April of 1984. Information was collected in several ways: through the standard anthropological technique of participant obervation, through extended discussions with several local healers and health care providers, seven of whom were Garifuna, through interviews with approximately one-hundred persons during or immediately following an illness episode, through a survey of one-hundred households in the community (representing approximately twenty percent of the total population of the town), and through the collection of information on a continuing basis from twelve individuals who suffered from a chronic or acute but reappearing illness, and from their families.

In Chapter VI I have presented information collected from four Garifuna healers. In a few discussions with these healers, I used a tape recorder, but, for the most part, these 'conversations' are based on notes taken at the time of the interview. If I have in any way misrepresented the thoughts of the individuals I interviewed, I apologize, though I believe I have accurately reported the content and the language of these conversations.

The spelling of Garifuna terms is my best approximation of pronunciations as employed by the Garinagu of Punta Gorda. Some pronunciations appear to have changed through time; certain terms seem to be known or utilized in one location or period and not in another (see, for example, Taylor 1951 and Coehlo 1955). A word may have more that one pronunciation (for example, *idáhadu*, *udahadu*), or more than one spelling (for example, *búiai*, *búiei*, *buyai*, *bóye*, *búye*, etc.) or change form through time (*mafia* [modern], *mapoya* [nineteenth century and earlier]. *Garifuna* is both the name of the language spoken and the singular and adjectival form of the plural *Garinagu*, though many researchers have used the term Garifuna in recent years to refer to the people.

CHAPTER 1

Defining the Boundaries of Medical Semiotics

In the last decade, semioticians have begun the task of charting a territory which I shall refer to as medical semiotics.[1] Yet the translation and interpretation of the physiological, behavioral, and linguistic signs which indicate health and illness are founded on a tradition more ancient than semiotics itself (Sebeok 1976), extending back to man's first attempts to make 'sense' out of illness. The list of contributors to this work grows according to the depth of our historical account. Many whose inquiries now define this field would have failed to recognize the term; yet the concept of the sign is central to the work of each. It is the multimodal, polysemous nature of the illness sign, its special communicative powers, its mythical and metaphorical qualities, which have through the centuries most intrigued and provoked us.

The discipline or doctrine of semiotics in general and medical semiotics (semeiology) in particular derives from a concern among the ancient Greeks with the translation or interpretation of signs of bodily dysfunction. The term *semeiology* still appears in some medical texts; it is generally equated with *symptomatology;* both terms are further linked to the terms *pathognomic* and *pathognomy*. *Pathognomy,* in turn, is defined as the "science of signs and symptoms of disease" and *pathognomic* as a sign or symptom which provides the basis for a diagonsis; the two terms are of Greek origin (as is *semiotic*, *semeiōtikos; gnomonikos* – fit to give judgment, and *gnome* – a means of knowing.)

Sebeok refers to semiotics as

> ... an ancient discipline, stemming from a pre-Socratic clinic tradition, which then led to the development of three fundamental semiotic traditions – the medical, the philosophical, and the linguistic – that have thoroughly intermingled at various periods in Western intellectual history, although there have been times when they strove for autonomy (Sebeok 1978:viii).

Baer (1982 MS) remarks that "[t]he art of healing, in Greek antiquity, was called *techne semeiotike*, a craft having to do with signs" (1).

Semeiotics, separated from the linguistic and philosophical semiotic traditions since at least the late 1700s, remains that sphere of the medical sciences principally concerned with diagnosis and the classification of signs of physical and mental dysfunction, although signs of disorder also point to a past (etiology) and a future (prognosis). But diagnosis, prognosis, and etiology constitute, at one level of abstraction, a single sign whose triadic nature has important sociological implications. These sociological and humanistic implications, however, have been ignored or minimized by a biomedical tradition which has failed to recognize the historical and necessary links between semeiology and semiotics.

In current medical practice, signs of disorder, both objective (produced or observed by the diagnostician) and subjective (offered by the patient), to the degree that observations and technologies are accurate and consistent and symptoms fully and honestly presented, are generally regarded as non-arbitrary in the relation of the sign (or more precisely, *representamen*), to "that for which it stands"; that is, the sign is *indexical*, directly motivated by its object. Determination of 'meaning' for such a sign then becomes dependent upon its inclusion within a system of signs (syndrome, symptom complex), produced synchronically or diachronically, which point to a 'disease' or labeled disorder. In the biomedical model of illness, signs are always regarded as empirically classifiable given sufficient information and the necessary technology to generate and evaluate that information. As Crookshank noted several decades ago:

> Teachers of Medicine... seem to share the implied belief that all known, or knowable, clinical phenomena are resumable, and to be resumed, under a certain number of categories or general references, as so many "diseases": the true number of these categories, references, or "diseases" being predetermined by the constitution of the universe at any given moment.... In this way, the diseases supposed to be extant at any one moment are capable – so it is thought – of such categorical exhaustion as are the indigenous fauna of the British Isles and the population of London. That our grouping of like cases as cases of the same disease is purely a matter of justification and convenience, liable at any moment to supersession or adjustment, is nowhere admitted; and the hope is held out that one day we shall know all the diseases that there "are", and all about them there is to be known (1938:342).

Biomedical science thus has as one of its goals the development of ever more sophisticated information gathering techniques. Such an approach to "sign" (the objective phenomenon) and "symptom" (the subjective phenomenon, the patient's presentation of his perceived state) leaves semeiology generally devoid of considerations of the social matrix in which all illness must occur. But illness is always a cultural event or experience, inseparable from social and political realities (see Eisenberg 1977; Fabrega 1972, 1974; Foucault 1965, 1973; Illich 1976; Kleinman 1973, 1980; Kleinman, Eisenberg and Good 1978; Sedgwick 1973; Sontag 1978 Szasz 1970, 1973, 1974, 1976; Janzen 1978a; Roberts 1981; Comaroff 1981). Illness may not only result from cultural practices and be treated within a specific cultural milieu utilizing techniques which derive from or conform to certain cultural expectations. but may 'express' or imply culture itself.

The experience called illness, the signs and symptoms as they are reported or expressed, the process whereby such signs are interpreted, are all semiotic phenomena, subject to a semiotic interpretation. That much seems unquestioned and provides us with the subject matter of a specifically medical semiotics. The question arises, however, – and it is a critical question in defining the limits of a medical semiotics – are biological processes equally subject to semiotic analyses?

In recent years, the distinction between *disease* and *illness* has been made frequently in the anthropological and sociological literature and is critical to a number of analyses. This separation of the social and personal experience and the concomitant behavioral responses from the biological has helped us to specify the precise nature of the phenomena discussed. Nevertheless, this distinction, while useful in many respects, perpetuates an ancient dichotomy – the separation of mind and body. This separation may ultimately inhibit our examination of the interpretive process for the dichotomy tends to deny the complex interweaving of physiological, emotional, and behavioral events. The subjective *experience* of dysfunction and disorder, for example, may well trigger the production of neurophysiological signs which are then attributed to the *disease* process. Further, biochemical and structural alterations may be differentially experienced and reported, and both the experience and the presentation may be affected by predominating cultural models of illness. Semiotics provides us with a model for treating the two phenomena separately, one the one hand, yet acknowledging the complex relations between the two, on the other.

Before further discussion of these semiotic assumptions, let us re-examine the question of the inclusion of biological processes in a medical semiotic.

The symptom, according to Peirce, is an example of an Index. The Index is defined as a "sign determined by its dynamic object by virtue of being in a real [that is, non-arbitrary] relation to it" (8.335). The symptom, further, "itself is a legisign, a general type of a definite character." The occurrence in a particular case is a sinsign [or token] (8.335). The appearance of a symptom in an individual is thus an indexical sinsign, while the symptom interpreted apart from its manifestation becomes an indexical legisign. Implicit in Peirce's discussion of signs is the notion that the symptom, as a variety of sign, may have qualities of firstness, secondness or thirdness. The symptom as a first, if I interpret Peirce correctly, involves nothing more than the awareness of its existence, a "feeling", though Peirce's notion of a first might allow for the existence of the symptom (more precisely, the physiological sign) apart from any thought of its presence. The symptom as a second involves a further recognition in the interpreter (in this case, the individual in whom the symptom is manifested). The afflicted or affected individual becomes aware of the symptom as an imposition upon the self, the ego. The contrast between self and non-self grows. There is ego and there is non-ego, and the symptom as a second is now clearly perceived as part of the non-self. The symptom as a third involves an interpretive process which moves the sign beyond mere perception or experience. The object is related to an interpretant according to a law or habit and the symptom gains meaning or significance in this triadic fulfillment. Thus the physiological sign exists as a sign to the extent that it has thirdness, that is, to the extent that significance is assigned to it. Peirce has further stated that a reaction is not a sign for it does not involve thirdness (7.531), a statement which would seem to exclude any sign or bit of information beyond human preception that is not amenable to interpretation. However, he further states that a "generalized reaction... is a law" (7.532). Since the transmission of information at the physiological level is governed by codes which function as laws in Peirce's sense, such signs become a part of Peirce's semiotic. The inclusion of physiological signs, however, remains problematic in that Peirce insisted on the involvement of an "intelligent consciousness" as a prerequisite for interpretation. I shall return to this point shortly.

The symptom (including here both the objective sign and the subjective sign) is treated elsewhere not as a variety of *sign*, but as a "morbid fact" existing prior to the sign.

> ...the word "symptom" does not carry... the idea of signification.... We believe that the symptom is something which is deciphered (Barthes 1972:39).

The symptom becomes the "unrefined fact offered in the work of decipherment prior to the commencement of work" (*Ibid.*). The symptom emerges as a sign only through the "organizing consciousness of the doctor" and through the "mediation of language" (*Ibid.*). The transformation of the symptom involves

> ...an operation that totalizes by comparing organisms...
> - an operation that recalls normal functioning...
> - an operation that registers the frequency of simultaneity or succession... - an operation which beyond first appearances, scrutinizes the body and discovers at the autopsy a visible invisible.... (Foucault 1973:93-94)

Since the symptom gains meaning (thirdness) only through its transformation by the physician, the emphasis is on the "correctness" of the physician's interpretation. The sign "is the result of an intellectual operation...." (Hecht, in Dechambre 1880:560). ..."all symptoms ... can and must be transformed into signs" (*Ibid.*). "It is the logic which presides over this transformation upon which the precision of the diagnosis and the value of the prognosis depends" (*Ibid.*) Foucault, drawing upon long established traditions within French medical thought, sees in modern technologies and diagnostic procedures the possibility of perfecting this process of transformation:

> Analysis and the clinical gaze also have this feature in common that they compose and decompose only in order to reveal an ordering that is the natural order itself; their artifice is to operate only in the restitutive act of the original. "This analysis is the true secret of discoveries because it makes us go back to the origin of things." For the clinic, this origin is the natural order of symptoms, the form of their succession or of

their reciprocal determination. Between sign and symptom there is a decisive difference that assumes value only against the background of an essential identity; the sign is the symptom itself, but in its original truth. At last, there emerges on the horizon of clinical experience the possibility of an exhaustive, clear, and complete reading; for a doctor whose skills would be carried "to the highest degree of perfection all symptoms would become signs", all pathological manifestations would speak a clear, ordered language (Foucault 1973:94-95).

Such an approach, however, in which the symptom becomes a sign only under the "gaze" of the physician, needlessly removes the symptom from the realm of the communicative act; the symptom may represent far more than an alteration in the organic state. Only in the psychoanalytic/psychotherapeutic literature is this communicative aspect noted and the symptom clearly disengaged from the limitations of the Peircian *index*.

In psychiatry, Fromm-Reichmann, in a little-known paper, pointed out the use of catatonic symptoms as communication, and in 1954 Jackson indicated the utility of the patient's use of hysterical symptoms in communicating with his family (Watzlawick et al. 1967:79).

The symptom is viewed as an action:

In general, we feel that a symptom is a piece of behavior that has profound effects in influencing the surroundings of the patient (*Ibid.*:45).

In his analysis of the work of the French psychoanalyst, Jacques Lacan, Baer defines the symptom in the following way:

A symptom is a substitution, a metaphor, for what is absent, and it is this absence, pushed by Lacan all the way from the perceptual level to the ontological level, which in frugal perception is filled, again and again, by the analyst's multimodal interpretation (Baer 1975:29).

The psychoanalytic symptom, however, is distinguished from the physiological in terms of its communicational qualities:

Lacan defines the psychoanalytical symptom as differing in kind from the neurophysiological symptom, and also from any natural form of expression, such as what has been called the language of bees. The main difference is that the latter two are natural signs with naturally fixed referents, while the psychoanalytic symptom is an artificial sign with no fixed referents. While the neurophysiological symptom is a natural index of some neurophysiological state or process, and while a natural mode of expression has a naturally determined code, the psychoanalytical symptom is an artificially coded mode of expression that has a meaning contrary to the conventional code, depending on the intentionality of the subject (*Ibid.*:37).

The psychoanalytic symptom is a "disguise."

...Lacan... has classified psychoanalytic data such as symptoms and dreams as metaphors in that they disguise original expressions of wishes by replacing them (*Ibid.*:62).

For Freud, the symptom indicated repression; it was, "...a sign of, and a substitute for, an instinctual gratification which has remained in abeyance... (1926:720). In all these formulations, the psychoanalytic symptom masks, the organic symptom reveals, the psychoanalytic symptom is symbol, the organic symptom merely index.

Baer has more recently emphasized the communicative powers of both psychoanalytic and neurophysiological symptoms. The symptom is described as a "paradigm of wisdom", a method for looking out on the world (1982MS).

The medical symptom is a sign in which existence – and this includes death – is "realized" in the sense of being an event with special communicative powers. Existence is – often suddenly – questioned, and often radically ... on the yawning background of absolute withdrawal.... In the symptom, existence often becomes oppressively concrete and at the same time frighteningly abstract. The medical symptom is the most bodily and simultaneously the most spiritual sign. There is no sign to match it in existential value and depth (*Ibid.*:1).

I return to the question posed earlier: are organic signs subject to semiotic analyses? Are they deserving of inclusion in our medical semiotic? Peirce has not provided us with a clear answer, requiring, on the one hand, the active involvement of a conscious intelligence, and, on the other, stating that a "generalized reaction" functions as a law or according to a law. Perhaps a rephrasing of the question will help: do physiological signs transmit information? Are they susceptible to transformation, and, if so, is that transformation equivalent to interpretation? Physiological signs contain and 'communicate' information. Further, they transmit information in a regular and systematic way: the transmission is governed by codes. If, however, the *meaning* of the information transmitted is inherent to the sign, then perhaps these "signs" do not exist as *signs* at all. Yet, their significance is not obvious. The body does not 'read' these signs and respond automatically and consistently. These data which are transmitted must be transformed into data of another sort for the body to make sense of and act upon the information, and that process of transformation or translation involves interpretation. That the body clearly makes mistakes in this interpretive process should further support this contention. "To err is human, we say, but we don't like the idea much, and it is harder still to accept the fact that erring is biological as well" (Thomas 1979: 23). Sebeok's statements on this point are important to the argument here:

The subject matter of semiotics – ultimately a mode of extending our perception of the world – is the exchange of any messages whatever and of the system of signs which underlie them.... The key concept of semiotics remains always the 'sign.'

Messages may be emitted and/or received either by inorganic objects, such as machines, or by organic substances, for instance, animals, including man, or by some of their component parts (e.g., ribonucleic acid, mRNA, that serves as an information-bearing tape 'read' by particles, called ibosomes, that travel along it, carrying amino acid sequence information....; one may also speak of information, for instance, in cardiovascular functioning, where messages are conveyed from peripheral vessels to the brain, relayed thence to the heart and back to the brain.... Then interaction of organic beings with inorganic things (such as communication between man and a computer) can also be treated as a semiotic problem (1976:1-2).

Communication involves sign processes. Physiological events are communicative events, involving the exchange of messages. Therefore, physiological events depend upon signs and become part of a medical semiotic. Any bit of code-governed datum involved in a message is a sign whether that sign is to be treated as an icon, index, or symbol; that is, it is a sign to the extent that it requires interpretation or transformation; furthermore, both its production and interpretation are code-governed. Symptoms, both intersubjective ("clinical signs", organic, physical, objective signs, etc.) and introspective (symptoms, the 'signs' presented by the patient, the subjective signs), may be indexical – that is non-arbitrarily related to their object. Their interpretants, in turn, may be either arbitrarily or non-arbitrarily linked to the manifestation of the sign, that is, the representamen. Neither statement denies their inclusion in a medical semiotic.

Communication and interpretation occur at various levels or within various domains of process and experience. They may be manifested strictly at the biochemical or structural level, in which case we are dealing with what is generallly referred to as proprioception and propriotransmission (Bateson 1968), endosemiotics (Sebeok 1976), or biosemiotics (Baer 1982 MS: Jandar 1981). The internally generated and internally intepreted signs are signals, which, by definition, mobilize a response which is, in turn, another sign. These signs generally remain 'invisible', often undetectable even with our sophisticated technologies. They are, in fact, not a part of our awareness, of our personal concept of self and body. This is not imply, however, as some have, that they are not susceptible to semiotic constraints.

Physiological signs which are not available to a "scientific intelligence" exist nonetheless as signs. They transmit information and require interpretation or transformation. The therapeutic response is constituted of a series of actions or events which result in the intervention in the patient's production of physiological and symptomatic signs. This response is initiated at the neurophysiological or biochemical level; organisms respond to indications of altered physiological states and attempt to maintain through such responses a normal or steady state. Only when the signs of disorder are consciously perceived and interpreted as discomforting or dangerous do individuals or groups or institutions undertake what I shall call sociomedical therapy. Sociomedical therapies, as the term is used here, include the many and varied ritual, religious, and other non-biomedically justified behaviors which are directed to healing. Such therapy cannot begin until physiological signs are further transformed or interpreted. That is, the representamen does not provide sociologically or technologically useful information until linked with an interpretant. But semiosis is, by definition, never static and the production of the sign (the unification of representamen, object, and interpretant) requires another sign. The display of signs or representamens, in a variety of domains (the organic, the technological, the social, and the cultural, among others) implies a series of progressively more complicated transformations and the sign becomes increasingly polysemous.

What is the specific value of semiotics in our analyses of disease and illness? Semiotics offers a unifying framework which cuts across the boundaries of many academic domains. It allows for the recognition of the analogies existing among the seemingly divergent fields of art, literature, biology, the social and medical sciences, and so on. It offers a metalanguage useful in the analysis of the production, relation, and manipulation of signs and for the transformation of one sort of sign into another, or for the recognition of analogous signs expressed in different idioms. Because semioticians aim at the discovery of conscious and unconscious codes, semiotics provides a potential schema for moving from one to the other, or for discovering the resemblances (or correspondences) between a biological (genetic) and a cultural (behavioral) code, or, for speaking, for example, of the transformation of an economic code (a code governing the production and value of material goods) into a social or ideational code (a code governing the production and value of human or human-object relationships). A *code* is defined here as any rule governing the production and signification of signs or the relations among signs, including their syntactic arrangement or the transformation of one sort of datum into another.

Semiotics further aims at discovering the codes or metacodes which govern the production of signs, the transformation of signs, the exchange values assigned signs, and the relationships among signs within a single sign system or multiple sign systems. Signs may be studied as they stand alone or as they come to refer within a specific context. But more frequently signs and sign behavior are recognized to be part of that persistent process we refer to as semiosis. Signs are embedded in other signs, they occur within a sequence of signs, they may have many referents which are activated singly or simultaneously, they are interpreted differently by different interpreters, they can be exchanged for other signs, they have a history, and they can develop or lose referents. Whether we are dealing with the physiological or the cultural expressions of illness, it is important to note that signs are not static phenomena, though there is often a tendency to regard them as such. This considerably complicates any attempt to define the illness sign and its significations. A description of the sign becomes impossible because "we can accede to the object only by means of signs...." (Baer 1982MS:4), each sign, in turn, requiring another sign. The sign, then, can be said to never exist, except as a process, a continual fulfillment and an "infinite regress" (*Ibid.*).

In the production of signs, signs newly generated are referred to one another or to other signs. Introspective or intersubjective signs are the interpretants of a prior sign. The action of supplying them with sociological or political or medical meanings becomes but one additional transformation in a chain of transformations. The sign thus moves from the body outward and back again, as the sociocultural and personal meanings imputed to a sign or series of signs re-express themselves through the organism.

The signs and symptoms which indicate illness and disease have communicative functions. They express culture and are culturally expressed. They provide a mode for the articulation of stresses and conflicts which might otherwise be inexpressible. They mobilize and reconstitute the social group. They verify, challenge, and, ultimately, reconcile basic cultural assumptions. They provide one means of revealing "significant truths" (Roberts 1981). They inform the afflicted individal, the social group, and the diagnostician, and provoke actions or reactions, both behavioral and physiological, which constitute the therapeutic process.

Some signs appear to be universally recognized as indicative of physiological or psychological disorders (Fabrega 1979); yet technological, cultural, political and other constraints imposed on the interpretive process lead to the excusion of others from the models that govern the distribution of health and illness signs. Not all possible signs of disorder are utilized within any single interpretive system. The objective and subjective signs of disorder are not presented and likely not experienced in the same way by all individuals. Both the presentation and experience are affected by the cultural values and practices which one accepts as a member of a specific ethnic or cultural group. The domains from which signs (etiologic and diagnostic) are drawn or generated are defined by other than natural parameters.

The signs and symptoms which constitute illness require further interpretation; they are not devoid of information for they motivate a variety of responses, but the interpretive process enhances, expands and transforms them into information of a different sort. This transformative process is determined by the various constraints imposed by a given medical theory, the social, historical, political and personal contexts in which the signs are manifested, the technologies available to the interpreter, the variety of alternative interpretations available and the degree of accessibility to those interpretations.

Illness functions as a communicative act, an attempt to inform self and others about general and specific concerns, an attempt to mobilize resources and to effect an environment which is advantageous to the afflicted individual and his social and political groups. At the very least,

> ...the healing process mobilizes potent symbolic resources; for in the attempt to redress the breaches made by illness, healers everywhere manipulate symbolic media which address a mutually entailed physical and social order. In the face of the doubt and anxiety which often accompany illness, healing processes powerfully reinforce the validity of meanings drawn from the dominant forms of knowledge in the wider culture (Comaroff 1981:369).

Illnesses are both social and personal experiences. They provide the occasion for reflection. They explain, exploit, and reinforce cultural, political, social, and technological models of the world. They occur not as single events, but as a sequence of experiences, decisions, reflections, and actions.

Therapy seeking is necessarily preceded by interpretive activities. This process may not involve the application of any disease or illness label, but rather a sorting of signs into broad categories which imply or limit the therapeutic alternatives. Signs may have communication-informational value within one therapeutic system, but not within another, leading the patient to seek out that system in which the signs are most likely to be regarded as significant or non-significant, according to his needs.

Illness is a semiosic act involving the production of signs which signify the intrasubjective perception, initially at some unconscious level, of changed internal relationships which must come to be regarded, at this same physiological level, as potentially harmful to the organism (for example, a quantitative change in the relationship between a pathogen and host organism). In other words, illness does not require a label for its existence nor that event called diagnosis nor even an awareness of the altered state.[2] The individual's information processing systems respond to these intrasubjectively perceived changes and initiate reactions which themselves constitute the majority of signs of disorder utilized by the diagnostician; but such responses may, in fact, be based on misinformation.

The definition of illness offered here does not require a distinction among physical, mental, and psychosomatic disorders; yet I have stated that illness involves the interpretation of changed *internal* relationships, a statement which would seem to exclude certain so-called mental disorders, at least those perceived to be precipitated by changing social or environment-self relationships. Nevertheless, mental disorders of this sort can be included within this definition if such changed relationships between self and environment (which includes other 'selves') are regarded as internalized. The self is a social product, a synthesis of interactions in which externally derived information becomes internalized (Shands 1970, 1978; Shands and Meltzer 1973, 1977). The individual integrates information about relationships with others, obtained through social transactions, and with the physical environment, obtained through person or organism-environment transactions, into a self, which evolves out of this process of integration and mediation of oppositions.

The signs signify a response, an *interpretant* in the language of the American philosopher Charles Sanders Peirce, which is, in turn, a sign of a perceived change; but such signs are produced according to a code which may not be devoid of cultural components save at the level of such events as the replication of DNA and the formation of protein chains; that is, the changed relationship was evaluated by internal information processing mechanisms which, I argue, may be culturally influenced; and the signs are *symptomatized*, that is, described by the patient according to a culturally mediated code (i.e., expressed through language, in terms of existing categories, and according to expectations associated with specific roles) and they are *inter*subjectively evaluated by individuals who are themselves social constructs.

I argue that the diagnostician and physician are also sign producers, both in terms of generating signs which signify illness and those which signify health, and that they operate under a restricted code in both their production and evaluation of signs. The physician's diagnostic role requires that he evaluate the state of the patient; this task he undertakes by identifying or eliciting certain objective and subjective signs which may point to illness. The patient's presentation of complaints (symptoms) may be symbolic (i.e., the relation between the *representamen* or what we normally refer to as the sign or symptom, and its *object*, or "motivating force" is constituted of an arbitrary link). But the physician is also a social construct who operates under a restricted code in supplying his interpretation. The diagnostic event, therefore, is also a symbolic act (in Saussurian sense), although the link between the *representamen* and the *interpretant* may be so conventionalized as to appear indexical. In fact, it is the conventionality of this link that allows the patient confidence in the practitioner. The underlying assumption is that several diagnosticians faced with the same sign or sign systems will 'see' the same event and provide the same interpretation.

If illness seems indicated the physician first seeks a label and then attempts where possible to intervene in the patient's production of signs. The physician's *therapeutic* role, by definition, becomes that of producer of signs (generally through reversal, elimination, or neutralization of existing signs of disorder), signs which point to the so-called normal (healthy) state.

In that set of verbal and non-verbal transactions which constitute the psychotherapeutic act, in the ordering of an X-ray, in the application of a visual sequential memory test, the diagnostician is, in fact, producing signs which he evaluates as pointing to a state of 'health' or 'illness' (or some incipient state) but which otherwise would not have existed had it not been for his production of them. The argument, or course, is that the 'signs existed, but were unperceived or 'invisible' and required the skill or technologies or "gaze" (Foucault 1973) of the diagnostician for their uncovering and illumination. Nevertheless, all potential signs are not interpreted within any one medical system. As Einstein once noted, "it is the theory which decides what we can observe." Thus, one task facing us is the discovery of the codes which govern the production, both by the patient and by the physician, of some signs but not others.

Once the signs are produced, or existing signs are 'observed' and noted, for them to take on meaning, to supply information, to point to a certain state which is conducive to therapy, they must be assigned to categories known as diseases or syndromes, or they must suggest an etiologic agent. This categorization is clearly affected by the diagnostician's 'philosophical' bias, whether that philosophy involves the notion that ancestors attempt to make their wishes known by inflicting disease or is the logical positivism underlying Western or biomedicine. Classification of illness is, then, "the first therapeutic act" (Kleinman 1973).

Because diagnosis normally involves communication, that is, a dialogue, the physician becomes inseparable from the 'system' that he attempts to observe. Moreover, the personal need for observations to coincide with the structured cognitive guidelines which are his cultural and intellectual heritage may interfere with his assessment; the diagnostician must, in Gregory Bateson's words, wish things to be as he knows they are. Additionally, the internal events taking place within the afflicted individual are not directly available to the diagnostician. He must, indeed, mediate them, either through verbal transactions, observations of intersubjective signs (which are not necessarily directly referable to a pathogen or to a changed relationship, but are the body's reponse to the perception or interpretation of such), or through the acquisition of those signs which are ultimately interpreted by the diagnostician but initially 'observed' or 'visualized' through the diagnostician's technological extensions.

Further, I believe the so-called objective signs of disorder as produced by the patient may be arbitrary in the relation of *representamen* to *object* (in other words, such signs are *symbolic*). The initial evaluation of change or process takes place *intra*subjectively (within the afflicted person); cultural mediation may affect this evaluation even at the level of the unconscious prior to the occurrence or manifestation of either introspectively produced or intersubjectively evaluated signs. I have thus far stated that the symptom (or introspective sign [Baer 1975]) is part of a communicative act. I have also argued that intersubjective signs are evaluated by individuals who are themsevles social constructs. But if certain signs are always motivated by certain *objects* and point to certain contents (*interpretants*) in a consistent way, such signs would seem to be *indexical*, in other words, the link is a 'natural' or non-arbitrary one. When there is a direct and consistent relationship between the sign (*sign-vehicle, representamen*) and its *object*, unmediated by the social self, the sign is *indexical*. Little is known about the mediating process, the intervention of a self, specifically a social self, in the process of perception and interpretation of sensory inputs. Nevertheless, correlational studies indicate an increasing array of links between 'predisposing' factors of a social, cultural, or personal nature, and certain illnesses or altered physiological states. Thus, the relation between *representamen* and *object* may be arbitrary, even in those cases in which we are dealing with organic or physical signs of disorder, signs which are supposedly immune to cultural or social interpretations at the unconscious level.

The system of internal codification by which sensory inputs (both exteroceptive and proprioceptive) are organized and made meaningful is not entirely available for examination. It is nevertheless clear that a codifying system exists and that this system reduces, summarizes, and organizes sensory impressions. The opinion is offered here that the reception, interpretation, and transformation of information is influenced or mediated by the self, which is primarily (but not exclusively) a product of the social and cultural milieu.

I have suggested that social and/or idiosyncrative factors may cause one to misinterpret an event, that is, the sensory impressions may be miscoded, the abstraction derived may bear no relation to reality, etc. That certain psychological or mental disorders are characterized by a response based on misinterpretation seems generally accepted; Bateson (1968) has said of psychosis, "the condition which the psychiatrist labels [as such] is essentially the result of the patient's misinterpretation of messages received." Illness of an 'organic' nature may be the manifestation of similar responses.

Signs utilized by the physician (or any other person making an evaluation of bodily or mental states) are secondary signs, or signs about signs. A pathogen or other supposedly 'causative' factor does not, in fact, usually provoke the signs which we label as designating disease; rather they are most often produced by the body in response to the perception of changing relationships; they generally refer to the body's attempt at self-regulation. Thomas (1974) provides an example of this sort of process:

> We carry brucella for long periods in the cells of our reticulo-endothelial system without any awareness of their existence; then cyclically, for reasons not understood but probably related to immunologic reactions on our part, we sense them, and the reaction of our sensing is the clinical disease (1974:91).

The concept of communication implies, as its obverse, the failure to communicate. Interpretation has as its opposite sign, misinterpretation, and both may play a critical role in illness. That the body makes communicative or interpretive errors is unquestioned. It is, for example, the occasional inability of DNA to properly replicate itself that has provided history with its remarkable evolutionary successes as well as its failures. "The capacity to blunder slightly is the real marvel of DNA", states Thomas (1972:23).

Humans, as all other organisms, possess internal mechanisms to process information. The internal and external *signals* which we receive generally prompt a fairly consistent response. That is, after all, what separates signals from other sorts of signs. Occasionally, however, the whole process is subject to error. We respond to these signals as though they were, in fact, signals of another sort. We misinterpret the nature and origin of the signals; we fail to properly categorize these signs. The high mortality rate connected with cholera is apparently the result of an error of this sort. Under normal circumstances, when food is delivered to the small intestine, a chemical signal stimulates the pumping of about two liters of alkaline fluid into the intestinal canal. When the cholera bacilli, however, invade and colonize the intestinal canal the body becomes confused. The disease itself is not an infection. The micro-organism does not invade the tissues; it merely comes to reside for a few days. Rubenstein explains:

> It cannot prenetrate or burrow between the cells that line the gut, it is incapable of

gaining access to the lymph channels and it does not enter the bloodstream. There is no microscopic evidence that it damages any tissue. The entire disease process, which kills half its untreated victims, is the result of the fact that the cells in the intestine respond to a chemical substance released by the bacteria as if it were a normal regulatory signal (1980:109).

This error stimulates the system into such overactivity that the cells pump from 20 to 30 liters of water into the small intestine.

Because fluid cannot be reabsorbed at that rate massive amounts of it are lost through vomiting and diarrhea. These huge loses of liquid account for the many deaths in cholera (*Ibid.*:109-110).

This characteristic of the body to occasionally commit errors, to misinterpret incoming or internally generated signals, to miscategorize such signs, may also account for the so-called placebo response or effect.[3]

When signs are manifested, either as symptoms or as intersubjective signs, made available for evaluation by self or others (the patient may also serve as diagnostician), the act is, in part, a communicative act, an attempt to order the disordered pronoun, the unstructured "I", to define and communicate a self. The sign, in this sense, is a metonym for the self and should be viewed as an *act* of social import, an attempt to communicate a self in opposition to the other ("I can describe my pain to you", the patient may be saying, "but you cannot suffer and, therefore, cannot understand my pain.") The sign is treated here not as a static manifestation of an organic state but as an event in a contiguous alignment of events.

It follows from the previous discussion that all illnesses are psychosomatic in that a self must always involve itself in the illness event at some stage, although perhaps only at the stage of symptomatization (the patient's presentation of the complaint, the creation and expression of the symptom). The possibility exists that the changed relationship was precipitated by the unconscious 'self' or that there was no change, but a misperception of such, triggering the signs associated with an illness state. I would argue, therefore, that all illnesses are psychosomatic in some respect, that the psyche and body interact, each having some effect upon the other. In the so-called 'true' psychosomatic illnesses, a social self initiates signs or intervenes in the process of interpretation in such a way that some sort of negotiation or 're-cognition' of events takes place. That there is considerable difficulty in deciding which of the above events has occurred should be obvious. I suggest, therefore, that the term psychosomatic as popularly used cannot distinguish among illness events in terms of their origin and, hence, serves no useful purpose.

I will use the term *sociosomatic* to refer to any illness in which the intersubjective or introspective signs are presented or manifested in a culturally condoned or channeled way, or in which certain disruptions in the social field or in interpersonal relations are expressed in specific somatic terms because this is a culturally sanctioned form of expression. Illnesses are sociosomatic to the degree that they conform to this definition: but to the extent that the self is a "social invention", any illness in which body and mind interact to produce some effect must also be sociosomatic in some regard.

Finally, medical signs or signs so classified are future-oriented (prescriptive) and past-oriented (appraisive or evaluative) and thus potentially exploitable for social ends, both self-serving and communal. The sick role which the patient fills, or attempts to fill, may also represent an effort to manipulate and control his environment, to alter in some way the sets of rights and obligations which define his positition within the society and his links to others in the social environment. The signs of illness may thus come to indicate some alteration in the individual's roles and can, in many cases, be manipulated to his benefit.

Innumerable studies have documented ways in which particular societies or political systems may also utilize or redefine signs to serve communal or state interests. Ruth and Victor Sidel (1972), for example, reported an interesting case in communist China. A woman had been admitted to a psychiatric ward suffering from auditory hallucinations. After considerable indoctrination into Maoist philosophy, she was pronounced cured. She still, in fact, suffered from hallucinations "but she quickly recognizes they don't really exist as result of an investigation based on the works of Mao" (1972:28). In such a case, the change in political philosophy has been incorporated into the sign, that is, the auditory hallucinations do not stand by themselves as a sign, but rather particular beliefs regarding the origin of the sign in "bourgeoise thinking" have become part of the symptom itself, and have, in fact, resulted in a negation of the symptom, from the diagnostician's perspective.

The tendency of physicians and administrative personnel in positions where decisions as to allocations of monies for research and applied medicine are made to define an ever broader range of signs as indicative of illness and thereby gain control over additional aspects of our lives has been fairly well described elsewhere. Alcoholism and drug addition, for example, are not defined as personal moral dilemmas, but as illness or disease states. What some have referred to as the "failure to learn appropriate communicative techniques" is interpreted elsewhere as mental disease, requiring the intervention of a physician and frequently the extensive utilization of psychotropic drugs, a move which, in its broader implications, has come to be known as the "medicalization of life" (Illich 1976). The tendency is toward a proliferation of named disorders which will require treament, almost invariably by professionals. As Sedgwick has remarked of the aging process:

> The natural causes of death are becoming, more and more, causes that we can control; so that the terminally ill, and their relatives, will be putting strong pressures on the medical profession to redefine the natural (and inevitable) causes of fatality, rendering them into medical (and hence controllable) pathologies which require the services of a doctor rather than a mortician.

The future belongs to illness; we are just going to get more and more diseases since our expectations of health are going to become more expensive and sophisticated (1973:37).

The signs that come to repesent illness are multireferential; they "stand for" a particular physiological or emotional state, but at the same time they indicate or point to a past event, some supposedly causative fact; they imply an etiology. Signs of illness, then, are appraisive or evaluative. The illness of a Mexican child may, for example, refer to its father's sexual promiscuity. A young African woman's failure to recover from an illness may be diagnosed as resulting from her lover's failure to complete marriage payments to her family (Janzen 1978). Since a diagnosis in many societies, including our own, is often a moral statement, a judgment about past actions of the individual and those who surround him, the evaluative aspect of signs is of considerable sociological importance. The same sign, however, points to the future. It implies certain expectations as to the future social status of the 'victim' as well as his future state of health or lack of it; this is *prognosis*, the code which governs *the expected course of events or sequencing of signs* It generally indicates a therapy, or, in other words, is prescriptive, and as medical science 'improves' almost all illness states would seem to indicate therapies.

Diagnosis is thus irrevocably linked to a prognosis and an etiology, even though those links have been shown to vary considerably from generation to generation and across cultures. Those links to the past and to the future are sometimes indexical (automatic, natural) and sometimes arbitrary (symbolic), but since signs of illness are polysemous, they may be both at the same time, making the illness sign a potentially powerful and manipulatable tool, leading to therapies which conform the patient to certain biomedical and social standards or to actions in which the patient attempts to conform the environment to his perceived needs and wishes.

The physiological sign, combined with its various interpretants, functions as a symbol, a "semantic unit" in a total semantic system (see Maranda 1972, Staiano 1979b). The organic and emotional signs of disorder unify "disparate significata" (Turner 1967:28). Thus, in a single sign may be manifested a set of oppositions – the organic and the normative, the natural and the supernatural, the libidinal and the superego – oppositions which must periodically be brought to awareness and commented upon. Because of the capacity of the illness sign to display these contradictions, such signs evolve as especially powerful ones. Illness episodes become narratives and the syntagmatic chain of signs takes on significance according to the etiological domain to which the signs are ultimately assigned. Illness episodes, as stories of personal failures and successes, of social and personal relationships, instruct; they provide models for and models of reality. Such episodes, occurring through time and across individuals become culture texts (Winner and Winner 1977; Staiano 1979b) constituted of critical cultural elements. Episodes develop as personal and social myths displaying important information about the sociocultural systems in which they occur and about the individuals who suffer them; they provide insight into the cultural realities which constrain and motivate personal behavior.

In general, it is not the mere presence of a sign which intrigues us, but the interpretive process whereby that sign becomes information of a different sort. *Interpretation* is defined here as the *process of transformation*, that is, a changing of form or structure. Information which is essentially 'meaningless' gains 'significance'; it is expressed in an idiom which allows for its 'clarification' and for its exploitation. In its altered form it provokes further action or response. Transformation, whether, for example, of carbohydrates to more usable forms of sugar or of the remembered forms of ritual to actual performance, are most commonly (though not always) governed by codes. A code was previously defined *as any rule governing the production and significations of signs or the relations among signs, including their syntactic arrangement or the transformation of one sort of datum into another.*

Whether we are speaking of behavioral codes or genetic codes, the process of interpretation is similar in several respects. The code functions to determine the arrangement of signs as information is transformed or reorganized to render it more meaningful or exploitable. This process occurs when thoughts spoken in one language are translated into the words of another. It occurs as well when mRNA determines the sequence in which amino acids are to be strung together in the creation of a protein. The more "introversive" (Winner and Winner 1977) the code, the less available for public use is the system whereby the signs can be decoded. That is, the code whereby data is transformed is not accessible; the relation between the type (code) and the token (expression) constitutes, in Eco's terminology, a *ratio difficilis* (1976). Two examples of "introversive" codes come to mind: the codes which govern the production of schizophrenic language and the codes which govern the array of signs referred to as poetry. Both are forms of communication, and, in some cases, the 'meanings' equally obscure. The message may be one which is fully understood only by the sender. It has, in fact, been suggested that the language of schizophrenia bears a resemblance to certain forms of poetry, particularly in the expanded use of metaphor. However, the code which governs the production of signs in one may be biological and in the other literary (and, hence, cultural). Such introversive codes, lacking ascertainable characteristics, are often highly inventive and produce statements which are highly 'meaningful', in the sense in which that term is used by information theorists.

Signs existing within one domain, that is, expressed in one particular idiom, may be transformed into signs of an entirely different sort, that is, expressed in another idiom. In the examples given below, signs are made more manageable through this sort of transformation. However, not all transformations function to increase the communicative power of the sign. The reverse process, in which signs are obscured in the transformative process, also occurs. Military codes and codes governing ritual performance are but two examples. Signs, in these cases, take on significance of several sorts. Communication is facilitated, but the audience is defined in terms of accessibility to the code.

The signs function not only as communicative devices within this 'elitist' group, but they serve to define and maintain boundaries. The exploitation of signs in such a manner, the transformation of data through a code which is generally not accessible, excludes from the communicative process those judged not be deserving of incorporation. Medical (and semiotic) jargons serve that purpose, though it could as well be argued that seemingly esoteric terms are convenient condensations of large quantities of information.

In the diagrams which follow, I have found it most useful to explain the transformation of information through the application of Peirce's tripartite division of the sign into its three components: the *object, representamen*, and the *interpretant*. The terms are used essentially as defined by Peirce. The *object* motivates, that is, causes or provokes, the *representamen.*[4] The *interpretant* occurs as the result of the presence of a representamen, and is said to be a thought, action, experience, or quality of feeling (Peirce 8:322). In a letter to Lady Welby, Peirce distinguished the relation of the representamen to the object from that of the relation of the representamen or sign to its interpretant. The first was said to be a relation of *denotation* and the second one of *signification*.

> Now a definition does not reveal the Object of a sign, its Denotation, but only analyzes its Signification, and that is a question not of the sign's relation to its Object but of its relation to its Interpretant (1953 [orig. 1919] :39).

The relation of the interpretant to the object is, in one sense, one of equivalence, that is, the interpretant is, or should be, nothing more nor less than the expression of the object in a different idiom or in a different form. Peirce's explanation of this relation is as follows:

> A sign therefore is an object which is in relation to its object on the one hand and to an interpretant on the other, in such a way, as to bring the interpretant into a relation to the object, corresponding to its own relation to the object (8:332).

Jandar suggests that the relation between object and interpretant is not necessarily one of actual equivalence:

> If semiosis is perfect, the two terminal sets [object and interpretant] are identical sets because a function and its inverse restore, by definition, the original state. In reality, however, we expect semiotic systems, acting as receivers, to be only partially capable of complementation or inverse symbolization, with the result that the meaning or restored set in the receiver is only a homomorphic model (instead of an isomorphic one) of the original set (1981:232).

It should be evident that any given interpretant may be but one of several interpretants existing as potential signigications of a sign. Neverthless, the individual (or institution or social group or organism) producing the interpretant believes or behaves as though it accurately represents (i.e., is equivalent to) the object or is the closest approximation possible under the circumstances. For example, a physician who observes a patient with intermittent fever who suffers from severe chills and in whom the presence of a certain parasite has been detected, believes that the term "malaria" as it is used by biomedical personnel to describe certain physiological processes, will most closely describe or 'stand for' the supposed etiology and will, at the same time, indicate a probable prognosis.

If the relation between object and representamen is non-arbitrary, the sign exists as an *index* or an *icon* according to Peirce. If, however, the representamen could as easily be replaced by another sign, the relationship is arbitrary and the sign exists as a *symbol*. Not only may various interpretants be signified by or exist as interpretants of a single representamen, but a variety of representamens may be provoked or motivated by a single object.

How can such semiotic principles be applied to the disease/illness process? The physiological event is an obvious starting point for this discussion. An antigen may function as an object motivating a representamen, for example, a fever. The relationship between object and representamen is depicted as one of cause and effect, and is, or is believed to be, non-arbitrary.

antigen ——————→ fever
(O)bject (R)epresentamen

The sign functions, in Peircian terms, as an index. But this dyadic relation is not yet a sign and requires an interpretant of some sort for its completion. I have supplied in the example below a sociomedical interpretant, is this case a disease label, though a physiological interpretant (e.g., profuse sweating) would have served as well.

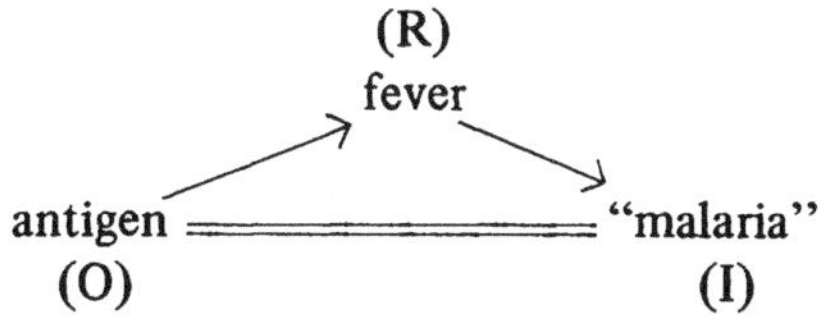

It is an assumption of biomedical theory that not only is the relation between object (antigen) and representamen (fever) non-arbitrary, which I have argued may not always be the case, but the interpretant (disease label, i.e., "malaria") is thought to be the only possible interpretant, or at least the most accurate given current medical knowledge and technologies for generating and evaluating signs (see Celan and Marcus 1973). In fact, one of the goals of biomedical experimentation is to be able to precisely link every object with a single interpretant. The relation between disease label and antigen in this case is implied to be one of equivalence and the label represents the transformation of the object into a more manageable idiom which implies a therapy and a prognosis. The object (antigen) may, however, provoke a variety of other physiological representamens (e.g., leukopenia, delirium, malaise). The existence and recognition of several representamens may be required for the determination of the appropriate sociomedical interpretant, which then, in turn, becomes a sign. Such a set of representamens is generally defined as a *syndrome*. An examination of these labeled syndromes may as much indicate the state of medical knowledge and the underlying assumptions which govern the creation of syndromes as it does to reveal the nature of illness. An interpretant may, in some cases, be derived from the appearance of a single representamen which then functions as a *diagnostic* or *pathognomic* sign. Such signs may, in turn, serve to trigger a search for additional signs also indicative of the same disease process.

Any interpretation involving the application of a disease label is ruled by cultural conventions whether that interpretation evolves out of biomedical theory or is one offered by the ethnomedical healer. The physical object has been transformed into a cultural one and the sociomedical interpretant itself now becomes another sign. The disease label as representamen is still believed to be linked in a non-arbitrary manner with the object and requires an interpretant (another sign) for its completion. The appropriate interpretant in this next transformation may be a series of etiologic, diagnostic, and prognostic signs. Just as a fever may exist as the representamen of an antigen, so too may the interpretant disease label (e.g., "malaria") become itself the representamen. The object antigen may also produce a representamen which is a complaint or symptom ("I feel feverish"); the complaint may also function as the interpretant of the fever and represent the transformation of the object into another (i.e., sensual) idiom.

But the assignment of the first sign ("fever") to an etiological domain, or the eventual negotiation of etiological domain based on additional information, will determine or limit the possible interpretants. Moreover, the interpretive model utilized determines other signs which will be generated and/or grouped with "fever." This inclusion of some signs and exclusion of others from the etiological chain or diagnostic syndrome, according to the interpretive model employed, determines or limits the therapeutic response. For example, a biomedical model excludes the afflicted individual's report of the appearance of an ancestor in a dream (a not uncommon occurrence among the Garinagu of Belize) from that set of signs which constitute the syndrome. Thus the propitiation of ancestors is denied by the biomedical model as a possible therapeutic response.

In Belize, the disease/illness label "malaria" is employed by medical practitioners, ethnomedical healers, and lay persons alike. This utilization of a single term to refer to a specific set of signs and symptoms appears to represent a case of the *articulation of codes*, a process which I shall further describe later in this book, and it does, in a limited sense, facilitate communication between and within professional and ethnic sections. However, examination of the full sign exposes the superficial nature of the supposed equivalence.

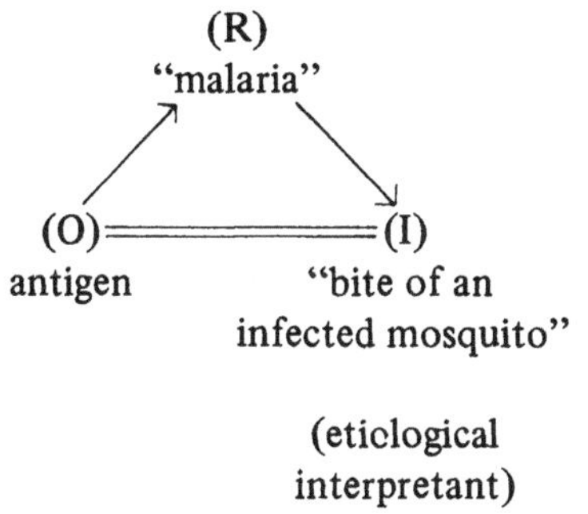

Biomedical Interpretive Model

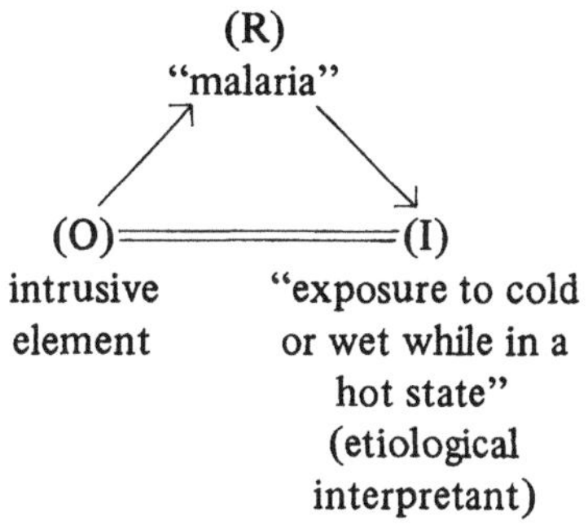

Garifuna Interpretive Model

Each of the above signs, though represented by the same term, "malaria", invokes a different interpretant and is motivated by a different object, or is thought to be motivated by a different object. Further, the assignment of etiological interpretant now determines the possible range of therapeutic responses.

Another question must be asked: Is the *therapeutic* response, either the physiological or sociomedical response, yet another interpretant? Morris' (1964) definition of the interpretant as a disposition to *behave* in a certain way would seem to allow for the incorporation of this sort of response into our illness sign. Peirce's statements on what can and cannot stand as an interpretant are not always clear. As Skidmore notes: "The chief difficulty in following, much less evaluating, what Peirce has to say about signs stems from the obscurity of the term *interpretant*" (1981:43). If the therapeutic response is to be included as a variety of interpretant, then it clearly does not stand in a relation to its object as the disease label, for example, stands for the antigen. Rather, it exists as the very negation of the object and in this relation validates the object. That is, it stands as the obverse of the sign disease/illness, and represents an attempt to invert or eliminate the object. As such, it functions as validation of the existence of the object and as one aspect of its signification. However, we must note that the relation between therapeutic response and object is governed by the code which assesses the relationship, supposed or actual, between object and representamen.

Medical ethnographers and physicians have attempted to define the cultual and physiological codes which govern the transformation of 'medical' data. While these codes have been and continue to be the focus of much attention, the pragmatic employment of codes has been little studied. Locker's (1981) exposition of the interpretive process employed by a small group of English housewives is a valuable contribution to this archeological exploration of mind. His work is important to the discussion here and is, therefore, reviewed at some length.

Individual constructions of social reality, according to Locker, or the ordering of impressions and events into meaningful experiences which allow for appropriate action emerge from "interpretive and definitional work." Social action, in turn, results from the way in which events and experiences are defined (1981:x). Thus to elicit from the data the rationale for action, one must investigate the interpretive processes through which action becomes constituted as a social object (*Ibid.*:133).

The interpretive process, the assignment of experiential phenomena to "socially available categories" and the behavioral response are not totally predicated on a priori notions of cause and effect relationships, for the construction of realities is unique to each individual and cannot be investigated apart from the consciousness of the actors who participate in these constructions. Further, interpretive decisions should not be examined without reference to the social, historical, and personal contexts in which they occur. Diagnoses "are not based solely on signs and symptoms but derive from a process in which other knowledge is employed to arrive at a decision". (*Ibid.*:77). Events and experiences are often ambiguous and cannot be interpreted, that is, assigned meaning on the basis of observation alone. Rather they must be located within a particular interpretive context (*Ibid.*:130). Moreover, meaning construction "does not take place within a vacuum but within 'actual and potential interaction with others'...." (*Ibid.*:13). Meanings are thus susceptible to negotiation.

Locker employs such phrases as "commonsense knowledge", "cognitive resources", "socially available categories", "systems of typifications", "recipes", and so on. Each indicates a process whereby unique experiences occurring in specific contexts can be made 'manageable' or 'meaningful' through reference to specific cultural domains. One of the aims of his book, he states,

> ... is to describe the way in which the cognitive resources contained within a commonsense understanding of matters of health and illness are used to make sense of experience and provide for the stable, orderly character of the world (*Ibid.*:x).

That is, the infinite range of experiences and sensory data has been divided and conceptualized to create socially meaningful categories which allow for the management of diffuse and unsystematic perceptions, feelings, and experiences. Yet Locker denies that the observations he describes should be generalized to other persons and groups. Rather he insists that reality is constantly created anew by participating individuals and that social reality always exhibits an "emergent and transient character" (*Ibid.*:178). Thus, logically, the individual functioning within a specific familial situation, rather than the larger social group, is treated in Locker's work as the locus of interpretive processes.

Problematic experiences may be defined as *illness*[5] in one context but not in another. Definitions may depend on social and psychological needs of the individuals supplying the interpretation. They may also be adjusted according to the biography of the afflicted individual or the historical moment (time-place context) in which the symptoms appear. That is, where critical information is lacking, reference may be made to previous afflictions or to known tendencies of the individual in question, the individual may be assigned to a "special status" (*Ibid.*:111) or reference may be made to events immediately preceding or following the appearance of signs or cues.

.... where the interpretive scheme available is insufficient to make sense of or identify a given object, then its context may be invoked and may furnish the grounds for imputing status and significance (*Ibid.*:13).

A claim to illness may be regarded as genuine, in which case the individual is expected to engage in certain therapeutic and sick role behaviors, or it may be seen "as motivated by anticipated gains" (*Ibid.*:14), in which case, the individual is denied access to the sick role unless other evidence contradicts this interpretation. Regardless of the initial interpretation and categorization of the illness sign(s), later events may result in a reinterpretation. Where discrepancies exist, as in the case where two signs suggest conflicting diagnoses, the facts may be presented "in a way that fits the pre-existent explanation" and are to be regarded as reinforcing that explanation. Where an unambiguous diagnosis is not forthcoming, a single event may be utilized to provide meaning to prior events and to allow for the redefinition of those earlier events in order that they be incorporated into the sequence of signs and cues indicative of illness (*Ibid.*:56).

Locker refers to an "inventory stage" within the sequence of illness events, defined as a "post diagnostic attempt to make sense of events" (*Ibid.*:63). Individuals or family members may also assemble a series of *cues* over a period of time; subsequent to the collection of such signs a *disorder*[6] may be redefined as an *illness* and dealt with appropriately. Diagnoses may require revision when new cues or events are identified as critical to the current state, a cue may suggest an alternative diagnosis (*Ibid.*:55), evidence that "does not fit an existing explanation may be selectively disregarded" (*Ibid.*:79) or aspects of a theory may be elaborated "so that the explanation continues to fit" (*Ibid.*:67). Moreover, individuals may not only provide interpretations "but provide for them by supplying the interpretive scheme to be employed" thus "denying the relevance of indicators which could lead to alternative conclusions"(*Ibid.*:111).

Certain cues or signs suggest professional intervention, but biography or assignment of the symptoms to a category of "severity" is often critical in making the decision to seek professional help. If personal knowledge is inadequate

> ... to make experience consistent with a familiar world then [the individual] may resort to consulting others, including professional problem solvers, who may offer solutions to the cognitive and practical problems with which [the actor] is faced (*Ibid.*:47).

Professional diagnoses may also assist in the process of determining moral responsibility for the illness.

As social constructs definitions of illness also function as moral constructs (*Ibid.*:6), that is, they involve judgments about responsibility and competence. As a member of a social group, an individual may exhibit *cognitive compentence* "by invoking socially appropriate causes to explain given events" (*Ibid.*:81). Communication is facilitated because individuals assume that every other member shares certain notions about the way in which the world of experience is organized. Individuals thus construct accounts which will allow them to be seen as "competent and adequate performers in particular social statuses and their experiences seen to be consistent with a known and routine order of things" (*Ibid.*:23). They must, moreover, present themselves as moral and responsible actors functioning in socially appropriate ways. Challenges forced by the physician on the patient's presentation of himself as a competent and responsible patient (or parent or spouse of a patient) thus threaten the patient-practitioner relationship as does the failure of the practitioner to take into account the biographic account of the patient.

When I first returned from Belize in 1980 after a year and a half of ethnographic field work, I was at least partially frustrated in my initial attempts to 'make sense' of my data, that is, to discover the underlying patterns or regularities in behaviors and interpretations which unified and ordered what otherwise often seemed to be disparate data. Eventually, I concluded that a substantial portion of the variability I have documented was real and not an artifact of the manner in which I had collected the data. Locker has illustrated that significant variability exists among the members of a single 'cultural' group whose members otherwise were quite similar in terms of sex, age, socio-economic status, role responsibilities and residence.

Variability is as important a phenomenon as the regularities we observe, but it is far more difficult to define models which account for variation than those which depict homeogeneity. Social scientists have most often chosen to deal with encountered variability in a statistical sense, showing, in the process, that most people behave predictably most of the time, or to relegate it to the margins or fringes of the social or cultural system. MacCannell (1979), however, describes this periphery as the locus of our most innovative enterprises:

> ...I want to suggest that pressure to get to the heart of culture has introduced into the field of anthropology a systematic bias which carries it ever further away from its subject; namely, a bias which favors conservative, particularistic versions of culture, which denies the creative activities that occur on the fringes of all cultures (149).

I would argue that such "creative activities" are to be found at the core of the cultural context as well.

Locker's focus on interpretive processes accords less significance to phenomena such as cause-effect notions and the outcomes of the interpretive process. Outcomes are of importance in Locker's scheme only in that they are logically related by the respondents to interpretations; notions about cause and effect relationships are essential only to the extent that they function as a resource in the interpretive process. My own field work experiences led me to believe – and this is again confirmed in Locker's work – few signs, events (which are constituted of sequences of signs) or cues are commonly assigned to a particular category of causation without consideration of a variety of contextual factors.

But if reality is negotiated anew according to the requirements of various participants, as Locker argues, how can we account for the fact that from those constructions emerge the patterns we commonly refer to as "culture?" How can the variability encountered be explained while we continue to speak of a "world view" or of "shared realities?" This is a critical problem for social scientists who remain convinced that the concept of culture is both valid and useful and that groups may be differentiated from one another on the basis of culturally prescribed behaviors or the culturally sanctioned use of symbols, yet do not wish to ignore intracultural variability. One resolution to this dilemma is to treat this phenomenon we refer to as culture as constituted of a set of possibilities, a range of interpretations from which we may select. *Culture* bounds our choices, but never totally determines them. The individual who wishes to function in a socially appropriate way recognizes, if unconsciously, the limits of his choices, the constraints upon his actions. The phrase "social construction of reality" is taken, in this instance, to refer to a reality which is created by individuals under a specific set of conditions and cricumstances utilizing a set of socially sanctioned and culturally appropriate resources, rather than a reality which is exclusively constructed by some social group and imposed upon its current and future members. This is not to deny that culture exists, but rather to state that culture defines and organizes the resources from which participants abstract their meanings. This view permits the reconceptualization of existing paradigms and innovative interpretations based upon new paradigms within the bounds of what we refer to as culture. I would further suggest that the new paradigms are themselves produced according to a set of governing codes or rules. In the face of the need to adapt to altered physical and social environments, transformative or interpretive codes are altered according to some metatransformative process.

But how is it possible to speak of "culture" as though it were autonomous, existing apart from the social beings upon whom it is dependent for transmission? According to Peirce, the subject is conceptualized by itself. The social self, therefore, is constructed from a series of conceptions. Every individual is unique not only in appearance, physical characteristics, experiences, and so on, but in terms of conceptualizations about subject and object which are always self-reflexive. We have come full circle to the original question: what is culture if all individuals are unique? Culture is not solely a system of constraints, for it has no life of its own. It is an *agreement* among a group of people that certain activities, objects, and relationships have symbolic importance, that they both unite and, at the same time, symbolize the unity of the group. Yet each individual within that cultural system maintains his or her own unique conceptions of those symbols. Therefore, no shared *understanding* of the symbols is necessary, but rather an acceptance of the belief that these symbols have a unique cultural meaning which serves as the basis for the unity of the group. These symbols produce certain actions, material products, and relationships because the production of such behaviors, objects, and relationships is necessary for participation in the group. The production of these behaviors defines membership in the group, not the conceptualizations of the symbols which remain unique and which define the subject. Yet, self is also defined by the production of objects, behaviors, and relationships. Therefore, symbol, 'meaning', self, and culture are interrelated and generate one another.

Individuals function as members of social and political units and they rely on other members of those units to assist them in the proper interpretation of signs. An initial diagnosis, offered by the afflicted individual or the family unit, may be determined to be self-serving and not conducive to effective functioning of the social or political unit. Individuals, groups and institutions are engaged in a continual process of negotiation. Signs are very often assigned meaning according to the benefit which accrues to the stronger.

Negotiation implies selection from among a variety of potential 'meanings'; it further implies a dialogue, an exchange of information. Negotiation need not, and most commonly does not, require the participation of a therapist. It may occur entirely within the context of the family, or it may involve friends or members of the social collectivity or the "knowledgable observer." The primary goal of negotiation is the achievement of an interpretation or an alignment and structuring of the relationships among signs which is acceptable in cultural (and other) terms and which leads to a therapy which is perceived as appropriate. The existence of alternative therapeutic systems both facilitiates and complicates this process by offering new medical paradigms.

In the process of reporting the signs and their effect, in the transformation from the physiological expression to the verbal (or non-verbal), information about observable or measurable physiological and behavioral changes in bodily or mental states may be transmitted as diffuse feelings or sensations. The *biomedical diagnostician* generally views his task as the transformation of these vague statements ("I don't feel well"; "I am tired all the time", "I am not myself", "I hardly knew myself", etc). to notions about organic change; that is, he attempts to determine the object which provoked the representament. This combination of object and representamen creates the sign which is referred to the proper 'disease' category. If, in fact, the patient's feelings cannot be reduced to such measurable changes or subsumed under some theory which would explain the patient's symptoms in physiological (even though not necessarily measurable) terms, the patient is generally not considered 'diseased' in the physician's usual sense of the term. The *healer*, on the other hand, often links these signs to *social* objects. That is, the healer sees in these signs information about alterations in the social milieu. If there exists a *biological* object, it may exist only as the interpretant of the *social* object. Like the symptoms verbally expressed, the biological object functions as an indicator of other and more important alterations.

Another sort of transformation is possible. The patient may also express diffuse and undefined or unstated or unstatable concerns (failing social or personal relationships; perceived personal inadequacies, fears, anxieties, etc.) in more concrete, i.e., physiological, terms. In this process of transforming the social into the physiological, the patient often makes reference to specific body-parts ("I have too much blood" "My blood is stagnating"; "There must be something wrong with my blood"; "I have heart distress"; etc.). Body-parts thus become metaphors, that is, they stand for perceived bodily or mental states or symbolize some changed internal or external relationship. The diagnostician and therapist, in turn, often come to regard such body-parts as metonyms, parts which stand for wholes; in this case they stand in place of the patient. The patient is conveniently excluded from the ensuing therapy which is directed toward the *metonymic* sign. This is most often true of biomedicine, but occurs in traditional forms of medical therapy as well. The X-ray, an analysis of blood, a removed foreign or intrusive object, come to represent the patient, or, in some cases, refer to some 'other' acting upon the patient.

In cases in which the patient's various social and personal concerns become manifest in physiological signs (for example, as in hysterical conversion, compulsive actions, and schizophasia), the diagnostician's task is to understand the concerns which provoked these statements, this concretization of the symbolic. He must come to some understanding of the total social matrix in which illness occurs. This is an area in which the healer excells. It should be noted that in biomedical practice, the division between practitioners occurs along the lines created by the two modes of transmission. Personal anxieties coded into bodily, physiological, organic changes are most often considered the purview of the psychiatrist, whereas physiological changes which are expressed as vague concerns are ultimately referred to the non-psychiatric physician. It is the object which determines the assignment of practitioner rather than the representamen. However, if semiosis is an infinite process, detection of a 'first' object becomes impossible. This is the basis for my opposition to the description of certain illness states as psychosmatic. My disagreement is not with the term psychosomatic, but rather its naive application to specific signs. All illnesses, as I argued earlier, are psychosomatic in that the mind and body interact at some point in the episode and this interaction produces further signs and symptoms.

The patient's production of signs, both "objective" and "subjective", may represent an attempt by the patient to conform the environment to his perceived needs and wishes. At the same time, the physician's or diagnostician's production of certain signs, and his evaluation of these according to culturally coded a priori decisions and categories (see Crookshank 1923) may lead to therapies which attempt to conform the patient to certain biomedical and social standards. The categorization or interpretation of signs is affected by the diagnostician's "philosophical" bias, and the structured cognitive guildelines which are his cultural and intellectual heritage may interfere with his assessment.

> When man perceives the world, he perceives without knowing it, the superimposed shape of his own mind, and entities can only be meaningful (or 'true') in so far as they find a place within that shape (Hawkes 1977:13).

> That is man constructs the myths, the social institutions, virtually the whole world as he perceives it, and in so doing, he constructs himself (*Ibid.*: 14).

Or, to paraphrase Peirce's dictum, man creates himself as a sign.

A variety of codes (i.e., models. conventions, "habits", "laws") govern the relation between the physiological representamen or the supposed physiological representamen and its potential cultural, political, personal, social, technological and biological interpretants. The disease label which exists as one sort of interpretant, and, in turn, becomes another sign, is as much a result of the application of one of these codes as is the therapy which it indicates, though biomedicine assumes that cultural biases have been removed from the labeling process. The symptom becomes symbol.

"All doctors", Kahn notes

...are participant observers, and as such they 'shape' by their idiosyncratic judgments, the very signs they 'observe'. Moreover, they weigh the degree of significance of such signs upon human scales of measurement that are readjusted, ad hoc, with each successive perceptual experience (1978:91),

Further,

..no diagnostic sign system can claim to be value-free. ...we master...culture-specific sign systems for defining and expressing "disease" and "health" (*Ibid.*:101).

Or, as Baer (1982 MS) remarks:

The organs of thought...are the reproductive organs of the world..., the genital organs of nature.... In thought, the self and the world are nested in one another. This mutual containment is *condensed* and made *existential* (Peirce's secondness) in the medical symptom, and it is for this reason, at least in part, that it is or becomes, properly perceived, *enigmatic* (5).

The body becomes a multileveled, polysemous source of information, the originator of conscious and unconscious signs which both influence the social and physical environment and are in part determined by it. For the diagnositician/therapist such signs allow interpretation of internal organic or physiological states. But for the patient, or potential patient, such signs may not only be perceived as signals guiding his behavior (his evaluation of himself as healthy or ill, in need of therapy or not in need of therapy), but may represent a culturally mediated response to non-organic or non-physiological changes. He may, in fact, find that only by talking about or symptomatizing his bodily or mental state can he express, or attempt to express, successfully or unsuccessfully, consciously or unconsciously, the personal and social concerns which may have provoked the production of signs. The verbalization or expression of the experience of illness stands not only as a sign made manifest for interpretation but as part of the therapeutic response itself.

The signs, outwardly manifested, serve another immediate communicative function. The sudden appearance or awareness of signs mobilizes both the resources of the individual and those of the social group. The illness episode becomes a critical event in which the victim attempts to apprise others of his situation in order that he may mobilize additional resources. His presentation of symptoms is constrained now by a variety of factors: the a priori categories of signs and diseases of which he is aware, the boundaries of his own language, his personal, social and psychological needs, and his understanding or lack of understanding of the interpretive models which govern the diagnostician's perceptions and procedures.

The transformation of a set of signs into something called *disease* has meaning for the diagnostician in that it leads to therapeutic intervention. Further, the experience of labeling the disorder has additional significance for the physician in that it confirms as well as conforms to existing or evolving models of organic processes and of the occurrence of specific diseases in specific places under certain designated conditions – that is, it supports the epidemiological model which governs the expected occurrence of signs and symptoms. The significance attached to the illness by the patient, the social group, and the ethnomedical healer, however, generally differs from that attached by the biomedical diagnostician.

In describing a portrait of Leopardi with the simple designation "Leopardi" written beneath, Peirce suggested:

> It conveys its information to a person who knows who Leopardi was, and to anybody else it says "something like Leopardi looked like this" (8.183).

The application of a disease label by the biomedical diagnostician is analogous to the labeling of the portrait. The label conveys the intended information only to the extent that the interpreter can supply the necessary links to the correct biological object. The sign points, instead, to an etiology which is phrased as a question – "What could I have done differently? – and to a prognosis which also occurs as a question – "What will happen to me?" In other words, from the perspective of the afflicted individual, diagnosis is an essential part of the sign called illness only in that it points backward and forward. The patient who has no knowledge of the appropriate links to the biological object may simply see in this sign (label) an indication of the perceived ability of the diagnostician to "know" and therefore manipulate the object.

For the patient, the biological-physiological domain of meanings generally remains inaccessible. The meanings attached by the patient, the social group, and the ethnomedical healer to the illness episode are retrieved from a variety of domains which are, in turn, often inaccessible to the physician. That is, the afflicted person generates his set of meanings from the culturally defined domains which account for all notions of causation and constitute an important part of his ethnomedical model. The patient frequently sees in his illness indications of alterations in both his interpersonal and intrapersonal relationships. The sign thus brings into question both his past and his future abilities to function in a series of personally accepted or socially imposed roles. The signs may refer as well to the domain of concerns wherein is found the patient's concept of *self*, and this too may be altered in the illness episode, often radically so. The patient may thus come to see in his disorder some failure of the organic or the social self in its relation with itself, with the community of social beings, with the community of spiritual beings, or with elements, living and non-living, in his environment.

Illness, for the healer, is both an organic process, in which the focus may be on specific body parts and on their relation to one another, and a social process in which illness is a metaphor explaining and supporting a larger universe of meanings. The meanings attached by the larger social group are metaphoric, reinforcing the cultural assumptions which bind together the group. The same set of meanings may reinforce stereotypes held by one group of another and may permit the exclusion of members of 'outside' groups from participating in the same array of cultural assumptions or from utilizing the same set of symbols.

The healer, even as a member of his cultural collectivity, is divorced to a greater or lesser extent from the experience of illness. His need to resolve the crisis caused by illness cannot be derived from the same set of concerns as that of the afflicted person. From the perspective of the healer, illness affects the social group; it threatens the social system in which the healer and patient operate. At the same time, illness validates certain philosophical principles, rationalizes the healer's specialization, unifies and mobilizes persons and resources. For the afflicted, illness threatens the very concept of self. It forces unacceptable alterations in image and role. Illness is necessary to the existence of the healer; it is the negation of existence for the sufferer.

Serious illness may not only separate an individual from his family and remove him from the contexts in which decisions are normally made, but may disrupt the assumption or resumption of normal activities. That is, the usual social roles in which he or she is engaged are, at best, temporarily altered, and, at worst, permanently threatened. For many, the concept of "self", of an 'I" separate and distinct from other *egos* is altered by the illness experience as well. This, of course, is true in any society, but the apparent close association between the concept and image of "self" and the roles which are pressed upon one during the normal life cycle in the southern Toledo District of Belize makes serious illness potentially devastating. To attempt to assume the sick role for one's own advantage for any period of time is a negatively sanctioned behavior. In fact, it is a behavior rarely seen. In a society in which every individual must contribute his share of work for the basic social unit to survive it is expected that individuals will give up the sick role as soon as possible and resume their usual roles. This provides us with one explanation of the patient's repeated failure to ask the physician for a name for his illness. Illness is regarded ideally as a transient event which leaves the patient minimally affected in his ability to resume normal activities. Illness is an abnormal and unacceptable situation. People do not identify with illness states; they do not incorporate illness into their personal identities. Individuals do not describe themselves as diabetics, for example, a move which would indicate that the illness had been integrated into a "self." Nor did I ever hear a patient describe himself as an epileptic, an asthmatic, and so on. There is, to my mind, an important distinction between the statement, "I am...." and the statement "I suffer from...."

The context in which signs are interpreted plays a major role in the determination of an interpretant and in the identification of an object; models governing the presentation of symptoms and the evaluation of signs and symptoms are context-specific. Signs which have meaning in one context may not be significant in another. Individuals in Punta Gorda, for example, frequently distinguish between "external" and "internal" fevers. The patient, in approaching the physician, may state that he has a fever. The physician, by taking the patient's temperature, produces a sign which he interprets as indicating normality or abnormality. The sign produced by the physician may contradict the symptom presented by the patient. But the apparent contradiction and negation of the patient's statement may be the result of conflicting models governing the production of signs. The model on which the physician's production of signs is predicated only allows for the observation of the "external" fever, thus denying the patient's production and interpretation of a sign which cannot be coded by the physician in a biomedical system.

The signs and symptoms presented by an afflicted individual or his therapy managing group (Janzen 1978) may be altered both according to the interpreter and the potential interpretations. There are specific illness states which the afflicted individual assumes will be properly understood only by other members of his ethnic group or by persons holding similar beliefs. This means that symptoms presented in the hospital or private clinic setting are necessarily restricted to those which the patient believes will be 'acceptable' to the physician and which, he, the physician, is likely to affect therapeutically. Patients limit their complaints to those which they believe will be understood. The language of illness is restricted and the entire social context as well as the sense of despair and loss of personal identity is omitted from any discussion of illness. The physician, on the other hand, believes that his patients are most often incapable of understanding the underlying paradigms of biomedicine; the cause of illness and its treatment, where an explanation is offered at all, must be explained in ways "they will understand." The physician generates signs or symptoms which the patient may not regard as having significance. The range of signs thus generated within the hospital/clinic setting and those generated within the family or in interactions with the healer varies according to the medical models governing the production of signs. The healer generates signs from domains beyond those explored by his biomedical counterpart.

Understandings of the body and its components differ as well.

> How an individual experiences his body and how he organizes perceptions of his body are culturally patterned. How a person perceives of the interaction of the body and distinguishes among its parts is a reflection of cognitive categories which are culturally determined. Culture and cognition filter, organize, and affect interpretations of all bodily structure, processes and changes (Shedlin 1977:1).

The body, in any social system, provides a set of metaphors for talking about social and political states or structures.

> ....societies take raw objects and transform them into artifacts pregnant with social meaning; and, of course, the body is the object *par excellence* for such an exercise for obvious reasons (Polhemus 1975:27).

Bodily experiences explain and reaffirm social experience. Concomitantly, social experiences impinge upon, define, and channel bodily experiences. "Society is the body; society is constraint", MacRae (1975:71) notes, or, in Mary Douglas' words:

> The body communicates information for and from the social system in which it is a part.... it mediates the social structure by itself becoming its image (Douglas 1971:387).

The body, too, provides the material whereby social and interpersonal problems may be redressed. That is, ritual acts upon and transforms the individual body and, in the process, transforms the social body as well.

The human body is, at one and the same time, vessel of meaning and source of experience; it engenders social significance and provides the medium for its expression. Cross-cultural analyses, however, clearly indicate that the appropriate modes of bodily expression vary; concepts about the nature of the body, its divisibility or indivisibility, its energies, its boundaries, and the meanings attached to its components and products differ. Cross-cultural data also provide varying models of the organization of the body's constituent parts and their interdependence (or lack of it). Even so initially obvious a notion as the extent and permeability of the body boundary differs within and between social systems. A semiotic approach to describing and defining bodily experience must focus on the body as a channel of communication, as an instrument utilized to convey feelings, intents, aesthetic qualities, disturbances in social relations, and political statements in a culturally appropriate idiom, and as a mechanism through which other states of consciousness may be reached. An explicitly semiotic approach additionally must examine the reflexivity provoked by conscious bodily experience. Confined by the body's boundaries and forced to deal with the limitations it imposes, every individual reflects upon the experience of illness. Such reflective behavior is, at least in part, governed by cultural models. While in some societies, persons are socialized into an acceptance of these limitations, in others, individuals are encouraged to transcend the body's boundaries. The body, in this latter system, is seen as an imposition upon or a confinement of one's 'true' nature. The most meaningful of all exprience thus requires the temporary negation of such limitations. Paradoxically, such a negation can often be accomplished only by those highly trained in control of the body's various functions.

The social, political and cultural concerns which are critical to the functioning of a social system both influence the personal experience of illness and are embedded in the models which govern the interpretation of signs. Illness episodes thus become communicative acts. A *post facto* analysis of the episode with its syntactic and semantic components produces a text with embedded cultural and personal statements about the world as it is and as it should be.

NOTES

1. Aspects of this field have been labeled "clinical semiotics", "diagnostic semiotics", and "biosemiotics,"
2. The term illness is used here to refer to what is often divided conceptually into "disease" and "illness."
3. See Brody (1980) and Byerly (1976) for recent reviews of the literature on the placebo effect.
4. The *representamen* is variously referred to as the sign, sign vehicle (Morris 1964), *signifiant* (Barthes 1972), and plane of expression (Eco 1976). Peirce often uses "sign" in place of representamen, while elsewhere insisting that the representamen is but one component of the sign.
5. Locker distinguishes between *disease* and *illness*, as have a number of medical anthropologists and medical philosophers in recent years. Disease refers to a biophysical state or event, whereas, "illness is a social state created by human evaluation; it is a symbolic ordering of given events or states of affairs by application of a label. Consequently, it is not an entity but a meaning used to explain, organize, and evaluate these events or states of affairs (1981:4).
6. A *disorder* evolves from problematic physical or emotional experiences.

CHAPTER 2

The Research Setting

The community of Punta Gorda, a town of approximately 2500 people located in the southernmost district of Toledo in Belize, Central America, was selected as the locale for research because it conformed to conditions necessary to the testing of suppositions concerning health seeking transactions and the interpretation of signs in multiethnic communities. Belize, formerly known as British Honduras, has an extraordinarily heterogeneous population for so small a country (approximately 150,000). Its citizens include several Mayan groups (Kekchi, Mopan, Yucatecan), Black Caribs or Garinagu (sing.: Garifuna), Mestizos, Creoles (non-Indian persons of African descent), and, in lesser numbers, East Indians, Chinese, Lebanese, North Americans, and Europeans. At least 1500 British soldiers of varying ethnic backgrounds (English, Scottish, Irish, and Nepalese Gurkhas) have been stationed in the country since the early 1970's and contribute in important ways both to the heterogeneity of the country and to the *awareness* of heterogeneity. Mackenzie described Belize as a "meeting place for the strands of history (in Grant 1976:xi), and Grant has suggested that Belize's uniqueness in the Pan American world lies in its cultural diversity (1976:6-8) see also Ashcraft 1973; Bolland 1977; Cosminsky 1976, 1977; Gregory 1976). While most ethnic groups have exhibited a tendency towards acculturation into either the Spanish or British (i.e., West Indian Creole) cultural complexes, each has generally retained elements of its indigenous medical model while utilizing, in varying degrees, the services offered by state controlled biomedicine.

Belize became a British colony in 1862, a Crown Colony in 1871 and an independent nation on September 21, 1981. It is, by almost any standard applied, a relatively impoverished country. Per capita income is under $1,000 U.S. The primary sources of income for the government are foreign aid and duties levied on imports. The taxation rate on salaries and properties is low. Most private capital enters the country from Canada, England, and the U.S. Little revenue is generated from industry, excepting large scale agricultural industries; the largest and most successful agricultural and industrial enterprises are foreign owned. No natural mineral or oil resources had been discovered at the time of my initial stay which might have encouraged development. As of 1975 only 10% of all arable land, the primary resource, was under cultivation (*Brukdown* 1978, No. 4, p. 8). According to Bolland, in 1971 3% of all landowners held 95% of the freehold land, foreigners owned 93.4% of all private land holdings over 100 acres and over 90% of all freehold land in the country (1977:7). Recent government policies concerning land ownership and redistribution have yet to result in significant changes.

The government of Belize, unlike that of many central American and Caribbean countries, has been extremely stable. The system of electing public officials and selecting a national leader is modeled after that of the British. There are two major parties, the Peoples' United Party (PUP), which held power from the 1950s to 1984, and the United Democratic Party which won the majority of seats in the National Assembly for the first time on Dec. 14, 1984. The same individual, George Price, had served as Prime Minister since the PUP came into power. While the stability of the country should prove attractive to foreign investors and entrepreneurs, the lack of a highly skilled work force, the inaccessibility of large portions of the country and the difficulty and expense of importing and maintaining equipment have discouraged many. In addition, until Guatemala's claim to Belize, and specifically to the Toledo District, has been resolved to the satisfaction of all parties, it is likely that investors will continue to be cautious.

Punta Gorda is located on the coast of the Gulf of Honduras. It lies approximately 15 miles north and east of the Guatemalan border though, at present, the only direct link with Guatemala is by sea, the Southern Highway of Belize extending no further south than Punta Gorda. The town is situated on a coastal plain; the Maya Mountains are located some 10 to 15 miles inland. That area of the coastal plain which has not been cleared for building or farming is covered with low growing, dense vegetation referred to as "bush." Even the more typical tropical jungle is often called "bush." Cleared land, left untouched, quickly reverts to one or the other.

The temperature ranges from approximately 55°F to over 100°F with humidity typically 80 percent and above. Rather than speaking of hot and cold seasons, Belizeans refer to wet and dry seasons as the amount of rainfall is far more critical to daily activities than the temperature. Punta Gorda receives, on the average, 180 inches of rainfall per year, though yearly rainfall varies from 140 to 210 inches. The so-called "dry" season, during which the tropical rainstorms occur infrequently, extends from February to the end of May. The "wet" season is characterized by sudden thunderstorms and showers, most commonly occurring at night or in the morning hours. The wet season makes agricultural activity difficult and often renders logging operations impossible. The soils are leeched of important minerals by the heavy rains and locating soil suitable to efficient crop raising is difficult. Heavy rains and high seas keep fishermen in port much of the time during these months. The rains additionally interfere with almost any outdoor activity though, most important, they stop the transport of people and goods back and forth from the villages to Punta Gorda and virtually halt the movement of supplies from Belize City to the southern towns. Punta Gorda and its oulying villages are the most severely affected.

One of the distinctive features of labor patterns in Belize is the tendency for adults, especially males, to migrate out, principally to the U.S., in search of jobs at better wages. One issue of *Brukdown* (1978, No. 4) reported that while 30,000 Belizeans are employed in Belize, an estimated additional 30,000 Belizeans are employed in the United States. Most are believed to be there illegally. The immigration/emigration figures for 1975 indicate 4,000 more persons left the country than immigrated. With births totaling 5,201 and deaths 733, the country showed a total increase in population for the year of only 569 (Annual Abstract of Statistics, 1976). But the tendency toward outward migration is not evenly distributed across all ethnic groups. It is the Garinagu and the Creoles who leave in the largest numbers.

The 1980 Census (Statistical Office, Central Planning Unit, Belmopan, May, 1982) shows an overall growth in the country's population of 21.2%, from 119,934 persons in 1970, to 145,343 in 1980. Further analysis indicates that the greatest growth occurred in the predominantly Mayan and Mestizo areas and the least in the predominantly Creole and Garifuna communities. Belize City, which is 76% Creole according to the 1980 census and the country's major city, grew by only 1.8% between 1970 and 1980. Punta Gorda, which is generally identified as a Garifuna town, grew by a modest 12.5% while the urban area of Corozal Town (59% Mestizo), the rural area of Corozal (58% Mestizo, 20% Maya), the community of Orange Walk (68.9% Mestizo), and the rural Toledo District (70% Maya, 10% East Indian) grew during the same period by 47.4%, 47.2%, 52.4%, and 36.6% respectively. Dangriga (70% Garifuna) actually suffered a loss of population.

Cosminsky (1976) estimated that in 1960 approximately 70% of the population of Punta Gorda was Garifuna. The 1980 figures show an increase in percentage of population for all ethnic groups with the exception of the Garifuna segment which had declined to 48.3% of the total population with a suggested absolute decline in actual numbers as well. This migration of the Garinagu and, to a lesser extent, the Creoles[1] rarely involves entire families. Rather, the younger adults leave in an attempt to find work at better wages.

A census of Punta Gorda conducted by the Town Board in 1960 indicated that 60% of the population was under the age of fifteen and 20% over sixty, giving evidence of the extent of out-migration of young and middle-aged adults (Avilez, personal communication). A survey of 100 households I conducted in 1979 and 1980 indicated that approximately 56% of the population was under the age of sixteen. The 1980 census shows 2396 person living within the township of Punta Gorda (Waight, personal commumication), an increase of only 265 over the 1970 figures. The greatest increase in population has clearly occurred in "rural" Toledo (an absolute increase of 2508), which is largely populated by East Indians and Maya. This is the result not only of a higher birth rate in the rural areas, but of inmigration of Kekchi Maya across the Guatemalan borders.

In one sense, the national government of Belize has relatively little impact on the lives of most residents of Punta Gorda, at least by comparison with the governments of industrialized nations. Freedom of the press is substantial, the right to assemble practically unlimited. There are few laws regulating the sale of goods, the provision of services, the rights and obligations of tenant and landlord, fishing rights, road use, and so on. There is no extensive welfare system, no unemployment compensation, and income taxes are minimal. There are few licenses to buy, permits to obtain, or papers to be filed, though individuals complained in 1984 that the "bureauracy" had increased. Property taxes are low and are collected once a year at the Lands and Survey Department. A social security system was instituted in 1982, but has had little impact thus far.

But, from another perspective, the government's role is considerable and increasing. The government regulates commerce with Guatemala and Mexico. It is responsible for the development and maintenance of major communicative channels. It controls Belize's only radio station. It prohibited the introduction of television for many years, though television programs from the States are now transmitted via a government-owned satellite. It provides a telephone system for Punta Gorda. though very few residents can afford telephones. It maintains the Southern Highway which connects Punta Gorda with towns to the north, but the Highway remains closed to traffic for several weeks of the year because bridges or roads are flooded and the country hasn't the necessary equipment to keep them open. Access to many villages, in any season, can be gained only by foot or by boat. Boats and barges which used to travel regularly along the coast are no longer in operation. The government is the provider of electricity, water, and health care, and partially underwrites and controls all primary school education. Upon my return to Punta Gorda I saw increasing evidence of government involvement in the District with the addition of several government offices in Punta Gorda.

Some food and other commodity prices are controlled, but inflation was a serious problem during my first residency in Belize. Belize must import most of its fuel and like most Third World countries was hard hit by the increasing cost of oil. The government has done little to encourage sudden expansive development and has cast a wary eye on certain potential foreign investors.

Lacking both visibility and exploitable resources, Belize has been unable to generate the foreign loans and capital investments on the scale to be seen in other Central American countries. In 1984 I found substantial evidence of increased American interest in the country. A local fishing co-operative had been established with funding from the U.S government and the number of Peace Corp workers had been increased. Foreign aid from the U.S government totalling ten to fifteen million dollars had been promised as part of the Reagan administration's Caribbean Basin Initiative. But it was the general consensus of those with whom I spoke in Punta Gorda that the Toledo District was now worse off economically than it had been in 1980.

Belize: A Multi-Ethnic Nation

The history of the settlement of Belize is an extraordinary story of migration, exploitation, and adaptation. The first inhabitants of Belize were the Maya whose occupancy of the territory seems to have begun some 3500 years ago (Hammond 1977:116). Rather than existing on the periphery of Mayan civilization as historians and archaeologists once believed, Belize now appears to have been in the very center of Early Formative to Late Classic Mayan activities.

The well-known site of *Lubaantun* and the lesser known site of *Nim Li Punit* are located some twenty miles to the west and north of Punta Gorda and a few miles from the Mopan Maya village of San Antonio. The minor Classic Maya sites of Seven Hills, Port and Doughboy Point, Wild Cane Cay, Frenchman's Cay, and Moho Cay are located from eight to fifteen miles north and east of Punta Gorda (Hammond 1975). *Lubaantun*, occupied from approximately A.D. 730 to A.D. 860, was a major ceremonial center with a population in its realm of up to 50,000, according to Hammond, supported by milpa farming of maize, beans and squash (*Ibid*.:133). The ceremonial centers appear to have been deserted by A.D. 900, though Manche Chol settlements persisted into the seventeenth century. Cortez reportedly passed through the southeast corner of the Toledo District in 1525 and found both scattered Mopan and Chol Maya settlements (Bolland 1977:18).

Both military incursions and religious conversions appear to have played a part in the disappearace of the Maya from the Toledo District.

> The Chol Maya were devastated by Spanish incursions, beginning in 1603, when Fathers Esquerra and Cipriano persuaded them to become Christians. Thirty years later, however, they revolted, burned all the churches, and abandoned the towns into which they had been herded. "For thirty-eight years the Chols retained their independence" until a series of missionary expeditions between 1671 and 1677 led to their repacification. But in 1678 "the Chols, irked by town life and the restrictions of Christianity, once more fled into the forests" burning the church at San Lucas Tzalac, which may have been near the Garcias a Dios Falls on the River Sarstoon. In 1685 Father Cano and other

priests rebuilt the church and again tried to control the Chols. That time the "pacification" lasted only four years, and the Chols once more burned the church in revolt. At that point the Spaniards changed their tactics. In 1689, 1690, and subsequent years they sent punitive expeditions to round up the Chols and transport them to the Guatemalan highlands, leaving the Manche area, which may once have contained as many as ten thousand people, a virtually uninhabited forest. The Chols were eventually absorbed by the expanding Kekchi Maya, some of whom returned to the area in the late nineteenth century and settled around San Antonio in the Toledo District. The south of Belize, which had been inhabited by Maya in the seventeenth century (a Dominican priest, Father Delgado, encountered many small Maya settlements when he crossed the area in 1677) was thus depopulated by Spanish action and remained practically deserted for a century, until the arrival of the Caribs (Bolland 1977:18).

The Maya who now occupy Toledo are recent immigrants to the area. The Mopan, with a population of approximately 3,000, inhabit the villages of San Antonio, Pueblo Viejo, Santa Cruz, and San Jose in the foothills and lowlands of the Maya Mountains. They are the descendants of a small group of Mopan who left San Luis in the Peten District of Guatemala to settle eventually at San Antonio around 1888 (McCaffrey 1967; Gregory 1972).

The Kekchi, numbering 3,700 in the southern Toledo District, arrived in the area from the Alta Verapaz region of Guatemala in the early part of this century. The first Kekchi entered Belize specifically to open up the bush on the Temash and Sarstoon estates of the Kramer enterprises (McCaffrey 1967:36). The Kramer estates were abandoned in 1915 but the Kekchi remained. Population pressures and the need for additional land for milpa farming led to the establishment of new villages. There were, in 1967, fourteen predominantly Kekchi settlements (*Ibid.*:34, 41). The vast majority of Kekchi still reside in Guatemala, although movement across the border has been common. The 1981 agreement between Britain and Guatemala resulted in a closing of the border between the two nations, prohibiting, or at least inhibiting, such migration for a time.

The languages of the Mopan (most often called Maya) and the Kekchi are mutually unintelligible and intermarriage between the two was for many decades uncommon. Now many Maya villages are ethnically mixed and children often bilingual or trilingual. The Kekchi generally live in the isolated "back" villages, off the main access roads, in Crique Sarco, Aguacate, Dolores, San Benito Poite, San Lucas, and Silver Creek.

The Maya are the largest segment of the district's population and its principal agriculturalists. While the land has the potential to support a wide range of crops, the Maya concentrate on the production of rice, beans and corn. These are sold to the district office of Belize's marketing board. The Maya bring small amounts of citrus fruit, plantain, and corn to the open market twice weekly, but rarely sell any other produce in Punta Gorda. Fruits and vegetables which are produced in or near the villages are usually consumed locally. The supply of fruits and vegetables which appears weekly in Punta Gorda is largely imported from Mexico via Belize City. Despite the potential productivity of the land, the Maya have been discouraged in attempts to produce vegetables for export because such crops are susceptible to spoilage and the roads to Punta Gorda and to the north are often impassable during the rainy season. The Maya raise some beef, and hog production has increased sufficiently to allow them to ship some animals to the north. Most of the "back" villages, however, remain largely isolated from the possibility of such commerce though hogs are sometimes herded out over jungle trails and sold in Punta Gorda or Aguacate (Schackt, personal communication). Hunting, fishing, and gathering additionally supplement the diet of corn tortillas and beans.

A small but thriving merchant class has emerged among the Maya offering goods to meet the relatively basic needs of the Mayan communities. But the requirements of these villages are changing with exposure to other cultures and the "urban" atmosphere of Punta Gorda and with increased cash income, a small proportion of which is earned as wages at Salamanca Army camp.

By 1638 or 1640, the British (primarily Scots) had established their first permanent settlement in Belize, likely on or near that spot where Belize City is located today. The earliest settlers in this land were not farmers or fishermen, but entrepreneurs and adventurers of the most exotic sort – the infamous pirates of the Caribbean who found the sheltered coasts and cays of Belize an ideal spot from which to conduct their raids against the Spanish merchant ships. The pirate Blackbeard was said to be among their number. Within a few years, the British had found it as lucrative – and certainly safer – to cut and ship their own logwood as to plunder the Spanish fleet, for the demand for logwood in England was high.

At first, these European settlers, pirates still, raided the small Mayan villages for concubines and, as the need for labor grew, for slaves. But the Maya had never proved to be the best of slaves and, in any case, they fled again – this time west and north into the interior. As the logwood trade declined and the demand for mahogany increased, the British were forced further into the interior where they occasionally encountered the Maya. The records of the day make reference to attacks by "wild Indians."

By the early 1700's, the British, now desperately in need of labor for the exploitaition of the forests, began to import African slaves from the West Indies and from Africa through Jamaica.

The earliest reference to the presence of black slaves in the Bay of Honduras is provided by a Spanish missionary who reported in 1724 that the British settlement consisted of "about three hundred Englishmen, besides Mosquito Indians and negro slaves, these latter having been introduced but a short time before from Jamaica and Bermuda" (Bolland 1979:5).

In 1779 Spain was successful in defeating the British at their main settlement of St. George's Cay, though their dominion over the northern portion of Belize was not to last for long. Those British who were not captured apparently took refuge on the Mosquito Coast of Nicaragua. In 1783, several hundred of these refugees returned from the coast to Belize, bringing with them their slaves. "In addition to their African and European heritage [these slaves] also displayed a strong injection of American Indian blood, the result of the Anglo/Mosquito alliance in various campaigns" (*Brukdown* 1979 6/7: 45). So strong had this alliance been that the Kings of the Mosquito Nation were crowned in the Bay territory in 1825 and again in 1840.

The Creole population of Belize is said to be descended from these earliest British settlers and the African slaves they found necessary to the conduct of their lucrative industry, but, in fact, the term Creole is used loosely to refer to almost any individual who is thought to have European and African ancestry. The Creole community of Punta Gorda is constituted of persons from disparate backgrounds who arrived in the town at different times. The Baymen, ignoring any treaties with the Spanish which confined them to the area north of the Sibun River, had moved as far south as the Moho and Sarstoon Rivers by the late 1700s. They brought with them slaves from Jamaica and the Mosquito Coast and they may have stopped briefly in the area where Punta Gorda is now located. There is no record of any permanent settlements in the area at that time; it was the nature of the logging industry that settlements were nothing more than temporary camps in any case. Perpaps it was knowledge of exploitable mahogany which drew some back to the southern Toledo when slavery was abolished and the period of "apprenticeship" finished. Whatever the motivation, by the mid to late 1800s, there was a small Creole population in Punta Gorda. Most initially came as laborers, but in subsequent generations established themselves in the community as merchants and civil servants. Punta Gorda was then principally a Garifuna settlement, the American Toledo Settlement (see below) was located approximately two miles to the north and west, as were the residences of their East Indian workers. According to one account, Spanish from Honduras arrived in the region as early as the 1850s.

It is unknown what commerce there may have been between these largely separate communities, but Americans had established a general store in Punta Gorda, known locally as the Planter's Store, before the turn of the century. The first major building in town was erected around 1890 and belonged to the German, Kramer, owner of the Kramer estates to the south.

While the community identifies certain families as Creole, the personal histories of elderly Creole residents of Punta Gorda illustrate that the term Creole refers to persons who do not share history, vocation, or physical appearance. One man, elder member of one of the town's most distinguished families and eighty-five years of age at the time of my stay in Punta Gorda reported that his great grandfather was French and migrated from Panama. His father married a Mestizo woman from Honduras; they settled in Punta

Gorda in 1892 where they opened a grocery and dry goods store. Another elderly Creole gentleman who was eighty-two in 1979 stated that he had arrived in Punta Gorda before World War II to work for an American logging concern. He purchased ninety acres of land with wages he saved, operated a small sugar planatation, and raised a few animals. He is the descendant of a Portuguese man married to a black slave and a Creole man whose wife was Irish. He claims Canadian Indians among his ancestors as well.

The Garinagu (Garifuna - sing.) or Black Caribs, presently constitute approximately fifty percent of Punta Gorda's citizens. They are descended from the union of fugitive slaves brought from the coast of West Africa and the "Red" or Island Caribs (Carib/Arawak) who occupied most of the Lesser Antilles and possibly parts of Trinidad and Puerto Rico at the time of the arrival of the first Europeans. According to Gullick, the Island Carib were slowly forced onto the islands of Dominica and St. Vincent (1976:6).

Slaves from the countries of West Africa were first brought to the Caribbean in 1517, however, no mention is made of them among the Island Caribs of St. Vincent until 1646, though escaped slaves may have arrived on the island of St. Vincent as early as the sixteenth century (Gullick, *Ibid.*). According to early records, one of two slave ships sank either near St. Vincent or the nearby island of Bequia in 1635 and the survivors took refuge among the Island Caribs. The nature of the relationship between the Caribs and the Africans in the early years is poorly documented. Some have argued that the Caribs took the Africans as slaves; other that Caribs engaged in warfare with the Black or mixed Caribs (mixture apparently having occurred early when escaped slaves first settled on the islands), and others still that they settled peaceably together and intermarried. Whatever the case may have been at the time of initial contact, only two generations later, European visitors to the Island reported that St. Vincent contained some 3,000 Negroes (Hadel 1972:3) and that 600 Black bowmen were counted among 900 Red Carib warriors (Kerns 1977:22).

> Whether the Indians acted as hosts or masters of the Africans, the intimacy between them was close enough that the Africans quickly adopted their language and many of their cultural practices. But the relationship was shortlived. By the end of the 17th century, the Reds and Blacks constituted two separate ethnic units. The nature of the breach between them has several versions, all written by Europeans long after the fact and perhaps appocryphal. What is clear about this period of the Black Carib genesis is that the Africans survived and multiplied, and that having gained their liberty from their European captors first, and later perhaps from the Red Caribs as well, they were loath to surrender any fraction of it thereafter (Kerns 1977:22).

Frequent hostilities seem to have been the rule rather than the exception in the century which followed. Gullick states that the mixed or Black Caribs sometimes took Blacks as slaves and occasionally killed Blacks during periods of hostility (1976:12). During this same period, he reports, "tribes [of Black Caribs] or even districts were frequently at war with each other in times of peace with or victory over the British" (*Ibid.*:22).

In 1795, at the instigation of the French, the Garinagu (or Black Charaibes as they were referred to at that time) attempted to regain control of the island from the British who had been granted jurisdiction over St. Vincent in 1763. The "Charaibes" were defeated in the following year and in 1797 were deported to the island of Roatan off the coast of Honduras. "[T] wo months after their arrival...., the Caribs peacefully turned over the island to the Spanish and set forth for the mainland, where they settled near Trujillo, Honduras" (Gonzalez 1969:19-20).

In 1802, the British admitted some 150 Garinagu into Belize, principally into the Stann Creek District to the north of Toledo. The main influx, however, did not occur until 1832 when many were forced to flee after siding with the royalist cause in an abortive attempt to overthrow the republican government of Honduras (Hadel 1972:4). According to Gullick, many fled to Punta Gorda in what was then British Honduras (1976:31). That event is now recognized as a national holiday in Belize, and on November 19 each year the Garinagu re-enact the original landing on the shores of the Bay Settlement.

> There is evidence that these early immigrants were not well received; ... for several years the British attempted to expel these Caribs from the Colony, believing them to be an extremely dangerous and undesirable elemet. Whether or not they ever succeeded in expelling them for a time, the Caribs kept returning, and finally in 1857 lands at Stann Greek were officially leased to the Caribs who had been settled there from about 1820 (Gonzalez 1969:24).

Gonzalez notes that "it is possible that the towns of Livingston (Guatemala) and Punta Gorda (British Honduras) were settled at about the same date" (*Ibid.*) Gullick remarks that Livingston was founded in the 1800's by a Carib "witchdoctor" (Gullick 1976:29). One of the older residents of Punta Gorda and mayor of the town during my stay suggested Punta Gorda was established by Garifuna settlers from Livingston, Guatemala. The town of Barranco to the south of P.G. was settled about 1860 by Garinagu who were "expelled by the 'white man' from their lands further to the north" (Palacio 1982:11).

Gullick states that the break-up of the Republic of Central America during the years 1839-1842 resulted in a multitude of frontiers. Many Garinagu fled to the more peaceful British territories of Stann Creek (Dangriga), Punta Gorda, and Mosquitia. Stephens, in 1841, described Punta Gorda as a "settlement of Carib Indians about a hundred and fifty miles down the coast ... with a range of low houses...." (in Gullick 1976:33). By 1882 Punta Gorda was said to have a population of about 400 and a resident district magistrate. A census conducted in the late nineteenth century indicated that the Garinagu were fully half of the population of the southern Toledo District. In the 1930's Thompson, who studied the Mopan Maya at San Antonio, reported that the inhabitants of Punta Gorda and other local settlements were all Black Caribs except for about six white people and twelve Ladinos (Gullick 1976:81). This conflicts, however, with the history given to me by several long-time residents who claim the area was far more heterogeneous, even at this early date.

The Catholic Church apparently lost little time in establishing a ministry for the Caribs. Buhler reports that by 1862, a Belgian Jesuit priest, Father Genon, had established a residence in Punta Gorda (1976:6). St. Peter Claver school was apparently built about 1890, the same year in which a Methodist school was built for the children of the Toledo Settlement and their East Indian workers.

The Garinagu who entered Punta Gorda in the first half of the last century survived and multipled because they had developed the techniques to exploit a variety of econiches and the social and ceremonial institutions which allowed for the efficient distribution of the products of exploitation. They were agriculturalists, fishermen, hunters and gatherers, and, according to Gullick (1976:33) occasionally smugglers as well. As the community grew and other groups appeared they sold their labor and as the church schools evolved they became the teachers to the community. Fishing today, while of symbolic importance, supports few families and provides only supplemental income for a few others. Interest in agriculture has diminished – except for the clearing of the fields or garden plots, it was largely considered women's work, in any case. The Carib Block or Reserve, 960 acres of land purchased by the Garinagu for the exclusive use of Garifuna people, is little used. In 1979, only twenty five persons farmed small plots of land; two men each utilized an additional twenty acres in a communal beef raising project. In 1984 I was told that approximately fifteen families utilized the Reserve lands. Some land had been rented to Spanish farmers.

The great majority of Garifuna families are supported by wages earned from the sale of their labor. As opportunities for wage labor decrease, the Garinagu are usually the first affected. The males, and, less frequently, the females, migrate out in search of work and better salaries, leaving behind the children to the care of aunts and grandmothers and sisters and wives. Flexibility and diversification are still the keys to the economic and cultural survival of the Garinagu. Children work in the streets shining shoes, running errands, selling home-made foods, gathering bottles for resale, etc. Women cook, take in laundry, sell frozen confections and ice, do sewing, and so on. Men may engage in various income producing activities while holding down full-time jobs, if such are available.

By the 1870's, Punta Gorda and its environs were already the residence of several distinct ethnic sections. But the diversity which characterizes Punta Gorda today had only begun to be established. The period from 1850 to 1900 saw the introduction of several additional ethnic collectivities. One of the least known but most interesting of the groups to settle in or near Punta Gorda was a small band of southerners who chose to leave the United States following their defeat in the Civil War. Induced by an "offer of 100 acres of land to every male at a 'gratuitous' price" (Grant 1976:34) the southerners migrated to Belize in 1867. Dobson's statement (1973) that the original settlement was at Cattle Landing (about one and one-half miles north and east of Punta Gorda) is in conformity with the account of a long-time resident of Punta Gorda who says the Americans first settled close to Punta Gorda, then, desiring to keep their community separate from that of the Garinagu, began to purchase land further inland, naming their new settlement Forest Home (Francis Martinez, personal communication).

Dobson's *History of Belize* gives the following account of the fortunes of the Toledo settlement:

> The life of the settlers was by no means easy; the virgin forest had to be cleared and few families had sufficient food or money to survive for a year until the crops could be havested. The cholera epidemic of 1878 killed several Americans and discouraged others, but, in 1880, a new group arrived to reinforce the settlement. It was soon realized that crops cultivated in the state of Mississippi could not be successfully produced in the colony; although bananas thrived, the distance from the market made them unsuitable as a cash crop. From 1870 onwards sugar proved to be the most successful commodity and within a short time twelve sugar estates were established, each with its own mill.
>
> Twenty years later about 600 acres were under cultivation and the settlers were employing about three hundred labourers. But 1890 proved the high point in the fortunes of the Toledo settlement. A determination to succeed, evident from the beginning of their enterprise, could not enable the Methodists to prevail against adverse social and economic factors. In the first place, theirs was a closed community which opposed complete integration with the community; once they reached adolescence the children were sent back to the United States for their education. In this way any question of miscegenation was avoided. But not only did the group regard itself as an exclusive community from the social point of view, it was equally unwilling to employ outside labor. As the sugar estates prospered the settlers had to change their minds on this point.... But the collapse of sugar prices on the European market meant the inevitable end of the settlement's prosperity and only those families who turned their attention to the mahogany industry survived. After 1910 there was a steady drift back to the United States, and the Toledo Settlement virtually ceased to exist (Dobson 1973:248-9).

Despite an early proclamation of total self-sufficiency, the American Toledo settlement was forced to import workers. Initially, Garifuna workers from Punta Gorda were employed on the estates. Whether the Garifuna males tired of agricultural work or the Toledo settlers found them unsuitable workers is unclear. Eventually, however, the Toledo settlers were forced to look elsewhere for labor.

In 1858, the British government had transported approximately one thousand Sepoy mutineers and their families to Belize following the India Mutiny. Other East Indians were brought in from the West Indies and from Calcutta to meet the labor needs of the growing logging industry and the sugar plantations. Form the 1870's on, the Toledo settlement utilized East Indian workers and small East Indian settlements appeared to the north of P.G. Though only a few individuals remain who claim descendency from the American settlers, an East Indian population of approximately 900 now occupies Forest Home, Mafredi, Jacintoville, and rural areas to the north and west. They prosper as merchants, wage laborers, teachers, and civil servants, Their primary ties, however, are to the land and they farm small to moderate sized parcels of leased or purchased land. Many raise cattle and some of the beef is sold in Punta Gorda. Dairy products are locally consumed and never reach the town. Rice, corn, and beans are sold to the Marketing Board. Women and children are expected to help in the fields, especially if the husband has another job. Men frequently rise before dawn to work the land and tend to the animals before leaving for jobs elsewhere. Some East Indians, generally merchants or the wives of other residents of Punta Gorda, now live in the town, though they probably comprise less than five percent of the total population of Punta Gorda.

East Indians and Maya may have profited most from what economic development there has been in the southern Toledo and both have developed a strong entrepreneurial sector. While the Maya seem to be relegated to an inferior social status and are often simply disregarded by other groups who refer to them as "backward", they have acquired considered political acumen and business skills. Certain Maya individuals are now recognized as having substantial political power, at least within the context of the Mayan community, and increasing wealth to support such power. The East Indians have developed a wide range of strategies in the exploitation of available econiches and are developing a potentially powerful merchant class. While the Garinagu often migrate out in search of new econiches, the East Indians and the Maya have strengthened their respective land bases and have sought new approaches to the exploitation of available resources. Since both Maya and East Indians have selected adaptive strategies which are similar in many respects, the possibility for competition over available resources exists. However, Belize's low population density and large areas of unexploited land mitigate against such competition in the near future though current farming techniques require an extensive land base. Some Mayan villages are experiencing population pressures which can no longer be relieved through the traditional techniques of fissioning and resettlement.

Another potential competitor for available land is the small Mennonite population of the District. There are Mennonite settlements at Blue Creek to the west of Punta Gorda and at Crique Sarco to the south and west. Unlike the Mennonites to the north who migrated from Germany through Mexico and Canada, those in Toledo have come from the United States in recent years. According to ethnographer Jon Schackt, American Mennonites first came to Belize in the early 1960's to provide relief to Belizeans following the devastation of Hurricane Hattie. In 1976, the "Pilgrim Fellowship Missions, Ltd." signed a contract with the village of Crique Sarco. In exchange for permission to settle in the village for a period of ten years, the Mennonite organization agreed to provide the village with a nurse. Schackt explains that, in addition to desiring the presence of a nurse in the village, some Catholic Kekchi hoped that the Americans "might prove a counterweight against the often unpopular 'hermanos' (Pentecostal Evangelicals)" present in the village since 1974. As the Mennonites chose to associate more closely with their fellow Protestants (often attending Pentecostalist services), these expectations were not fulfilled (Schackt, personal communication).

The efficient agricultural techniques and relative wealth of the Mennonites have, in some areas, attracted Kekchi Maya converts to the Mennonite faith. Market day in Punta Gorda brings an interesting mix of Mopan and Kekchi women in their traditional and distinctive clothing and a few Kekchi women dressed in the conservative Mennonite style. No intermarriage between American and Maya Mennonites appears to occur as the result of religious conversion. While there are presently few Mennonites in the District their presence is likely to become increasingly significant. The Mennonites of Blue Creek are responsible for the only large-scale production of chickens in the district and their introduction of farm machinery represents an agricultural technique previously untried in the southern Toledo. What fresh dairy products there are in the country are generally supplied by the Mennonites, though sales of such products in Punta Gorda are negligible.

The small (less than one-hundred persons) "Chinese" population of the Toledo district is scattered through Punta Gorda and some of the outlying communities, and forms no distinct community in most respects. While the Chinese first arrived in northern Belize as indentured servants in the 1800's, the families of Punta Gorda are descendants of those who immigrated in the early part of this century from the province of Canton. They came as merchants and traders and continue in these trades, though members of the younger generation have taken up other professions, such as teaching. No Chinese women were allowed in the colony in the first decades (it was believed they were prone to tuberculosis [Octavio Castillo, personal communication], and the Chinese males of Punta Gorda married Spanish or Mestizo women exclusively. The current generation of Chinese are therefore of mixed ancestry. As Chinese women were allowed into the country, the preference for marriage with Chinese women was expressed.[2]

The history of the Spanish or Mestizo settlement of Punta Gorda cannot be so clearly written. Spain failed in its several attempts to colonize Belize, though it continued its efforts to dislodge the British settlers. The last of these attempts was defeated in 1798 at the Battle of St. George's Cay where the Spanish were repulsed by a combined force of British settlers and African slaves. Spain, of course, succeeded in colonizing the remainder of Central America and there has been a gradual influx of citizens from the surrounding countries since at least the middle of the last century. The majority of

Spanish-speaking Belizeans still live in the northern districts of Belize. Many are descendants of the refugees from the Guerra de Las Castas (1847-1853). Others have arrived in more recent migrations. But there is at present a considerably larger Spanish population in Punta Gorda than Cosminsky found during her periods of fieldwork in Punta Gorda (Cosminsky 1976, 1977), indicating the migration of Spanish-speaking people in recent years into the Toledo. Some of Punta Gorda's Spanish residents have come to P.G. from the north. Others have arrived from Guatemala and Honduras, though the principal migration of Spanish-speaking people from these countries appears to have occurred in the latter part of the last century as the result of political disturbances there. It is as difficult to describe in cultural or physical terms those who refer to themselves as Spanish (the term Mestizo is rarely used by anyone in P.G., but appears in the Census) as it is to define those categorized as Creole. Most appear to be more European than Mayan in appearance while, in some, Indian features predominate "Urbanized" Maya often adopt a "Spanish" identity, though recent migrants to Punta Gorda have difficulty legitimizing this identity if they continue in the use of a Mayan language.

The Spanish of Punta Gorda, like the East Indians, have effectively adapted to a wide range of econiches. However, few farm and fewer still live in the isolated rural areas. One or two families appear to supplement their wages with income earned from the sale of produce from small "plantations" located outside of Punta Gorda. The Spanish serve within the community as merchants, civil servants, landlords, teachers, and laborers. A number of stores within the town are owned by persons of Spanish descent. There is a strong tendency for intermarriage among members of Spanish, East Indian, Creole, and Chinese ethnic groups, particularly within these "merchant" families.

Ethnicity and Ethnic Groups

The development and conceptualization of ethnic group boundaries is a process. Ethnicity is a reaction to categorical ascription by others as well as to the creation and incorporation of symbols into the collective identity. Ethnic groups do not evolve in isolation; they are a response to interaction. Ethnic boundaries are fluid yet capable of persisting despite a flow of personnel across them (Barth 1969). Nevertheless, boundaries, like other sign systems, are subject to reinterpretation and may be adjusted according to the interests of those within or those without. Clearly, however, conflicts of interest impose limitations on the extent to which these boundaries may be redefined.

Most individuals in Punta Gorda identify with a single ethnic group though many are of mixed parentage. There is, as might be expected in any situation in which power and advantage accrue to the members of specific groups, a degree of situational ethnicity, that is, the renegotiation or altered presentation of one's ethnic identity for a period of time and within a particular context. The size of the community, however, mitigates against frequent alterations. Assignment to ethnic groups is not highly problematic; that is, ethnic self-reference and referral to an ethnic category by others generally coincide.

The soliders of the British army have not been included in the census nor listed as an ethnic group within the country; yet their interaction with the "locals" of Punta Gorda is often intensive, though limited to certain sorts of transactions. Because the soldiers in the area (numbering approximately 450) are replaced every six months, they represent, in fact, not one ethnic group but several. A large contingent arrived in Punta Gorda in 1975 when the Guatemalans made their first serious threat against the southern border of Belize. Their presence has been significant for a number of reasons:
1. They have brought a considerable amount of money into the community, both as cash outlays for goods and services and as salaries paid to the fifty to one-hundred "locals" employed at the three area bases.[3]
2. Local townspeople and rural villagers alike have developed a new set of adaptive and exploitative strategies in their dealings with the soldiers.
3. In an already heterogeneous society, they have increased both heterogeneity and awareness of the phenomenon of ethnicity by exposing local people to customs and beliefs often unlike their own.
4. Their continued presence in the region is gradually altering the gene pool of the town.

There are other recent immigrants, generally arrivals from America and Europe, who form an almost insignificant portion of the population but whose effect has been considerably greater than their numbers would suggest. The reasons for their impact are varied; they come as entrepreneurs (many fail and return home), as teachers and Peace Corps workers, as missionaries and anthropologists. They bring skills often lacking in the country and, perhaps more important, they very often bring badly needed capital. In a community in which diverse appearances and patterns of behavior are the rule, they are easily integrated into the town and their presence and actions an accepted part of the ebb and flow of daily life.

Ethnicity and Adaptive Strategies

Ethnicity, viewed as a process, implies the development of a series of adaptive strategies in the exploitation of a changing variety of econiches.

Such strategies come in many shapes though groups have historically been restricted to certain strategies and niches through competitive interaction with dominant groups. There is a tendency to regard the adaptive strategy as resulting from those shared beliefs and behaviors attributed to ethnicity, the signs which define ethnic boundaries. In fact, the reverse may more commonly be the case, that is, that strategies result from ascription and the processes which follow. Shared culture, in Barth's view, is the result of ethnic group organization "rather than a primary and definitional characteristic" (Barth 1969), or, in Bennett's words, "an ethnic self need not be founded on a genuine native tradition at all; it is a 'collective representation' imagined out of needs for assertion and defense, for maintaining one's boundaries in a world of competition and usurpation of resources" (Bennett 1975). Cohen describes this process as the adjustment of a group to a new situation through the reorganization of its own traditions or through the development of new customs under traditional symbols, "using traditonal norms and ideologies to enhance its distinctiveness within the contemporary situation" (Cohen 1974).

Adaptive strategies both evolve from and constitute markers – signs – of ethnic identity; they are related to but not necessarily determined by other sign systems. They are susceptible to change and negotiation. The adaptive strategies employed by the various ethnic groups in southern Toledo are, in part, the result of historical circumstances and the limits imposed by the exploitability of the environment. The production of goods and services, the manner in which such products are utilized, and the benefits derived from production are all determined by and determinants of human relationships.

The environment imposes limits on the range of adaptive strategies which may be effectively employed. Large scale exploitation of timber resources is a thing of the past throughout Belize, though a few persons, mostly American and only part-time residents, continue to generate substantial income from logging operations in the region. While water is in abundant supply for most of the year, water shortages occur regularly during the dry season and there currently exists no effective method of supplying the water necessary to any sizeable industry. Some once believed oil would become the salvation of the Toledo District, but Esso's attempts to locate off-shore oil were reportedly unsuccessful, an assessment which many of the residents of Punta Gorda do not accept, believing the oil companies will return when Guatemala has given up its claim to the Toledo.

The sea has never been fully and effectively exploited, but such exploitation requires equipment which few can afford. The fishermen of Belize are concerned that the Guatemalans are encroaching on their fishing territories and it was rumored that the President of Guatemala maintains a vacation home on one of the cays off-shore from Punta Gorda.

Hunting and gathering are often not worth the caloric cost and time expended except for those who are closest to resources. The land requires either labor intensive techniques or the expenditure of large sums of capital to which few have access. Perhaps more than any other condition, it is the lack of locally available capital which hinders further economic development. The potential for the development of a tourist industry is currently limited. While game fishing could conceivably attract a number of tourists, most prefer the beaches, cays, and amenities to the north. As one writer stated of Toledo:

> There are no major sources of employment and one never hears of anyone going to Punta Gorda for work. In fact, one rarely hears of anyone going to Punta Gorda for any reason (Bullard 1973:94).

Stratification, Ethnicity and Resources

> Economic structure tends to coincide with ethnic stratification. There are basically two classes in Punta Gorda: an upper class of merchants and government officials, who are non-Carib, and a lower class which is made up of the rest of the population. Within the upper class there are ties of marriage, kinship, and friendship. There is virtually no middle class although much individual variation exists. The teachers tend to form a separate clique and often associate together and one might view them as an incipient middle class. The few Caribs who are either store owners or officials are *not* part of the upper class or elite (Cosminsky 1977:241).

This characterization of social strata, based largely on fieldwork conducted in the mid-1960's, remains an essentially accurate picture of Punta Gorda at the outset of the 1980's. The town is still dominated by Creole, Creole-Spanish, and Chinese-Spanish populations, with growing Spanish and East Indian influence; the Garinagu, despite their numbers, are still without broad political and economic powers. Nevertheless, while Belize once fit Furnivall's description of a plural society, dominated by a single ethnic/racial minority, the current political and economic structures allow opportunities for all groups. There is today an emerging middle class, though they control little wealth by U.S. standards. The influx of British soldiers and, on a smaller scale, American and European entrepreneurs and professionals, has meant the creation of additional jobs and the circulation of additional currency. Growth has affected every group and changes are evident in each ethnic section. This is not to imply that dramatic economic and social progress has been made in recent decades or that growth has equitably affected all ethnic sections, for the country remains underdeveloped and its population impoverished by any international standard.[4] Even the elite are not conspicuous in their wealth, at least not in Punta Gorda. Nevertheless, the material signs of a middle class are in evidence and they given indication of relative changes in the distribution of wealth. Class, as determined by access to and control over various resources, including education, land, capital, health care, positions of authority, and so on, is of growing importance in determinations of future alliances and distribution of power. Despite some obvious changes, however, ethnic group membership is still a primary determinant of an individual's status within the community as a whole. That is, ethnicity and class remain in many ways inseparable.

Cosminsky described the "hierarchy of ethnic groups" within Punta Gorda from the perspective of both the Garinagu and the Creoles (1977) as follows:

From the Garifuna perspective, the relative status of groups was:

Spanish
Creole
Garifuna
East Indian
Maya

From the Creole perspective, the arrangement was somewhat different:

Creole
Spanish
East Indian
Garifuna
Maya

This assignment of position within the hierarchy of ethnic sections has evolved from a complex history of relations among sections and the competition over resources and the right to exploit specific econiches. In turn, the adaptive strategies employed by each section have been, in part, determined by the structure of relations among ethnic sections from the earliest period of the exploitation of land and sea to the present. Further, adaptive strategies remain consistent with values, beliefs, and the nature of social relations within ethnic sections, though clearly the ethnic specific exploitation of econiches has been determined as much by denial of access to other econiches as by the values and social structures which supposedly define and separate sections. It has long been argued by some researchers that such values and structures are, in fact, determined by, rather than determinant of, relations of power, access, and obligation among ethnic sections.

Increasing power derived from the acquisition and effective exploitation of a land base by the East Indians and the Maya and the development of an entrepreneurial sector within both ethnic sections can be expected to result in alterations both in the nature of the social strata and in the type and frequency of transactions. The Garinagu place high value on education but have difficulty, for largely economic reasons, gaining access to educational institutions beyond elementary school. They generally have not exhibited a real interest in the establishment of business enterprises and haven't access to the capital to finance them, in any case, nor do they effectively and fully exploit either land or sea. They serve as wage laborers to the community, for the most part, though many migrate out in search of new econiches. It might be noted that so many Garifuna people now live in New York City and Los Angeles that Carib Settlement Day is said to be celebrated annually in both U.S. cities.

Despite an arrangement of strata based on ethnicity, a number of factors mitigate against a total coincidence of political, class, and ethnic boundaries. Several institutions cut across and negate sectional distinctions. Creole, Creole-Spanish, and Chinese merchants, for example, exert considerably unofficial influence in town matters. This is largely due to their position as the chief merchants to the community and to the fact that much of Punta Gorda's wealth is concentrated in their hands. However, many of these families are linked through affinal and consanguineal ties, which, in turn, means that much of the control over resources is in the hands of one large 'corporate' group composed of members of not one, but several ethnic groups. A survey of store ownership which I conducted in 1979 and 1980 indicated that twenty-seven stores, of a total of fifty-six, were owned by Creole, Creole-Spanish, Chinese-Spanish, or Creole-Spanish-Chinese individuals. Even this figure understates their control over certain economic resources in that the remaining twenty-nine businesses are generally smaller enterprises. Those twenty-seven businesses control an estimated seventy-five to eigthy percent of all cash which flows through the community, excluding salaries paid by the government and monies paid out by government departments to farmers for their produce. In addition, these merchants are often involved in other business enterprises, such as logging, transportation, the lottery (the *boledo*, which is responsible for a substantial flow of cash through the town weekly), and so on. Yet, locally, the political power of these ethnic sections is less obvious. In fact, cross-cutting alliances – political, economic, regional, ethnic, and familial – work against the control of town affairs by any one group. The Town Board, which controls limited aspects of the town's affairs and operations, is largely Garifuna and most board members are members of the opposition United Democratic Party (UDP).[5] All are long-term residents of Punta Gorda with extensive and intensive social and kin networks in the town. The two powerful elected national representative positions are held by a Creole and a Maya. Both are UDP members. The appointed Senator for the District is Garifuna and a member of the majority People's United Party (PUP).[6] While her position is admittedly not as powerful as that of Representative, she does have access to the Prime Minister.

The majority of businesses and much valuable property are controlled by permanent residents who, as stated, are Creole, Creole-Spanish, Spanish, Chinese-Spanish, and Creole-Spanish-Chinese. In general, these individuals are UDP members or members of the recently established Toledo Progressive Party (TPP) which argues for the unification of the Toledo District with Guatemala. The positions of judicial and administrative authority within the

District offices are held largely by Creoles who were born outside the District, who are generally PUP members, who have far fewer ties of kinship, friendship or mutual interest within the town, and who control little property.

The Catholic Church cannot be ignored in any discussion of control over resources. They are major landholders within the community and responsible for the education of the majority of the youth of Punta Gorda. Large sums of money are channeled through the church, and while the church must remain technically apolitical, its priests exert considerable influence. But a coincidence of power, religion, and ethnicity does not occur. The priests in charge of the two major churches in Punta Gorda and in San Antonio are American, while the next-in-charge at San Antonio is Garifuna and the one in Punta Gorda is French.[7]

Nor is sectional distinctiveness based on participation in a religious group possible. According to the 1980 census, 72 percent of the residents of the Toledo District describe themselves as Roman Catholic. The only major ethnic group which remains substantially outside Catholicism is the East Indian section, the majority of whom are Methodist. While most remain Methodist – the religion of the American founders of the Toledo Settlement – there has been a gradual shift toward Catholicism in recent years. Many East Indian children are currently being educated by the Catholic Church in a school some three or four miles outside Punta Gorda in a predominantly East Indian enclave.

The Anglican Church claims a few members in town, but they meet only infrequently and not at all in recent years. There are, or have been, several independent missionary (generally Pentecostal) families in the area; the number fluctuates. A number of Maya in the outlying villages have converted to Pentecostalism. In San Antonio where, in 1969, James Gregory found that villagers could not imagine being anything but Catholic, a large Nazarene church now stands at the center of town. There is another Nazarene center between Punta Gorda and San Antonio and a small Baptist Church at Big Falls. Some Kekchi have adopted Mennonite practices, as have a few persons of Spanish-East Indian descent (Francis Martinez, personal communication). Clearly the introduction of these religions or sects into the Toledo[8] has made inroads into the membership of the Catholic Church.[9] However, members of each of these newly established groups have been drawn from all ethnic sections and there is no one-to-one correspondence between religious group affiliation and ethnic group membership. The Roman Catholic Church continues to provide a basis for the unification of culturally disparate groups.

Transactions between and among members of ethnic groups serve a variety of functions. They alter (or verify) the stereotypes held by members of one group of another. They allow for the regularization of channels whereby goods, services, and information may be transferred. They facilitate the development of mutually intelligible codes. They create or reinforce social networks, configurations of cross-cutting interpersonal linkages based on kinship, friendship, mutual interest, economic ties, and so on. In addtiton, all transactions, from the exchange of goods to the exchange of gossip, offer an opportunity for the expression of the relative status of each participant. Transactions may occur between participants whose relation is symmetrical, that is, both participants (assuming all interactions can be reduced to sets of dyads) stand in an equivalent relationship to one another. The relation between participants may be asymmetrical, in which case one individual stands in a subordinate position, at least for the duration of the transaction. Finally, the relation between participants may be nonsymmetrical; each assumes a particular role required for the completion of the transaction. In this last sort of transaction, the relation between the participants is defined by role rather than status (as, for example, in an employer-employee relationship) (Barnes 1972).

Personal, i.e., ego-centered, networks are constituted of all three types of relations. In general, symmetrical relations in Punta Gorda obtain among members of the same ethnic section, and the *density* of the linkages within any portion of a personal network is dependent upon the ethnic identity of the persons with whom *ego* interacts. That is, 'interconnectedness' generally increases in proportion to the number of members of a personal network who are also members of the same ethnic group. Multiplex relations among members of Punta Gorda's "elite" are the rule rather than the exception, for the "elite" is constituted of individuals from several ethnic groups. Given the limited number of potential mates available within any one of these sections, an exchange of women has been essential for biological reproduction. Since even the larger 'corporate' group is not of sufficient size to maintain itself biologically, it can be expected that future transactions will continue to include the incorporation of women from several ethnic sections.

But interethnic mating appears to be relatively common among all groups, though less so among those which remain geographically separate from the community. Cosminsky (1977) said she could identify only fifteen households in which partners (married and unmarried) were from different ethnic groups. However, my survey of one-hundred households indicated there to be clear evidence of interethnic mating in forty percent of them. That is, in forty of the surveyed households, one or more of the adults in residence indicated they were of mixed parentage, or an adult couple in residence were members of different ethnic groups and so identified themselves, or children present in the house related consanguineally to a resident adult were of mixed parentage. The extent of such mating suggests Punta Gorda is a far more 'intergrated' community than pervious assessments suggested, while preferential mating patterns support the hierarchical arrangement of ethnic groups. It appears that East Indian, Garifuna, and Mayan males generally establish sexual relationships only with women from their own ethnic sections, though there are exceptions to this, while Creole, Creole-Spanish, Spanish and Chinese-Spanish males have access to the women of all ethnic groups.

Crossing lines of authority may be more difficult than penetrating ethnic boundaries for the conduct of transactions. Such actions are facilitated if both participants in a transaction are members of the same ethnic section and are more difficult where participants are not only members of different ethnic groups, but the ethnic section of the subordinate or petitioning person is lower in the hierarchy of ethnic sections. Simple economic transactions which should, in theory, be based on a non-symmetrical relation between buyer and seller, in fact provide opportunities for the expression of status differences and become constituted as transactions based on asymmetrical relations.

The somewhat ambiguous status of Americans and Western Europeans actually facilitates transactions across authority lines since participants are relatively free to act as though ethnic group membership had no place in determining the relation between participants. In part this ambiguity results from the generally temporary nature of their residence in Punta Gorda. It is this ambiguous status which often allows Americans to function as brokers in transactions involving persons from different positions in the hierarchical arrangement of ethnic sections. But Americans and Europeans, in particular the British soldiers, are not only brokers, but also resource; that is, they are viewed as a potential niche in the "opportunity structure" (Hannerz 1975). Many residents of the southern Toledo have, as a result of their interactions with these individuals and groups, developed a new set of exploitative strategies. Those least likely to profit from their presence are also the least likely to develop new strategies for use in transactions with these individuals.

Where social distances are great it is not uncommon for persons to seek brokers. This was frequently true in the hospital setting where East Indian and Garifuna patients would issue complaints or make requests through aides or lower ranking nursing staff of the same ethnic group. The Maya had no access to such brokers, as the only Mayan nurse in the hospital did not work in wards. Had she worked among hospitalized patients, her identity as Mopan would likely have affected her ability to function as a broker for Kekchi patients. Though the members of Punta Gorda's community generally make no distinction between Maya (Mopan) and Kekchi, the Indians regard those distinctions as considerable importance. When townspeople do take note of the differences, they often speak of the Kekchi as "backward" by comparison with the Mopan, though both groups carry on substantial commerce with the town.

The nature of the strategies used by members of ethnic sections to exploit niches in the opportunity structure at least partially determines in advance of any transaction between individuals the roles which each must play. Hence, strategies may define the relation which is manifested in any given transaction. Certain values which are an important component of ethnic world view or critical to the structure of social relations inter- and intra-culturally are both producers and products of the strategies utilized to maintain the ethnic section biologically and socially. Moreover, values come into play in the economic and social transactions which transpire between sections or members of sections. The symbols which constrain personal behavior, define the boundaries of any ethnic section and distinguish that ethnic section from others may determine or influence the attitude of one member in an interaction to the other. That is, values, beliefs and culturally defined expectations may subtly (or not so subtly) affect personal behavior in interethnic transactions and thus create complex variations on the three types of relations mentioned above. Either partner in a transaction may select certain diacritica or indicators of ethnic identity to classify or categorize the other partner and may react to the other participant according to assumed ethnic characteristics rather than personal characteristics displayed in the transaction. This phenomenon of categorical interaction (Mitchell 1974) is clearly manifested in transactions between members of certain ethnic groups in Punta Gorda, in particular those who have had the least contact with one another.

Let me offer one example of the manner in which behaviors and values derived from membership in an ethnic group affect interactions. East Indian males almost always marry, the marriages are generally stable, and it appears that East Indian males have few if any sexual relationships outside their marriage. Certainly they do not speak of "outside" children casually. The structure of the domestic unit is an important aspect of the strategies they utilize to exploit available econiches. The stability of family or household units allows for stable relationships among many such households of affinally and consanguineally related persons. The wife and children contribute in significant ways to the maintenance of these relationships and to the effective exploitation of the land base.

Garifuna males, on the other hand, generally do not marry (this is especially true of the younger generation), they will most likely move through a series of sexual liaisons, sometimes maintaining two or more at the same time, they may not contribute significantly to the household of their 'spouse' and often speak proudly of the number of children they have fathered, both within and outside the confines of a legal arrangement. These practices are again inseparable from the adaptive strategies they employ for, as Meillassoux (1981) has clearly pointed out, relations of production and relations of reproduction are interdependent.

What emerges from this dynamic interplay are ethnic specific notions about appropriate masculine behavior in male-female and male-male interactions. Concepts about the nature of "masculinity" for the members of each of these groups thus varies sufficiently that it is difficult to establish a mutually agreed upon basis for conducting transactions entailing symmetrical relations. It is hardly surprising, therefore, that British Army employers found their East Indian and Garifuna laborers had difficulty in working together. The British, failing to understand the origins of the conflict, were frequently forced to take sides in what appeared to be simple labor disputes in which divisions 'happened' to coincide with ethnic group membership. The British, whose view of male-female and male-male relations is more akin to that of the East Indian males, tended to be more sympathetic toward the East Indians, though those attitudes were never phrased in terms of "world view" or social structure.

NOTES

1. The Creole population of Punta Gorda may well have increased. Cosminsky estimated, based on a survey of 1574 names from the Malaria Health Survey, that approximately 17.5% of population of Punta Gorda was Creole. The Creole population in 1980, as reported in the Belizean census, was 23.6% (Statistical Office, May, 1982). My impression on my return to the town in 1984 was that the ethnic compositon of the community had changed in my four year absence with an increase in the East Indian, Maya, and Spanish populations resident in the community. However, no survey was conducted to verify this impression.
2. Within the past two years another Chinese family has migrated from China to Punta Gorda. They are related to a Chinese-Spanish family already resident in the community. Punta Gorda now boasts three Chinese restaurants.
3. There are now only two British Army bases in the area. The third has been turned over to the Belize Defense Force.
4. During my initial stay in Punta Gorda, there was little evidence of extensive or intensive production of marijuana. According to various residents with whom I spoke, however, the Belizean government had been unable at some point to pay the Mayans for their rice and beens and the Maya, deprived of their most dependable source of income, turned to growing marijuana. In the last year, these marijuana fields were sprayed with Paraquat. The consequences to the District were substantial. Many Mayan families had apparently invested a considerable sum in the plants. That investment was lost, as well as any potential income from that crop. There were several individuals who claimed that the Paraquat was sometimes sprayed indiscriminately and that other crops were destroyed as well. The flow of cash within the community of Punta Gorda was slowed. There were a number of indications that several East Indian farmers had turned to the production of marijuana as well during this brief period. Throughout the District, whether individuals were involved in the growing of marijuana or not, there were increased expectations of an improved standard of living. At least one individual expressed to me the feeling that the government had unfairly allowed the spraying of these crops and that the Toledo District should have

been allowed at least one good year before the crops were destroyed.

5. The party which was the opposition party at the time of my fieldwork in 1979, 1980, and 1984 is now the majority party, while the PUP is now the opposition or minority party.
6. This woman is now deceased. I did not determine if a replacement had been selected.
7. The priest now in charge of the Punta Gorda Catholic Church is Garifuna.
8. Percent population by religion, as reported for the Toledo District, (Statistical Office Belmopan, May, 1982):

Roman Catholic	71.8%
Pentecostal	7.9%
Methodist	4.5%
Nazarene	4.5%
Anglican	1.7%
Mennonite	1.5%
Jehovah's Witness	0.6%
Seventh Day Adventist	0.4%
Baptist	0.3%
Other/Not Stated	6.7%

9. In 1970, 94% of the residents of Punta Gorda and 90% of those in rural Toledo described themselves as Roman Catholic.

CHAPTER 3

Therapeutic Resources and Pluralistic Medical Systems

Healing knowledge is always prized and often protected. Such knowledge, combined with the technical aparatus and skills necessary to the effective operationalization of a medical paradigm, is a resource, susceptible to the same relations of production which determine access to land and the tools required for its exploitation. That is, just as relations of production govern the right to exploit resources and the distribution of the products of that exploitation (Meillassoux 1981) so too do they formulate therapy as a resource. Within Belize, access to specific skills, apparatus, and the medical paradigms which allow for the specialized production of signs and their interpretation is largely controlled by an ethnic or otherwise constituted (professional) community, as are the products of the exploitation of that resource.

The notion of resource carries with it the implication of inherent exploitability. Medicine or medical systems or therapeutic systems are exploitable resources utilized in the battle against suffering. But illness must also be regarded as a potential resource, the basis for the accumulation of "profit and power" for a select few (Waitzkin and Waterman 1974) and the validation of moral convictions communally held, providing the key elements in a social myth continually replayed.

There is no doubt a struggle for control of both medical and "illness" resources among professionals and specialists in Belize. Nevertheless, the existence of alternative therapeutic systems provides afflicted individuals and their "therapy managing groups" (Janzen 1978) with options. These multiple therapeutic systems are, therefore, to be treated as sets of resources which are available for utilization or exploitation by a client population.

Therapeutic resources are constituted of certain "primary medical resources", defined by Unschuld (1975) as medical knowledge, medical skills, medical technology, including drugs and medical equipment and facilities; but the concept of resource includes as well the various roles occupied by persons possessing medical knowledge and skills, the ideological system which underlies and, in theory, renders coherent a complex set of beliefs and practices, and the mechanisms for the delivery of care which include the private and public networks which may be utilized during the course of an illness. Such resources are both tool and prize in a struggle for control. Professionalization becomes simultaneously strategy and outcome in the process. The differential access to technical knowledge serves as one source of the professional's power.

Therapeutic resources must be located as well within that infrastructure which results from relations of production and reproduction. Medical knowledge and behavior are, in Young's words "determined by social relations" (1981:384). Even the effectiveness of the spiritual intermediary is dependent upon a set of social relations, publicly acknowledged. That is, as Young perceptively points out, the authority of the spiritual healer is the product of relations among people rather than relations between people and spirits (*Ibid.*).

Therapeutic resources thus consist minimally of a set of therapeutic roles, the set of social relations which determine ownership of and access to skills, facilities, and products, the therapeutic practices, facilities, and materiel necessary to the diagnosis and treatment of illness, and those beliefs which render logical the relations among perceived cause, effect, and therapy and which generate behaviors designed to protect or encourage health.

The system of therapeutic resources within Punta Gorda is pluralistic, as opposed to plural, in that no one ethnic section or professional sector totally dominates the others. This statement must be qualified by the observation that the nation's official medicine is biomedicine and there are sanctions which are aimed at ensuring its dominance. However, these sanctions are not consistently effective.

Ownership of health care resources in any democratic country with socialized medicine theoretically lies in the hands of the populace since members of the government are simply representatives of the electorate and responsible for the efficient management and distribution of resources. The ability, however, of the individual to exploit to his own benefit these "commonly owned" resources is, in large part, dependent upon his recognition of the nature of the network controlling distribution and an awareness of the intracacies of its functioning.

Within Belize certain mechanisms for distribution are controlled by the government and the 'beneficiary's' receipt of health care is not voluntary. It is law, for example, that all homes must be sprayed with D.D.T. annually in an attempt to eliminate or control malaria-carrying mosquitoes. Both the tuberculosis sanitarium (Hattieville) and the asylum for the mentally disturbed (Seaview) admit the majority of patients involuntarily and function to assist in the enforcement of health regulations and behavioral standards.

The mechanisms for the delivery of care, which include the private and public networks utilized during the course of illness, exist as an aspect of therapeutic resources and yet can be analyzed apart from them. If *network* is defined as those systems of interconnections which guide persons to one or more medical resources or which lead to a confrontation, voluntary or otherwise, between resident and resource, then it becomes clear from a review of case studies (Chapter VII) that the utilization of networks exists always as an element in the process of exploitation. Certain networks are relatively "public", that is, their utilization does not require considerable esoteric knowledge. Such networks render health care more accessible. The government's attempts to make biomedical care available through the establishment and publicizing of nationally subsidized programs, such as district hospitals and outpatient clinics, prenatal clinics, and innoculation programs for children, increase their accessibility. Both ethnic group membership and class, as we shall see later, affect access to and utilization of such networks.

Private networks may be activated under specific conditions even though based upon a permanent and structured set of relationships, such as the network of kin ties. Networks normally utilized to facilitate other sorts of transactions may be put to use for the purpose of bringing the resource and the potential utilizer together. Informal, non-structured, symmetrical relationships, usually based on friendship or prior acquaintance, are frequently the basis for the network, though in many cases, networks involve symmetrical. asymmetrical, and non-symmetrical relationships simultaneously.

A brief history of a single illness episode illustrates how a network may be created as the result of an individual episode and may persist and be utilized only for the duration of the illness (see Boswell 1969 for a more elaborate example of a similar process). In this case, participation in the network was based upon shared national identity. Participants had differential access to various therapeutic resources and attempted to exploit those resources in different ways.

The events described occurred when I first arrived in Punta Gorda and was still resident in a local hotel. I was introduced to Cindy, an American tourist, and her three American companions by Tom, another American tourist. Tom and I had met the previous week through a mutual American friend and he had assisted me in a move from one hotel to another while I searched for a house in which to live for the duration of my stay. That evening, Cindy and her friends invited me to join them for dinner at a local restaurant. We were to be the guests of an American couple who had flown to Punta Gorda in their private plane for a few days of deep sea fishing. We were joined during the course of the evening by Jim, an American logger, and Allan, an American raising cattle in Belize.

Early the next morning, Tom approached me while I was shopping downtown and reported that Cindy was seriously ill. I returned to the hotel where several of us were staying. Cindy was suffering from severe and frequent vomiting and diarrhea. I explained that I had no medicine except for aspirins and antihistamines. Anne, one of her companions, went to the pharmacy to see if she could purchase Pepto Bismo, but returned empty handed.

I left for the Police Station a block away to ask when the hospital would open. In addition, I had hoped I might be able to prevail upon the police to drive Cindy to the hospital which was almost a mile away. I based my assumption of assistance on my previous meeting with the District's Inspector of Police who had been most cordial. However, the Inspector was not available; the policeman on duty informed me that the doctor's residence was nearby and that the doctor would be at home at this hour. I walked to the physician's residence; the maid informed me that the doctor could see Cindy in the afternoon.

I returned to the hotel. Cindy was no better, but informed me she did not want to see the doctor. She feared she would be hospitalized. At about that time, Allan came by to look in on the group. We described the course of Cindy's illness and explained that Cindy did not want to see the doctor though her symptoms had not abated and she was becoming increasingly dehydrated. Allan remarked that the two men who had accompanied Cindy and Anne to Belize were at the logging camp and would return in the afternoon. Jim, the American logger, would be with them, he said, and he suggested we wait to see if he might be able to help.

At 2 P.M. I returned to the doctor's house, hoping I could obtain either advice or medicine. The doctor, whom I had not met previously, said I should ask Cindy if there were either blood or mucus in her stool. If either were present, I should return to his house. He told me there would be no charge for my visit.

I returned to the hotel. Jim had just arrived with the others and was taken to see Cindy. He later returned with an impressive array of medications which, he explained, he kept for treatment of illness and injury among the members of his logging crew. He reported that he had a larger supply of medicines than the physician and could treat a wide range of illnesses. Jim offered Cindy Lomotil and Sandoz.

During the day several Americans, all recent acquaintances of Cindy's, dropped by to offer advice and to see how Cindy was progressing. They discussed similar cases and attempted to identify an etiology and diagnostic label for her state. They spoke in terms of problems of the 'stomach' as this was thought to be the locus of the problem. Bad water and bad food were mentioned as possibilities and the previous evening's meal was suspect. For North Americans and Europeans in Belize, the skin and the stomach are regarded as the most susceptible organs. The major model of illness causation expresses the common fear of 'invasion.' Models of imbalance or stress, common in the States, are quickly set aside here. The preventive model is based on avoidance. Food and water which may contain bacteria or "germs" are the principal culprits (although Jim offered the following explanation: "These people cook with coconut oil and that destroys all the bacteria in your stomach so you have to replace the bacteria.") Snakes, scorpions, mosquitoes, and all the varieties of insects which abound in Belize are considered dangerous. The skin becomes a major organ whereby invasion may be accomplished.

On his second visit, Jim suggested that Cindy's illness was "just one of those things that Americans get." This seemed to satisfy the assembled group for it placed Cindy's illness in the category of 'normal' illness (Locker 1981) and relieved all present of moral responsibility. This categorization carried with it the implication that Cindy would recover, that no extraordinary measures were called for, and that Jim understood this illness and therefore had prescribed an appropriate treatment. Further, culpability was either of no concern or lay with the community which failed to protect Americans. Finally, Cindy's suffering could now be shared by the group in that it had been defined as an illness which all Americans had or would experience.[1]

The following morning, Cindy was considerably improved and I last saw her waiting with her friends for the boat to Guatemala. The network which had formed to provide assistance was never reconstituted, though dyadic relations which had evolved as a result of Cindy's illness persisted for a period of time.

Syncretism, Pluralism, and Therapeutic Systems

The 1980 Census of Belize identifies eight different "racial" groups in Punta Gorda. Ethnic diversity is even greater than this categorization would suggest. Included in the category "white", for example, are individuals from Australia, Germany, the British Isles, and the United States. Diversity in medical beliefs and practices is obviously to be expected, as is a certain – and sometimes considerable – degree of syncretism. Moreover, the beliefs and practices introduced into the country with each ethnic section often reflected the historical influences of other cultures. Mayan concepts about health and illness were influenced by Spanish medical beliefs and Roman Catholicism. Spanish beliefs, in turn, as introduced into Spanish Central America in the 16th to 19th centuries emphasized humoural balance concepts evolving out of early Greek medical thought, modified by Arabic influences. Garifuna beliefs were likely at least a mixture of West African and Carib/Arawak Indian ideologies. The Creole medical system, evolving first in the bush camps and port cities of Belize, was West African, West Indian and British. East Indians, divorced from commerce or exchange with their country of origin, were strongly affected by American and British medical theories and practices and whatever mix of beliefs had prevailed in the West Indies at the time of their emigration to Belize. Biomedicine was introduced by the British, modified by continuing international biomedical research and evolving concepts of etiology and therapy, and adjusted to the local cultural, economic, political and ecological situation. To speak, therefore, of "traditional" ethnomedical systems is misleading.

No simple division of the total set of all therapeutic resources is possible.[2] The people of Punta Gorda and the southern Toledo, while recognizing linguistically the distinctions among certain 'systems', move back and forth across the boundaries of these domains without awareness of the anthropological significance of their actions. They conceptually distinguish "hospital" or "doctor" medicine from "bush" medicine, but the first is described by its users according to ownership of resources and the location of its facilities, while the second is necessarily linked securely to ethnic identity and intra-ethnic social relations. Thus the two 'systems'[3] are not equivalent. There are other resources which are identified as neither "bush" nor "hospital", yet they function as sources of healing. But the concept of 'healing' is imposed by the observer on an otherwise disparate set of resources.

While their potential to produce healings gives the categories of "bush" and "hospital" medicine unity from the anthropologist's perspective, basic premises concerning the nature and cause of misfortune, the sources of healing power, the method whereby healing is effected, and the means by which one gains access to such resources are sufficiently different to render them incomparable in other respects. They are combined as members of a set within a single domain (healing) only in that each offers some technique for relief of suffering. As the case studies will indicate, distinctions between bush and biomedicine are of little importance in the "quest for therapy" (Janzen 1978).

If, on the other hand, our examination of "illness" and, by extension, the techniques utilized to "cure" it, and the explanatory models which make sense out of signs were based on some clinical paradigm, that is, if we use a biomedical definition of "illness" or disease as our starting point, we necessarily ignore a wide range of "illnesses", for there are those signs which are interpreted as abnormal as the result of the application of one explanatory paradigm, but not another. Further, there are alterations in the human organism which are manifested clinically, but which result in no change in social role or ability to function in a routine and culturally accepted manner and are, therefore, not necessarily constituted as a form of suffering within many if not most medical paradigms. Finally, if illness and its relief defined the total domain of our examination, then we would necessarily overlook all those techniques and paradigms which are employed to maintain health.

People define themselves, or are defined by others, as "sick." Whenever such an event occurs, medical semiotics locates the material for its analyses. But the notion of what is signified by the term "sick" varies across cultures and, just as importantly, within cultures. The analysis presented here does not examine the appearance of specific physiological indicators of altered biological states (though that too is the subject matter of a medical semiotics), but takes, instead, as its material the signs of suffering as presented, produced, and interpreted within specific contexts. That the label "sick" may be imposed externally does not alter this approach. The concern, then, is with the various significations of signs which have been categorized as indicating "sickness" and the resources which are utilized to provide explanatory models and to effect an appropriate therapy. Those behaviors which are consciously utilized to prevent future occurrences of "sickness" (which can only be imagined and are therefore not available for analysis) are also included.

Therapeutic resources are divided according to ownership of the resource and the manner in which the resource is integrated into the infrastructure of social relations. This division does not allow for the superficially clear-cut distinctions which are characteristic of many ethnomedical studies. In fact, it leads to a confusion of the usual categories. But it does permit an understanding of phenomena which otherwise might remain inexplicable. Therapeutic resources incorporate models which provide both for the generation and interpretation of signs, but other therapies neither condoned nor explained by these models may be utilized to deal with the same set of signs and even with interpretations generated by these models. Therefore, the concept of therapeutic resource is not necessarily linked to or dependent upon the concept of the sign. That is, we must make a distinction between the notion of sign and the notion of resource. Our examination here is of resources and the explanatory models which exist as a part of these resources and which used to generate and interpret sign.

Ownership, Access, and Exploitability: Categorization of Therapeutic Resources

Lay Therapeutic Resources

Just as in the domestic community described by Meillassoux (1981) individuals have rights to the use of land as a result of their membership in the community, so too are certain medical resources available to all members of an ethnic community. Further, all aspects of these resources are subject to exchange through interethnic and intraethnic transactions, resulting in a pervasive "system" of medicine which is separated from other resources on the basis of the nature of the relations of production and distribution obtaining among its users I shall refer to this "system" simply as lay therapy.

Lay therapeutic resources are those resources which are shared among the members of an ethnic group and frequently between members of different ethnic groups. Ethnic boundaries are of little importance in the determination of accessibility and ownership. Lay therapy is characterized by common ownership of the needed skills; medical materials are usually easily accessible. Such materials, in fact, often acquire no exchange value because they circulate through the community and the 'identical' product is returned to the first producer. No special facilities are required. Technical skills are simple and divorced from metaphysical concerns. Role and status are lacking or unimportant in any transactions. The information which is exchanged is non-esoteric and secular. The paradigms which govern the use of medicines are unsophisticated and may integrate elements from several sources. These models may be ethnic specific, but there is some articulation of models among groups. Common concern for the techniques of healing and the maintenance of health draw together individuals from different ethnic sections, allowing for the development of mutually intelligible codes, which, in turn, provide the basis for future transactions. It would be exceedingly difficult for individuals or institutions to control skills, materials or explanatory models, especially in view of the inherently dynamic nature of these models.

Much of what is referred to locally as "bush medicine" can be categorized as lay medicine, though important segments of "bush medicine" must be located elsewhere in this scheme. The state recognizes the pervasive and persistent use of bush medicines and makes few serious attempts to discourage their use. While the government cautions the public,

> ...a great many of our local medicinal plants are listed as recognized drugs or medicines in the Pharmacoepia, the official "bible" of the pharmacist; and a surprising number of present-day drugs come from natural products; [however] it must be pointed out that "bush medicines" are in no way recommended for serious illness. While many are harmless; there may be some that could be dangerous if used indiscriminantly. It goes without saying that medical help from qualified doctors should be sought (*New Belize*, Vol. VII, No. II, Nov. 1977, pp. 2-5).

the sale of bush medicines continues unabated in the markets of Belize City, and the government licensed pharmacy in Punta Gorda sells many of the components of popular remedies. There are literally hundreds, if not thousands, of widely used treatments and practices which constitute this category of lay therapy (see, for example, The New Belize [op. cit.]; Cosminsky 1976; Sanford Ms; Palacio 1982; Gonzalez 1963). *Contrebo* is commonly used to "cleanse and purify the blood", boiled corn water and Red Fanta (a strawberry flavored soda pop) to reduce fever during measles or chicken pox[4], Red Lavinda, a bottled product imported from Guatemala, is said to "cool the blood", lime juice is used for nausea or to "cut phelgm" in the stomach, sienna, castor oil and a variety of purchased and herbal medications are used to "purge the system" or to "remove the cold" from the body, various oils and salves are used in "nointing" (massages) or for treatment of sores, "tonics" (a term which usually refers to liquid vitamin supplements varying considerably in actual vitamin and mineral, as well as alcohol content) are said to be good for the blood and for general health, alcohol is rubbed on the skin to reduce pain and to relieve other discomforts, Hammond's leaf is said to lower blood pressure when served as a tea, fever grass reduces fevers, sorocee and Jackass bitters are used to lower blood sugar levels, antibiotic ointments are used in the treatment of sores, and so on. This brief list provides only a suggestion as to the variety of medications, herbal and otherwise, and the uses to which they are put. Medicines such as antibiotics which are acquired only as the result of the intercession of a physician in the States are readily available "over-the-counter" in the local pharmacy in Punta Gorda. No sophisticated model of body functions or organic interactions is required for their use. Thus medicines whose efficacy is explained through a biomedical paradigm come to constitute one portion of the materiel of a lay therapeutic system.

All lay healing resources do not conform fully to the characteristics described at the beginning of this section (common ownership of skills, accessibility of materials, etc.), yet none varies sufficiently to remove it from this category. Nevertheless, there is considerable variation which must be taken into account, and the divisions among categories as described here are not always clear-cut. For example, the pharmacist has been descibed elsewhere in this chapter as a "therapeutic specialist", yet the pharmacist and many of the town's other small store owners serve as purveyors of a range of patent and other medicines. Local remedies which are a component of lay therapeutic resources are often concocted out of materials which must be purchased (e.g., sweet oil, blue soap). Further, much "bush" is no longer readily available and must be obtained from individuals who know where the appropriate plants are located and how these plants are to be harvested and prepared. Such persons may or may not be identified as herbalists. The preparations they make are sometimes sold for cash and sometimes simply given away. In any case, there is generally little profit in their sale. Nevertheless, it should be recognized that "medicines" under such conditions as described here and above acquire exchange value and the system of distribution is altered.

I have identified the healing "cult" of Esquipulas, located within the Catholic Church, as a lay therapeutic resource for several reasons, despite the fact that its healings are sacred rather than secular. Access to this therapeutic resource is limited only by the requirement that one be Catholic. The explanatory paradigms are easily assimilated; necessary materials are few; no technical skills are required and facilities are non-essential. Most importantly, no "intermediary' or professional intervention is needed.

On January 15th of each year members of each of Punta Gorda's diverse ethnic groups assemble at the Catholic Church in Punta Gorda to celebrate the Feast Day of Señor Esquipulas. Esquipulas, also known as the Black Jesus, has a prominent position both visually and symbolically in the church.[5] Infertile women claim to have become pregnant and both males and females claim miraculous cures after petitioning Esquipulas for the cessation of suffering. There are, however, obligations imposed on those who recover. Each individual blessed with a healing must fulfill any promise made to Esquipulas and must engage in a significant and sometimes financially burdensome way in the ceremonies which begin ten days before the Feast Day. The Feast Day of Esquipulas has become one of the most important of all religious holidays in the community. Initially celebrated only in the homes of a few of Punta Gorda's citizens, the day became an official local Church holy day in 1979. Much of the activity was transferred to the Catholic Church.

The priest in 1980 explained that he saw the adoption of the Feast Day and associated "cult" (though he does not refer to it in those terms) as a means of uniting the many ethnic groups in the southern Toledo. Some, however, viewed his actions in less positive terms, believing the Feast Day was adopted as a Church holy day and the major portion of the ceremonial performance removed from the control of individuals to that of Church officials in order to channel funds previously utilized in private celebrations into church coffers. Local perceptions of Esquipulas and the content of the "cult" vary considerably. It is clear that the priest's understanding of the full significance of this "black Jesus" to the members of the community was not comprehensive. Seeking a clearer statement on the meaning and origin of the cult, I sought out the local American priest. He kindly loaned me a book on Esquipulas published in Guatemala. The book was written in Spanish and it was necessary that I have portions of it translated. The priest, aware that I had requested a translation, asked that I pass that translation on to him as he had never read the book and knew little of the history or local interpretations of the role and significance of this "black Jesus."

How the recent elevation of the cultic celebrations to the status of a locally recognized Holy Day of Obligation will affect access is, at this point, unclear. Many individuals continue to hold private ceremonies in their homes. Further, the priest had, at the time of my research, not yet fully comprehended the power to be derived from the effective transfer of 'ownership' of the resource. It is easily conceivable that the mediation of a professional spiritual guide will alter the nature of cult performance and limit free access to this therapeutic resource. It should also be noted, in justification of the placement of the cult within that category of resources referred to as lay therapies, that the distinction which is generally drawn between sacred or spiritual and secular healings is not one which underlies the distinctions that citizens of the southern Toledo make between and among therapeutic resources. Many herabalists and bush doctors, for example, collect holy water from the church for use in their preparation of herbal medicines. Yet none would refer to the healings which result as spiritual healings.

The government is least effective in affecting the lay system because of the lack of therapeutic specialists, distribution sites, the limited exchange values attached to the therapeutic materials, and the generalized sharing of medical paradigms.

Therapeutic Specialists

This second category of therapeutic resources in characterized by the following: individual ownership of skills, transactions based on non-symmetrical relations between individuals, medical or explanatory paradigms which are accepted by users but not necessarily fully understood by them, private ownership of materials having exchange value, increasing variety in therapeutic roles, and both secular and sacred healings. Facilities are generally not of great importance, except in the case of the pharmacist and the physician in their entrepreneurial roles, among the secular healers, and for the *búiai* and the priest, among the spiritual intermediaries. Secular specialists include the herbalist (though herbalists are not highly specialized and are, in many respects part of the lay therapeutic system), the bush doctor, the pharmacist, the midwife, and the private physician or government physician in his private clinic, although his activities are, to some extent, controlled by the state. Sacred specialists include magic men, the *búiai*, the gifted bush doctor, the diviner, and a variety of other spiritual intermediaries or guides. Among the sacred specialists, the therapeutic *means* is pre-eminent over the therapeutic material.

The usual reference for persons who deliver medical care for a fee outside the biomedical or state system is "bush doctor" or "snake doctor." There were perhaps ten to twenty such persons, including midwives, within Punta Gorda and in the immediate vicinity at the time of my stay. There are many more persons who might be classified as herbalists. The acknowledged skills of both herbalists and bush doctors vary considerably and not everyone is in agreement on what constitutes evidence of role legitimacy. A number of bush doctors also practice in the Mayan and East Indian villages, though not every village has a bush doctor. There are some villages which also have no midwife and, in these cases, the husband assists with the delivery. The majority of bush doctors in the Mayan villages are said to be Kekchi, rather than Mopan. Concomitantly, the Kekchi are also accused of having greater knowledge of magic and the evil uses of medicine.

All bush doctors practice within their homes though both midwives and bush doctors commonly travel to their patient's residence. Few if any have accumulated much material wealth as a result of their practice, and none practices full-time. Materials and diagnostic tools, when there are any at all, are generally simple. It appears that Mayan bush doctors share less of their governing paradigms and rationale for treatment with their patients than do the bush doctors of other ethnic groups.

Snake doctors are generally regarded as specialists in the treatment of snake bites though they are known to treat other illnesses as well. Access to bush or snake doctors generally requires only knowledge of their existence. Fees are usually far less than those one pays to see the government physician privately. Individuals rather commonly cross ethnic boundaries to seek care; it is unlikely that services would be refused to anyone because of their ethnic group membership. Most bush doctors pride themselves on the fact that they treat persons from all ethnic groups and social strata. Nevertheless, class and ethnicity play a role in therapy seeking decisions.

Some bush doctors will treat almost any form of suffering, while others specialize in the treatment of no more than one form of illness. Individual bush and snake doctors are known for their skills in treating certain disorders and they will be sought out when those disorders are suspected. One East Indian bush doctor used a mixture of drugs and therapies – antibiotic injections, vitamins, and so on – obtained from pharmacies in Guatemala, as well as local herb perparations. He was referred to as the "private doctor" to distinguish him from the government physician and other bush doctors.

In general, bush doctors charge only for the medicines they provide and add a small fee for their services. Some charge no fee at all and provide medicines at cost. A midwife might ask no more than $10 B.H ($5.00 U.S.) for her attendance at a delivery. That charge, in many instances, also includes prenatal and postnatal care. The local snake doctor, whose skills in this sometimes dangerous country are highly valued, reported he had no set fee, but asked patients to pay what they could. No bush doctor can expect to do more than supplement his or her income with the money made providing care. The one exception to this is the few remaining notable and highly respected *búiais* of Belize and Guatemala.

Ownership of the means and models for the achievement of spiritual healings is not restricted to the *búiais* of the Garinagu. Medical missionaries are frequently found in the cities, towns, and back villages of Belize. Most come for brief periods of time, claim a biomedical model of illness and therapy, conduct routine examinations, and dispense biomedically rationalized advice and medications. The Mayan village of Crique Sarco signed a contract with a Mennonite organization. One of the provisions of the contract was that the Mennonites would provide to the villagers the services of a full-time American trained nurse. An American-born lab and x-ray technician who was stationed in Punta Gorda and who worked in the local hospital, was sponsored by a medical missionary organization headquartered in the States. The missionary group provided her with medical supplies. She, in turn, frequently furnished medications and supplies to the Peace Corps nurse in San Antonio and the Mennonite nurse in Crique Sarco.

None of the individuals or groups mentioned above claimed spiritual healings, and all, including the Peace Corps nurse, were, at least in theory, under the supervision and authority of the Minister of Health and the District Medical Officer. However, there were missionary groups which operated largely free of government control and which offered therapy to any who sought it. They provided sacred rather than secular healings.

Several missionary families, usually American, have settled from time to time in the area, many come with unrealistic expectations about villagers' religious needs and their own capacity to cope with life in south Toledo. Consequently, few have remained for long. Some appear, however, to have become permanent or semi-permanent residents of the southern Toledo. Most of these missionaries are "charismatics" and claim affiliation with a Pentecostal group; Pentecostalism has spread rapidly through some Mayan villages and political and social conflicts have become manifested in a religious split between Pentecostal and Catholic factions in at least one Mayan village. Almost 8% of the residents of the Toledo District now identify themselves as Pentecostalists.

The most visible of Punta Gorda's "charismatic" families offers religious services several times weekly. A healing ceremony is performed at the request of individuals. These family members report that not only are cures frequently achieved but that they have knowledge of Indians in the villages who have been brought back to life through prayer. They state that they personally never use a physician for any member of the family and discourage others from doing so, though they believe that in the case of injury, the services of a physician may be required. Disease is said to be an unnatural state, the "work of Satan." They state that both Satan and Jesus may heal but one "pays the greater price" for the former sort of healing. In their opinion, the healings attributed to Esquipulas are Satanic, as is the work of the *búiai*. They speak openly against the *búiai*, though even Catholic priests hesitate to publicly denounce the *buiai*, and they condemn the *dugu*, an important Garifuna ceremony through which healings are accomplished.

According to their teachings, Psalm 91 may be repeated for protection against disease.[6] Occasionally, however, God will remove even this protection against misfortune in order to provide proof of his power. Hence periodic illness among loyal followers is further validation of the model of health and illness. Belief in the healing power of Jesus and in the importance of faith in the maintenance of health is founded upon an interpretation of several Biblical passages.[7] Thus far the influence of the Pentecostalists has been the greatest among the Maya and perhaps the least among the Garinagu.

Midwives stand on the sometimes vague border between bush and biomedicine, or between therapeutic specialist and state medicine. Legally they are required to obtain a license and must first complete coursework and practical training. All licensed midwives have received training in the Belize City hospital and most now work in the country's public hospitals. However, the great majority of midwives in the rural areas were trained by unlicensed midwives and practice without a license. Technically, they practice illegally. The government attempts to update their training where possible, but otherwise takes no action. Unlicensed midwives have simply been redesignated "traditional birth attendants" by a government which cannot hope to provide obstetrical and pediatric care to all isolated rural areas. Lay midwives (unlicensed) not only deliver infants but provide prenatal care of the mother and postnatal care of mother and child. It is clear that even within Punta Gorda unlicensed midwives are called upon privately to help with both though the mother almost invariably gives birth at the local hospital. A licensed midwife may legally deliver babies within the home. However, a licensed midwife who works within the hospital is prohibited from delivering babies outside the hospital. Because there are no licensed midwives in Punta Gorda who are not employed in the hospital, very few babies are delivered outside the hospital. Occasionally, a local unlicensed midwife will "sneak" a case. In the villages, however, most women remain at home for the birth of an infant and are attended by an unlicensed midwife or by their husbands. The Peace Corps nurse stationed in San Antonio delivered babies, charging a fee of $10B.H. for a service which would otherwise have been free, thus avoiding charges of unfair competition from "traditional birth attendants" who ask $10 for their assistance.

The local pharmacy offers a wide range of therapeutic materials from antibiotics and tranquilizers, medicines whose efficaciousness is explained by a biomedical paradigm, to the materials which serve as components of "home remedies" and bush medicines, such as baby aniseed, mansinilla, pericon, alucema, culantro, romero, aloes, spice seed, and almond oil.[8] The pharmacist is as knowledgeable in the use of these as he is in the utilization of biomedically rationalized preparations. The dispensing of some medications (those explained by a biomedical model) is, in part, controlled by the state, while sale of others is not. The pharmacist is licensed by the state to fill prescriptions given patients by the District Medical Officer, but most prescriptions are filled by the government doctor out of his personal stock during private office hours or they are filled by a nurse or pharmacist at the local hospital pharmacy.

Individuals frequently seek out the pharmacist for advice, a service for which he charges nothing. Afflicted individuals present him with symptoms such as constipation, diarrhea, toothache, headachie, itch, fever, cough, backache, and so on. They rarely offer or demand diagnostic labels and even less commonly ask for an explanatory model which details the relationship between the anticipated benefits of suggested therapeutic materials and the symptoms presented.

There are other resources and therapeutic specialists available to the citizens of the district. Towards the end of my stay, I was told a famous healer from Guatemala was in town and that he was conducting interviews and prescribing therapies. A North American who had lived in Punta Gorda for many years provided several services to residents, usually at little cost. For twenty-five cents B.H. he would read cards and consult on various problems. Among other things, he offered analyses of dreams and medical advice. He said his analyses were based on certain skills he had acquired, on the signs generated by the cards themselves, and on common sense. He played a significant role in one of the cases reported in Chapter VII.

State Medicine

The final resource, or more accurately, system of resources, is defined here as state medicine. The characteristics of state medicine are as follows: facilities and therapeutic materiel are of increased importance; the governing paradigm (actually, paradigms) are esoteric and ownership of such paradigms is restricted to a small cadre of 'experts' or biomedical specialists; relations between therapist and afflicted individual are non-symmetrical or, more frequently, asymmetrical; the system of distribution of facilities, materiel, access to paradigms and skills, and persons possessing skills is under state control and decisions regarding distribution are most commonly made at the national level. In any system of socialized medicine, such as exists in Belize, a portion of the labor of the citizens of the state is, in theory, converted into medical materiel, facilities, skills, and so on. Thus, again in theory, ownership of all state resources is shared equally by all citizens of the state who, on the basis of shared ownership of means and materiel, have equal access to resources. As we shall see, such is not the case.

Overall responsibility for the delivery of health care belongs to the Minister of Health who establishes policy for the Ministry of Health in conjunction with the Prime Minister. The Chief Medical Officer heads the Medical Department (a subdivision of the Ministry), and has authority over each districts' hospitals, clinics, and medical staff. The personnel employed by the Ministry at the District level are responsible to the District Medical Officer though certain jurisdictional ambiguities have sometimes resulted in unclear lines of authority within the districts.

Belize operates ten hospitals, including an institution for the mentally ill (Seaview), a tuberculosis sanitarium (Hattieville), and some twenty-five clinics scattered throughout the country. All services and medications are essentially free, though there are charges for certain items (e.g., blood); a small fee is collected when an individual is hospitalized. There are no charges to the indigent. The Medical Department of the Ministry of Health reported in its Annual Report of 1972 (the most recent report available in 1980) that $119,669 in revenue had been obtained from the delivery of health care in the previous year, less that $1 B.Z. per person. In the same year, the government reported that per capita expenditures on health were $16.39 B.Z. (approximately $8.20 U.S.). By 1976 this amount had risen to approximately $30 B.Z. (*Belize Annual Abstract of Statistics*, 1976). However, this increase likely reflects little in the way of improved services given a proportionate rise in costs. Total expenditures on health in 1976 were $4,233,000 B.Z. This included monies spent for salaries, maintenance, supplies, drugs, capital improvements and all other services. It is apparent that the government of Belize must indeed stretch its health care dollar.

Within the town of Punta Gorda there is a government run and supported hospital (approximately 30 to 35 beds) with only limited quantities of the equipment, facilities, diagnostic materials, and drugs one expects of a hospital in a more industrialized country. There is an obstetrical ward for maternity patients and a pediatrics ward, but all surgical patients are transferred to Belize City. Within the hospital are located a laboratory equipped to do simple tests and an X-ray machine which was functional no more than three to four months out of the seventeen I was there. Also attached to the hospital is an Outpatient Clinic and pharmacy. Several programs operate within the District, including a malaria eradication program and a prenatal clinic. Medical care provided by the government is largely free, though there are charges for special services.

Those citizens who can afford to do so seek out private medical care. Government physicians are also allowed to establish their own practices and are given some flexibility in setting office hours. Belize City abounds in private and government physicians operating privately who can be consulted for a fairly sizeable fee. At least one private laboratory is also operated in Belize City. A private hospital, Holden Memorial, was closed a few years ago and the building renovated for use as a hotel. Another private hospital now provides for the needs of those who can afford such care.

The government salaried physicians in Punta Gorda (there was, until 1980, only one in the District; another physician was stationed temporarily in one of the Mayan villages; there were in 1984 two physicians in P.G., but apparently none in any of the villages) also operate private clinics where patients are seen and treated. The District Medical Officer present in the Toledo District when I first arrived had chosen not to operate a private clinic, but the two physicians who followed did. The fee charged generally ranged from $10 B.Z. to $20 B.Z., depending on the medications provided. This is a considerable amount in an area where most individuals earn no more than $50 B.Z. per week. However, patients are allotted additional time if they see the physician privately, with time, in theory, for 'negotiation', they are afforded considerably more privacy, and their chances of obtaining the medications prescribed are enhanced since the physician maintains a stock of medications at his expense, or did so at the time I was resident in Punta Gorda, and is not dependent upon government supplies. These are among the reasons that many choose to pay the fee rather than attend the local public clinic.

The government's policy toward "bush" medicine does not specifically declare that the delivery of health care by bush doctors is illegal. Rather the law states that medical treatment can only be rendered by a licensed practitioner and all bush doctors are denied licenses. Nevertheless, bush doctors continue to practice openly, as do other therapeutic specialists, and no person within this district has ever been prosecuted for delivering medical care without a license.

Suppression of therapeutic specialists in competition with those who utilize, or claim to utilize, biomedical models of intepretation and therapy is attempted in two ways: 1. laws probibit the delivery of health care by all except licensed persons; all 'bush" doctors, as stated, are denied licenses, and 2. there is no mechanism for the allocation of national resources to support ethnomedicine or any other non-biomedical form of therapy.

There seems to be little overt competition among ethnomedical healers, regardless of ethnic group membership. Specialization appears to have lessened the likelihood of competition. Primary competition for non-biomedical therapeutic specialists, both sacred and secular, comes from state medicine, and, in addition, from the Pentecostalist cults which not only provide their own healings but directly and openly oppose the *búiai* of the Garinagu and the cult of Esquipulas. While also opposed to biomedicine, their opposition is hardly so vehement. It appears that any therapeutic system which incorporates into its diagnostic procedure or therapy the intervention of spiritual beings is viewed as in competition with the healings of the Pentecostalist sects and therefore constitutes their gravest threat.

Non-biomedical therapeutic specialists not only continue to practice, but their practices often thrive for a variety of reasons, not the least of which is that biomedicine offered through the state cannot meet all the health needs of Belizeans. State medicine is, for example, often inaccessible. Seventy-five percent of the residents of the Toledo live in rural, often isolated areas. It is often difficult or impossible to obtain transport into town, even from the more accessible settlements. One young Mayan woman whom I interviewed in the hospital walked barefoot over thirteen miles of jungle trails carrying her seriously ill one-month old infant in order to reach a village where transport to hospital (still over two hours away) was available. A young boy of thirteen had come out on the same trail the previous day in order to obtain treatment for his abcessed foot. Both left the hospital "without medical approval" after a few days when they heard that transport back to an intermediate spot would be available that day. The nurses' response to their unauthorized exit was: "Well, that's the way the Indians are." Another man from the same village laughed when asked what residents of that village normally did when seriously ill (there was no bush doctor in that small village) and replied, "We die." Toledo is often referred to as the "forgotten district"; the inaccessibility of these villages and the government's inability to deliver basic services to them reinforces that image.

Even when villagers did reach the clinic, care was often inadvertantly denied them. The trucks carrying the Mayans arrived early in the morning on market days and left by noon or 1 P.M. The last District Medical Officer (DMO) to serve in the District did not arrive at the hospital until 10 A.M., as he saw "private" patients from 8 A.M. to 10 A.M. He visited his patients who were hospitalized and then appeared at the outpatient clinic about 11 A.M. This made it extremely difficult for the villagers to see the doctor and, as was usually required of them, to have a prescription filled and return to the trucks, some three-quarters of a mile away, before their departure.[9]

Many of the Maya believed they were discriminated against in any transactions occurring in town. Attempting to gain access to the state controlled therapeutic resources was but one sort of transaction. There is no government policy of discrimination directed toward the Maya; however, many of the observations I made on health care delivery during my seventeen months in Belize suggested that their attiude was, at least in part, justified.

Not only is health care physically inaccessible to many, but when accessible, it may be "culturally inappropriate." Given the large number of ethnic groups in the southern Toledo, cultural appropriateness is likely an unrealistic goal. However, representation of the Maya on the nursing staff might have helped for the Maya are the group whose cultural assumptions about illness and its treatment most highly contrast with the emerging "Creole" culture of Punta Gorda.[10]

There is, moreover, often a lack of continuity and consistency to the therapy and preventive care that are delivered. People are encouraged to come to the clinics, yet, upon arrival, may find diagnostic equipment nonfunctioning or the pharmacy lacking in prescribed drugs or closed without warning or explanation. Two District Medical Officers utilized a system whereby only a certain number of out-patients would be seen in the clinic each day. This invariably meant that those arriving late in the morning would not be given a "ticket." Because of the competition for tickets, many arrived early in order to obtain a ticket, though the physician could not be expected to arrive until approximately 11 A.M., thus necessitating long waiting periods. Many who worked could notafford to be absent from work for such extended periods.

The British Army has at least one physician and several medics in the District. The Belizean government's policy toward delivery of care by army personnel to Belizean citizens fluctuates. One of the representatives from the Toledo District told me he was asked by the British Army when the soldiers first arrived in the area in the mid-1970's what they might do to ensure their acceptance by the people of the District. The representative suggested that they deliver medical care to the villages which otherwise had little medical attention. This was done, either with the support of the government or with its knowledge. Free clinics were established at the local army camp and persons from Punta Gorda or the surrounding area were free to consult with the British physician two mornings a week. The same physician also made visits to the clinic at San Antonio once a week. Eventually, for reasons which were never made clear, the government changed its policy and prohibited the delivery of health care services by army personnel. Later, it again altered policy and gave permission for the delivery of limited care, but this was publicized neither by the army nor the government. The physician at the army camp confided that when the DMO established a private practice in Punta Gorda, he (the DMO) apparently regarded the British clinics as an infringement upon his potentially lucrative practice. To avoid further problems, the British physician stopped holding regular clinics at the army camp, though emergency medical care was still provided.

The greatest harrassment of practitioners seems to be directed to those individuals who provide biomedicine in some form but who remain outside the government's immediate jurisdiction. The only bush doctor who, to my knowledge, had been questioned by the police was the East Indian "private doctor" who includes vitamins and antibiotics in his pharmacopeia and sends his patients to Guatemala to obtain medicines.

The government of Belize attempts to deliver adequate medical care to its citizens; that is often fails is due in part to a lack of adequate funds. However, the government prides itself on its preceived ability to provide for both social and economic development without the large-scale intervention of foreigners. This and other policies sometimes result in fragmented and ineffective health care, as does the competition for scarce resources.

A measles epidemic in early 1980 devastated the villages surrounding Punta Gorda, resulting in the deaths of approximately thirty infants and young children. I was told that an American medical missionary team had, some six months prior to the outbreak of measles, offered to vaccinate the villagers. The government, according to reports I received, refused on the grounds that it had sufficient personnel and supplies to deliver adequate medical care to its people. As the epidemic grew in intensity, the government was forced to send in teams to inoculate individuals in almost every village in the Toledo District, expending in the process, a very large portion of the total health care budget for the year. The American lab and x-ray technician referred to earlier received medications and diagnostic supplies and equipment from organizations in the States. In 1980, the government initiated a policy whereby all such supplies arriving in the country were to be given to the local district medical officer before being sent on to their original destination. Convinced that the government would thereby confiscate a sizeable portion of her supplies, if not all of them, she left the country shortly after the implementation of the new policy.

NOTES

1. As Jim had predicated, within two weeks I had contracted a similar illness; though my symptoms were not so severe, the illness was of considerably longer duration. No medication I tried and no therapy which was suggested seemed to help. Eventually I was looked after by a Chinese-Spanish-Creole family who insisted I stay in their home for several days during my 'therapy.' They fed me lime juice (a common remedy for a variety of symptoms), tea, and toast. After a short period I recovered.
2. It is impossible, for example, to examine all behaviors or beliefs which have medical or health implications.
3. The use of the term *system* here is not meant to imply that these diverse resources constitute a system in any rigorous sense (see Press 1980 for a dicussion of the concept of medical systems).
4. Red Fanta was commonly used by the Maya for treatment of fever. When many Mayan children became ill with measles and needed to be rehydrated, the American lab technician had the hospital kitchen prepare large batches of strawberry Kool-aid which children readily accepted and parents approved.
5. The statue of Esquipulas had, in 1984, assumed the central position in the church.
6. Psalm 91 includes the following passages:
   Thou shalt not be afraid for the terror by night; nor for the arrow that flieth by day; Nor for the pestilence that walketh in darkness; nor for the destruction that wasteth at noonday. Because thou hast made the Lord, which is my refuge, even the most High, thy habitation; There shall no evil befall thee, neither shall any plague come nigh thy dwelling.
7. Including the following: Mark 16:16-20; I Peter 2:24; Mark 11:12-24; James 5:13-16; Hebrews II:1; II Corinthians 1:20; Matthew 8:16-17 Exodus 15:26; and Deuteronomy 7:15.
8. In 1984, there was a new pharmacy and pharmacist in town. The pharmacy

appeared to carry a greater array of biomedically justified medications than the pharmacy mentioned here.

9. This routine appeared to have been changed by 1984. The District Medical Officer was said to hold private office hours later in the afternoon.
10. In 1984, there appeared to be at least one Mayan nurse or aide who had been added to the staff.

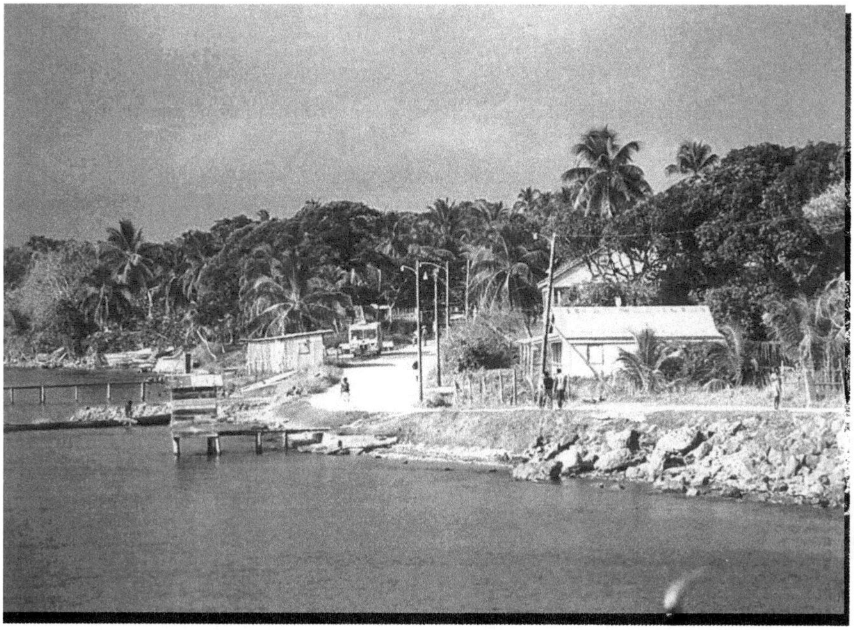

Punta Gorda Town

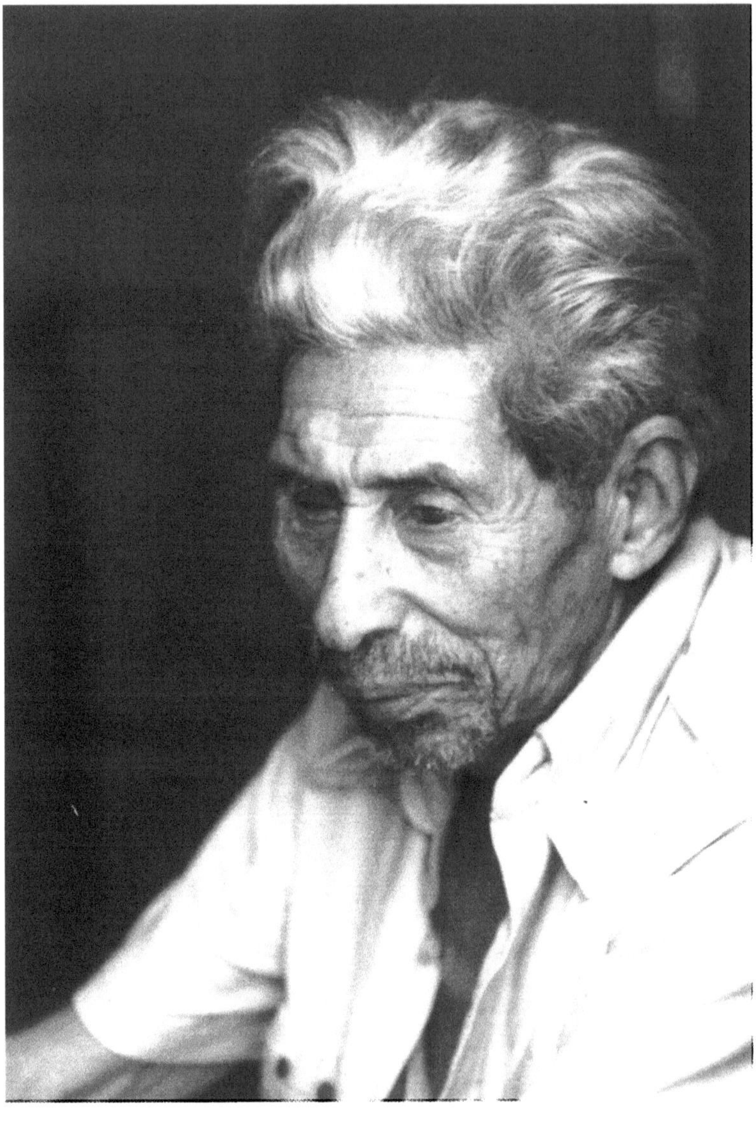

Domingo Gonzalez

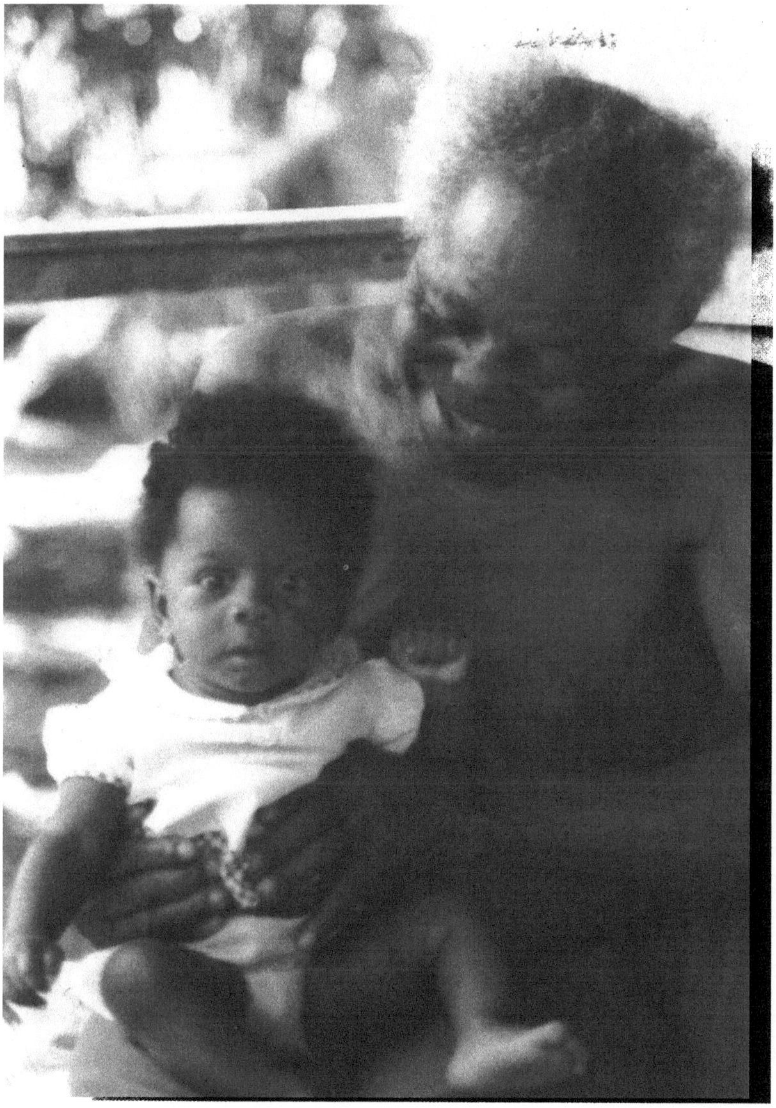

Mr. Peter Benguche and his great grandchild

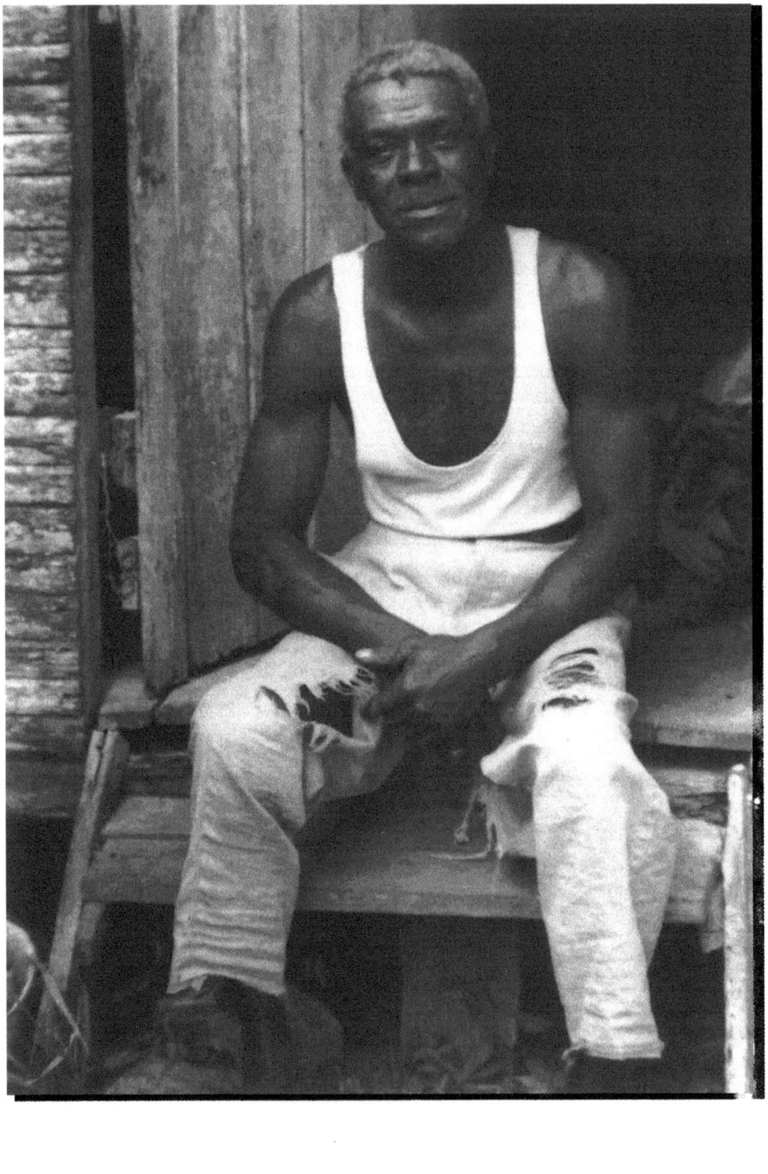

A well-known Garifuna healer

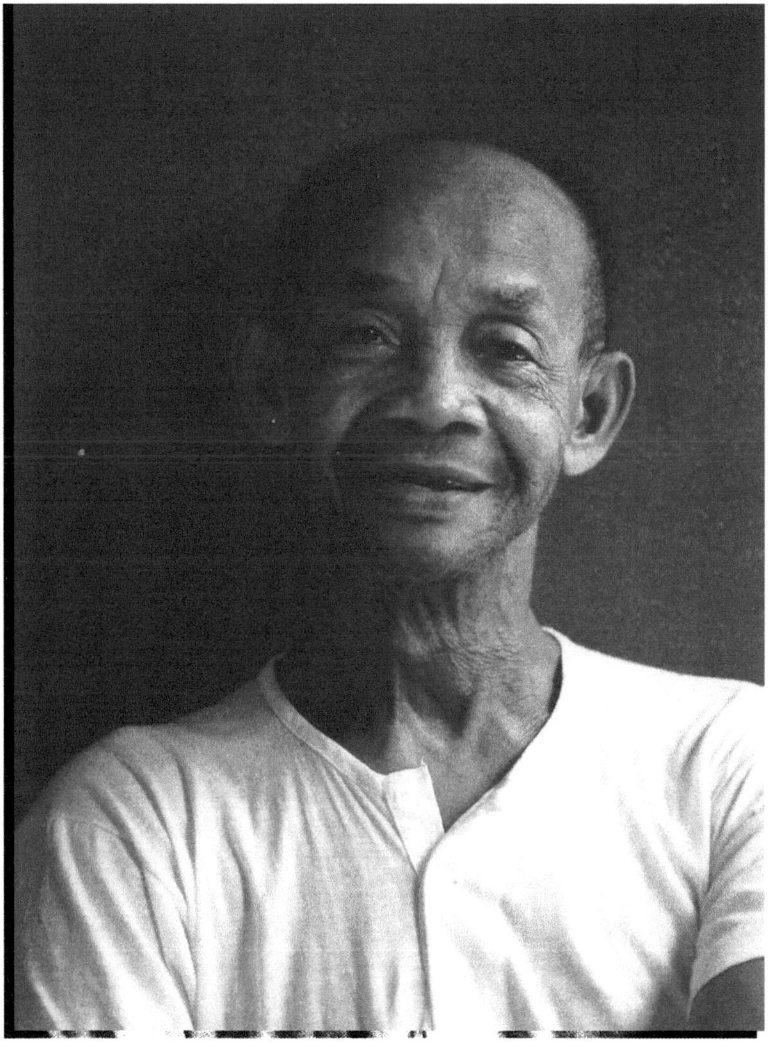

A prominent Garifuna healer

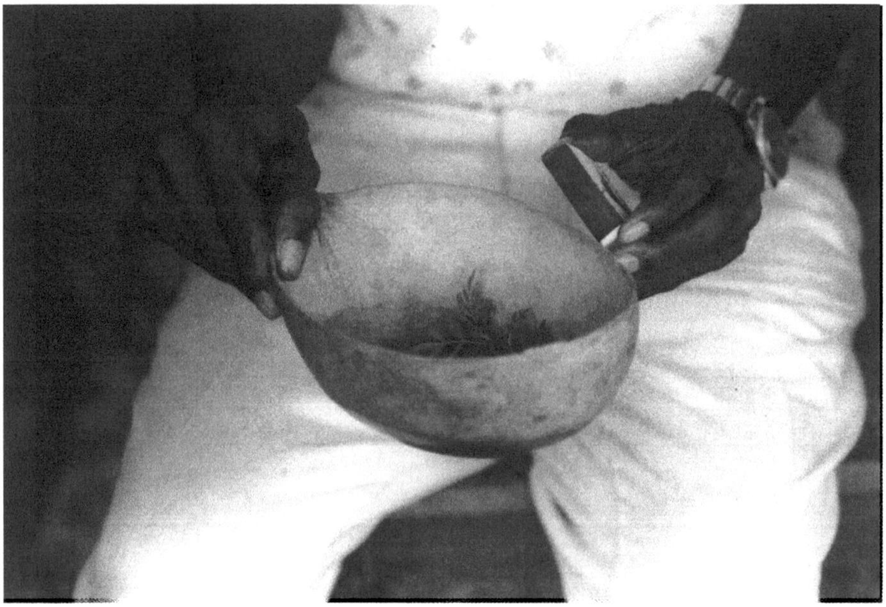

A Garifuna bush doctor prepares medicines in a calabash

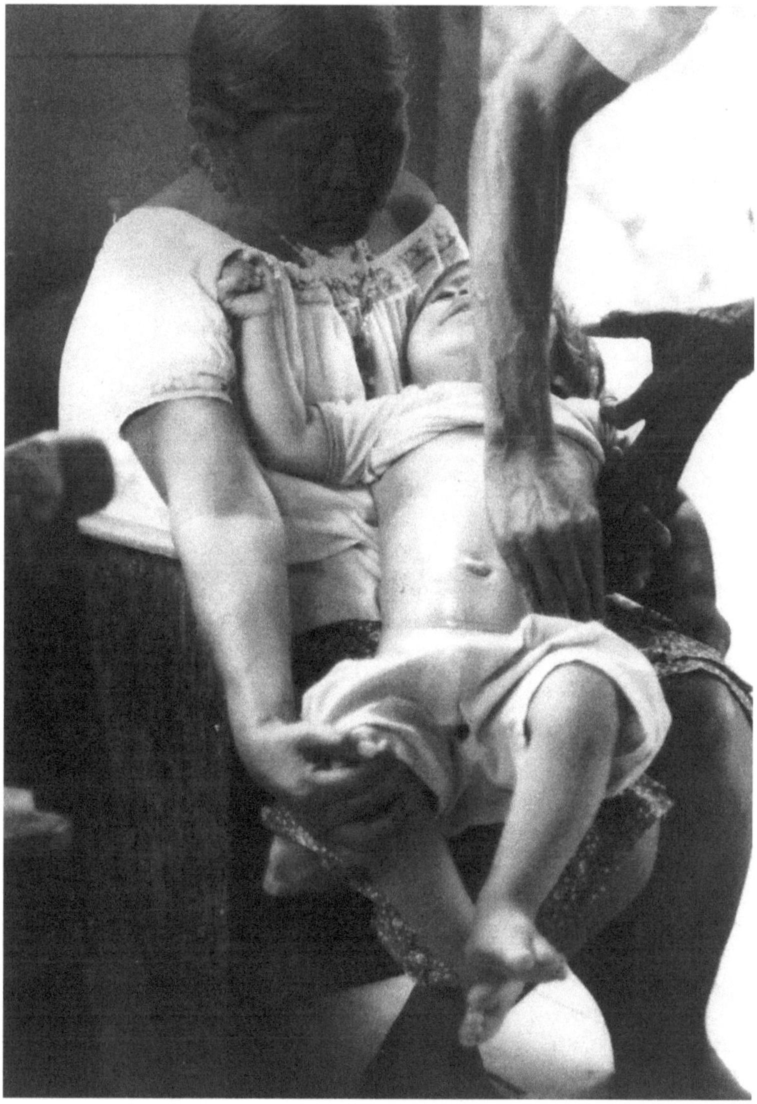

A Mopan Mayan child is treated by a Garifuna bush doctor

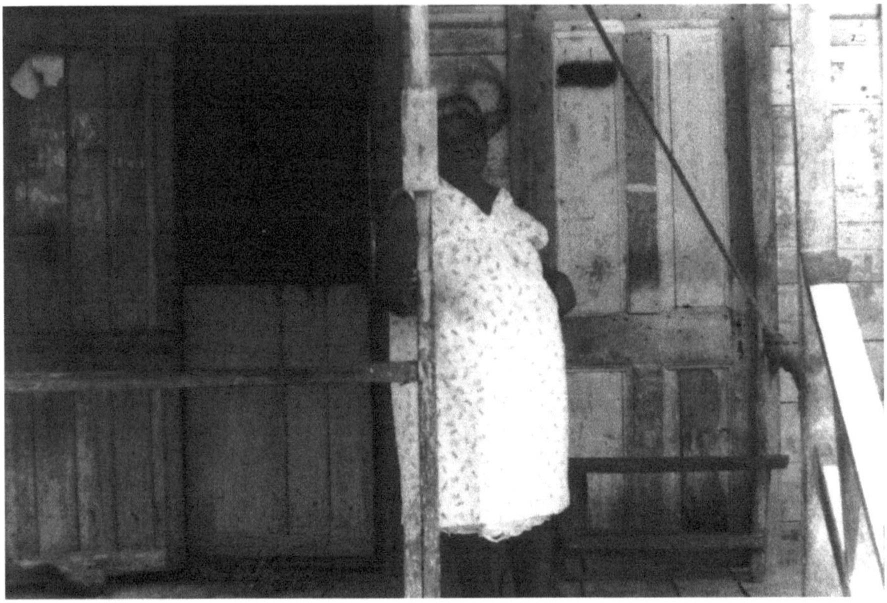

Mrs. Mary Sentino

CHAPTER 4

The Garinagu of Punta Gorda

In the preceding chapters I have argued that intraethnic diversity in the interpretive schemes or in the employment of paradigms is an important and all too often unexamined phenomenon. As social scientists we seek out and memorialize the regularities, creating models which depict and explain the behavior we refer to as culture and, in the process, often de-emphasize intraethnic diversity in order to focus on differences between sociopolitical systems or to support statements concerning the logical relations among components of a system. But models are icons, our best approximation of reality. They are useful only to the extent they do not substantially inhibit our observation and description of actual behavior. The creation of explanatory paradigms may do more to signify the Western need for systematization, for analysis and resynthesis, than to explain or predict the behavior of individuals in other societies. Or, in other words, they may better explain the cultural assumptions of the anthropologist than those of individuals within the social system under examination. Culture functions not to determine our actions, but to provide us with a set of 'meaningful', that is, logically related and socially and historically appropriate choices. Culture offers an integrated, if not always interdependent, range of resources and explanantory paradigms from which individuals draw in making sense of historic events and life crises. As social scientists, we must continue to ask questions concerning the culturally bounded understanding of the natural and spiritual worlds in which individuals live and by which they are affected. Yet, we must simultaneously acknowledge the extent to which each individual is the author of his own story. Each person, at any given moment in time, is, in Peirce's words, a sign, composed of all the signs which preceded, with a unique perspective of a world which is, in turn, constituted of a set of signs created and interpreted according to a model which is not totally available for evaluation.

Garifuna culture offers a wide range of solutions to specific and universal questions. Hadel has said of the Garinagu: "If there is any generalization that can validly be made of the Black Caribs, it is that they do not all think and act alike" (1972:vi). But, while diversity in interpretation may be the rule rather than the exception among the Garinagu and healers pride themselves on their autonomy, sufficient similarities exist across geographic regions and through time to speak of a broadly based paradigm of health and illness. Though distortion may result from the creation and employment by the social scientist of synthetic models, there is much to be gained from an examination of the broad parameters of the dominant medical paradigms which manipulate both physical resources and notions of cause and effect, and which render coherent the majority if not the totality of beliefs, therapeutic practices, and personal and social (group) responses to illness.

The Garifuna interpretive paradigm was selected for this study for several reasons. From among the various interpretive models available in the southern Toledo, the largest body of information was collected from Garifuna healers and lay persons during the course of my fieldwork. Additionally, substantial data from other researchers provided information on stability, or the lack of stability, adaptability, and intraethnic diversity. (see Cosminsky 1976 MS, 1976, 1977; Gonzalez 1959, 1963, 1969; Gullick 1976a, 1976b, 1979; Hadel 1972; Jenkins 1980 MS Kerns 1977; Palacio 1973, 1982; Macklin 1976; Sanford 1976 MS Taylor 1951; Wells 1980, 1982a, 1982b, Whipple 1976).

The "explanatory models" (Kleinman 1980) which render logical the total medical model of any given group cannot, of course, be examined apart from the context in which the system functions. As Comaroff notes:

> ...it is becoming increasingly difficult to sustain the view that 'medical' facts constitute a 'natural' system which may defensibly be bounded and excised from their total context for purposes of exposition and explanation (1981:387).

Before proceeding with the description of the parameters of the Garifuna medical model, the socioeconomic and historic context in which that model is located must be described.

The Garinagu: The Ethnographic Context

The Garinagu are the largest of Punta Gorda's ethnic groups, constituting almost fifty percent of the town's population. Garifuna households are located throughout the town; there is no section identified with any specific ethnic group though related Garifuna families tend to live near one another. The Garinagu are the descendants of escaped or captured West African slaves and the Carib and Arawak Indians who inhabited the Lesser Antilles in the fifteenth and sixteenth centuries (see Chapter Two). The language they speak is refered to as Carib or Garifuna; it is a derivative of the languages spoken by their Island Carib and Arawak ancestors[1], with an admixture of Spanish, French, English, creolized English (Creole) West African, and Miskito lexical items. All adult Garinagu are fluent in Garifuna though many children speak only English or Creole. The common language of the streets, especially among the children, is Creole, though a good portion of the adult Garifuna population continue to use Garifuna in the home and in public when with other Garifuna adults. All adults are also English speakers, though degree of fluency varies considerably. Many speak Spanish and some speak Mopan or Kekchi as well. Cosminsky has referred to this multilingualism as:

> ...one of the few Carib characteristics that are praised by the Creoles and others. It is regarded as something inherent in the Caribs, as a native ability or racial trait. The high degree of multilingualism may be related to, and reinforced by, the social and psychological rewards it provides for the Caribs, since it is one means by which they can feel superior to others (1976:100).

The household is the basic social and economic unit. Researchers have generally emphasized the use of consanguineality in the recruitment of members into the Garifuna household. Gonzalez describes these consanguineal households as matrifocal and states that such household are:

> ...an alternative type of domestic group that develops during the process of acculturation of neoteric societies in which the primary mechanism of Westernization is recurrent migratory wage labor with low remuneration (16).

Helms (1975) suggests that:

> ...these household types facilitate the necessary *diversity* of economic pursuits *at any one time* and/or the necessary *flexibility over time* to move between different types of economic activities as external economic conditions or personal inclinations may require. The closely knit cores of consanguineal women also provide *social continuity*, solidarity, and security to counteract whatever relational stress and social tension may result from male or female absenteeism in general and/or discongruities between traditional subsistence economic pursuits and those of the market economy (6).

Helms goes on to state, however, that the consanguineal household does not necessarily represent a new form of household structure arising as a response to Westernization, but the persistence of earlier forms:

> I would also suggest that among the Black Caribs of today the permanent nuclear family houshold fails to work in many cases not only because of current economic problems but also because it is still socially prestigeful for a man to have several wives and to father several families of children. The failure of the nuclear family household so far can traced to the traditional (i.e., "Red" Carib) residence pattern in which men and women resided in separate lodging, women remaining close to female consanguines while men centered their interests on the men's house (12).

Despite the relative importance often assigned to consanguineality and matrifocality among the Garinagu, the data collected during my stay indicated that two-thirds of the Garifuna households[2] of Punta Gorda were headed by an adult couple and, therefore, not constituted as consanguineal households in the sense in which Gonzalez defined the term, though consanguineal relatives other than children are often present. This figure of 66% can be compared with the 54% of households headed by an adult couple reported by Gonzalez in Livingston, Guatemala (1969) and the 47% reported by Palacio for the town of "Lisurnia" (1982). Of greater importance than the presence of a "consanguineal core" is the overall diversity in the structure of the domestic unit and the range of variation exhibited by the units of production and distribution.

Thirty-nine Garifuna households without evidence of inter-ethnic mating were identified in my survey of one hundred homes. Twenty-six of the thirty-nine households were comprised of an adult male and female who had established a sexual/economic liaison. Of these twenty-six, however, only six were constituted of nuclear families along. Three additional households were comprised of an elderly couple living alone without children. The remaining seventeen were constituted of a couple living with individuals other than their children, though children of that union and of previous unions might also be present. With the exception of three cases in which the spouse of a child was present in the household and one case in which a non-related individual had been adopted into the household, almost all individuals in residence were related consanguineally to one of the adult members, though not neccessarily to the female. Thirteen of the thirty-nine households were headed by women.[3] Men attached to the female-headed households were most likely to be the sons of the females residing there. The children of the daughter of the adult couple or of the female partner of an adult couple were present in seven of the twenty-six households. The daughter and her spouse were resident in two of these households. The children of the son of an adult couple or of the female partner were present in three of the twenty-six households. The son and his spouse were present in only one of these households, along with the children of a previous union of the son's spouse. The children of a daughter were present in two female-headed households; the children of the son of the female were present in one female-headed household, along with both the son and his spouse. In two female-headed households, an adult female cared for the children of a sister who was not present. To properly categorize all thirty-nine households would have required twenty-five distinct categories.

Descent is reckoned bilaterally; both sons and daughters may inherit property from either parent. The question of "legitimacy" as defined in Western· terms is of little importance in determining right to inherit; "legitimacy", in fact, occurs when the father choses to recognize his paternity and bears no relation to the performance of a civil or religious ceremony. The term used to refer to the other member of a sexual/economic union is *umári*, regardless of the legal status of the relationship or the sex of the individual referenced.

In nuclear units the man may well dominate in some household matters, but women are usually outspoken and have a major role in most decisions. Though fishing, with its inherent risks, is no longer the important economic activity it once was and most men are now employed as wage laborers rather than fishermen, Coehlo's remarks on the relation between men and women still ring true:

> The position of the woman in the family is in no way to be conceived as subordinate, the principle involved being one of partnership under equal terms, not of one person

commanding and the other obeying. It should be noted, moreover, that though greater social prestige is associated with the position of the men, since masculine activities demand the esteemed traits of daring, cunning, and resourcefulness in the face of danger, his position does not in itself entitle a man to the services of a woman (1955:86).

If the man lives in the same house as his *umári* he will usually provide funds for food and other items. Men are generally not expected to help with household duties though some will as the situation demands. Men who have publicly accepted the responsibility for a spouse and children are, ideally, expected to provide financial support for both and to furnish a house and keep it in repair, regardless of their place of residence. The male's status in the community is, in great part, determined by his ability to father children *and* to provide for their support on a continuing basis. However, men who do not reside in the house on a permanent basis may provide little or no support, even when there are children. If a man chooses not to recognize his children or to accept the responsibility for a wife, little social pressure is actually exerted on him to provide anything but minimal and irregular support for the children. A woman's status is generally based upon her ability to properly care for, and, if necessary, provide for her children. The source of support and the number of lovers or husbands she has had are of far less importance, though loose sexual conduct by women is not condoned.

Sons, brothers, husbands, and lovers may be permanent household members and the principal support of the household, but where they are absent or unemployed, the women must manage for themselves, obtaining whatever support they can from temporary mates or the fathers of their children or from their own economic activities.

Garifuna females generally begin bearing children by the age of sixteen or seventeen, some reportedly as early as twelve or thirteen. Most commonly, the girl's *umári* is also young and may not have sufficient employment to allow him to establish a separate household for her and any children of their union. She often continues, even after the birth of a child, to live with her parents or with her mother. The spouse provides what support he can for the child and makes "visits" to his "wife." He will likely continue to live with his parents, though he may also choose to live with his spouse in her parent(s)' home. Birth control is only infrequently practiced in Punta Gorda and additional children usually arrive. The man, often still without adequate employment, may find himself unable to provide more than irregular support for the additional children. He may eventually migrate out in search of better employment and, if he is successful, he may send back small amounts of money. Ideally, the couple eventually establish their own home if local job opportunities allow the male to remain in the same village. The comparatively large percentage of households headed by couples in Punta Gorda may be due to increased wage labor opportunities available locally for both men and women as the result of the establishment of three army camps in the region and the recent (until 1980) presence of Esso Oil.

In my sample of thirty-nine households, there were forty-one males over the age of eighteen (the approximate age at which they begin to establish permanent or semi-permanent relationships) and sixty-two females over the age of sixteen (the approximate age at which they begin to establish permanent or semi-permanent relationships) indicating the shortage of eligible males and the prevalence of outmigration of males. There were, in these same thirty-nine households, sixty-three males under the age of eighteen and seventy-two females under the age of eighteen. This sizeable discrepancy in number of males and females under the age of eighteen may be result of a higher male infant mortality rate and/or the outmigration of males before the age of eighteen. I suspect the second explanation accounts for the major part of the discrepancy. In fifteen cases (not included in the thirty-nine households referenced above), a Garifuna male or female had established a union, legal or extra-legal, with an individual who was not Garifuna. The number involving a Garifuna male was four. It is clear that one strategy which Garifuna women employ to offset the shortage of eligible males is the establishment of relationships with males outside their ethnic section.

Among young adults relationships are often unstable, dependent as they are on available work and adequate wages, and the young adult male may give up the task of caring for his spouse and children altogether. He may migrate out from the community or he may begin a relationship with another woman, perhaps one who has her own house. His first *umári*, left without adequate support, may work to make money to support the children and/or may establish a sexual/economic liaison with the "next" man from who she may hope to obtain some support for her children and herself. But resources are scarce, good jobs are difficult to find, salaries are low, employment irregular and unpredictable, and the temptations of the "outside" world too great, and her hopes are often not fulfilled. Further, the man may also be required to provide some support to the household of his parents or earlier 'spouses', placing an additional burden on the male who hopes to establish and maintain his own household.

An individual may develop, over the course of time, several sexual and economic liaisons. Women may become involved in a relationship with a man who is willing to provide support for any children of the current union, but not for children of her previous unions. Those children may then be left with the grandparent(s) or other kin. Grandparents are often relied upon to raise children when parents migrate to seek employment elsewhere or when a daughter takes a new 'husband' (see, for example, Palacio's study [1982] of social structure and food relations in the Garifuna village of Lisurnia). The respected and responsible male ideally establishes separate households for his "wives" and provides support for all his children. The ideal, however, is often not achievable. There is greater pressure on the male to provide a home if there are children, but the female may continue to live with her mother or her parents. When possible, she will establish her own house where she may live with her children with or without male companionship. The establishment of a variety of household structures which is, in part, a response to the inability of males to provide adequately for their children and the mothers of their children, is one adaptive strategy which allows for the more equitable distribution of scarce resources.

Where marriage or acceptance of a more or less permanent sexual/economic liaison occurs, the couple usually move to their own household, finances permitting. Actual marriages, however, appear to be infrequent. No Garifuna individual, to my knowledge, was married within the town of Punta Gorda during the seventeen months that I resided there. The 1970 Census showed that of 1062 adults then residing in Punta Gorda, 613 had never been married. I do not mean to imply that stable relationships do not exist and that no Garifuna individuals marry. In fact, the data I gathered suggest that at least fifteen of the twenty-nine adult couples in Garifuna households had married. But such stable relationships are generally found among the older generations of the town and most commonly among those who have managed to obtain secure employment in the area. According to Coehlo (1955): "Marriage is not conceived as an abrupt change in status, but is rather the final step in the stablization of a sexual union" (74). Even though a man may eventually establish a more or less permanent liaison with one woman, the likelihood that he will have "outside" children is high. It should be pointed out that the "old heads" are somewhat disturbed by the instability of many of the liaisons among those of the younger generations.

Women left without adequate support are generally forced to find a job or to establish small businesses within their homes, baking bread and sweets, doing laundry, selling ice, and so on. Women who are not able to work are often forced to turn to the sons, daughters, parents, and the father(s) of their children for whatever support those individuals will provide. Some receive money from relatives who have secured employment in the States or in Belize's larger towns, but the reliance on such forms of assistance has been vastly overestimated by some who have written on the Garinagu. The Social Development Department provides only minimal support to the indigent. At the time of my research, the maximal amount available to an individual classified as indigent was $7.50 U.S. per month.

There are no corporate groups based on either agnatic or uterine ties. First and second cousin marriages are prohibited though they may occasionally occur. Taylor (1951) and Gullick (1976a) suggest cross-cousin marriages may have been common in the past. Relationships are generally not calculated further back than three or four generations. There is also a clear tendency to lump relatives under the terms cousin, aunt, or uncle, when English is employed, rather than to specify the precise relationship; the Garifuna language forces terminological distinctions between mother's sister and father's sister, between older and younger brothers, older and younger sisters, older and younger sons, older and younger daughters, and so on, depending on the sex and relationship of the speaker. Such distinctions are lost with the increasing use of English.

The basic economic unit is the household.[4] It is the primary unit of production and distribution, though mechanisms for distribution of resources beyond the limits of the household exist and are fully operative. For the most part, goods and services flow outward to consanguineal kin, though there is sharing among persons related affinally and among neighbors and friends who are unrelated. When goods and services are distributed to unrelated persons, the expectation is that such an action will eventually be reciprocated, though reciprocity may not take the same form. Cooperative labor arrangements based on lineal ties, such as are common to the Maya, are rare among the Garinagu. There are few activities which require help beyond that available within the household. As we shall see later, preparations for the *dugu* are an exception to this and involve many individuals from within the entire cognatic kin group.

In a society in which individuals must constantly cope with irregular employment, low wages, and unpredictable natural resources (such as variations in the supply of fish affected by daily fluctuations in weather), food becomes an extremely important resource and the exchange of food serves several functions (see Palacio 1982). The presentation of food to another is, among other things, an action of great social import. It may serve as an expression of gratitude, but even more importantly, it may function as the 'mortar' which helps hold an intricate social network together. We see in Peter's case study in Chapter VII that the failure of an older son who was living with her father to give her some portion of the fish he had caught, caused Peter's mother to re-evaluate her entire relationship with her children and to take Peter back from the old couple with whom she had left him. In Chapter VI we will also see how the Garifuna ceremony, the *dugu* allows for the distribution of food beyond the boundaries of even the larger collection of related households.

Women are responsible for the maintenance of home and children, even though the children are often not their own. Women do the cooking, cleaning, shopping, laundry, and sewing. They may also tend a small garden and care for chickens. Few women have plantations any longer, but some still walk several miles each day to reach the Carib Block where they continue to raise cassava, yams, plantain, tomatoes, bananas, cucumbers, ginger, wangla, coconut, sweet potatoes, beans, okra, banana apples, cocoa, rice, and pineapples. Many women also take on small jobs which can be done at home to earn cash. In some cases, this may be the only income for the household. A sizeable percentage of Garifuna women now work full-time as store clerks, waitresses, cooks, maids, nurses, laundrywomen (at the local army camp), secretaries, school teachers, and in civil service positions. A few make small sums of money selling the Boledo (the lottery) for the town's more prosperous merchants.

At the age of two or three children are assigned simple tasks such as picking up their own clothes. Soon after, both girls and boys take on more responsibilities: sweeping, "backing" water, running errands, shopping for specific items, gathering firewood, coconuts, breadfruit, and so on. It is more common to see girls engaged in most of these activities than boys, but these are all chores done by boys as well. At the age of five or six, children enter school, but are still expected to help with work both before and after school. The care of younger children is often assigned to the older children, especially if the mother has many children, and it is quite common to see a child of nine or ten carrying a younger child on his/her back or guiding the child through the streets. Children of nine or ten may also be expected to help the mother by selling baked or cooked items in the streets or door to door. A girl of twelve might be expected to cook for and look after all other children in the mother's absence. In some cases, young or adolescent children take on certain jobs, such as running errands, shining shoes, and chopping grass in order to provide income to the household. Boys are responsible for chopping grass and clearing bush and may be expected to help their fathers or related males with care of boats and fishing nets as well. Some children in Punta Gorda also help with work on the "planations", but this is far more common in the Mayan villages and in the East Indian communities since comparatively few Garinagu farm, even on a small scale. Children gradually take on more and more responsibility, though the burden is heavier on girls than boys. There is no sudden transition to adolescence or to adulthood for the children of either sex.

The child of any ethnic section is generally considered an adult at about the time he or she leaves school. The fact that some children continue in school longer than others means that they may delay taking on the full responsibilities of adulthood. In general, girls of fourteen to twenty and male of fifteen to twenty-one are expected to begin the search for a mate. Many have had previous sexual experiences. Few Garifuna girls reach their 20's without having had children.

Those men who can find employment most commonly work as laborers and are employed by the town or the national government on public works projects, by private businesses, or by the British Army. They work as mechanics, masons, carpenters, painters, cabinet-makers, electricians, and plumbers; they repair roads and clean the streets, and chop the bush. Many are also employed in skilled or semi-skilled positions as teachers, clerks, policemen, civil servants, cooks, hospital aides, and so on. Some function as managers or foremen. A few operate their own small businesses (sales of dry goods or products, tailoring, a restaurant, a tavern, etc.) In the past, a number of men were employed by the Esso Oil Company, but the oil company closed down its operations in 1980. The relatively high salaries paid by the oil company created, at least temporarily, a sense of prosperity among many of the town's residents and the departure of the oil company has had serious consequences. When and if the British Army leaves the area, as it has long said it would do eventually, severe economic stresses will occur within the community.

Perhaps a dozen men continue to fish on a regular basis and a few others supplement their income by fishing from time to time. A fishing co-op failed in the late 70s, and attempts to establish a fish processing and distribution center in Punta Gorda in 1980 with private U.S. financing also failed. By 1984 a new fishing co-op had been established with a sizeable loan from the United States. It was unclear at the time of my second visit whether the co-op would succeed.

The town, district, and national governments now regulate many aspects of individuals' lives which were previously dealt with by institutions within the ethnic collectivity or the extended family. For example, Punta Gorda now has a relatively large police force and arrests, though not frequent, do occur. The most common causes for arrest in 1979 and 1980, in approximate order of frequency, were use of indecent language, assault, housebreaking, stealing, rape, and indecent assault. With the growth of the marijuana 'industry' in the Toledo District, there appears to be an increasing number of arrests connected with the sale of marijuana.

Punta Gorda also has a court which is most often presided over by the District Officer who is the chief judicial and administrative official residing in the district. A magistrate from Belize City is present on a somewhat irregular basis to hear more serious or sensitive cases. While imprisonment is not uncommon, the majority of cases tried in the lower courts result in fines levied against the guilty party.

Only upon a few rare occasions does the Garifuna population of Punta Gorda function, in either a social or political sense, as a collectivity, though they may occasionally appear united on certain issues of importance to them and they have a strong sense of their separate and unique identity. The household is the locus of much decision-making, though during crises, a larger social network comprised primarily of consanguineally related kin can be mobilized.

Children can be expected to be under the authority of their parents or guardians only until about the time they graduate from school. Parents and guardians have few techniques for successfully dealing with obstreperous young adults, though they may still be living at home. Many decisions, such as the decision to set up a household separate from that of the parent(s) may be made by the individuals involved without consultation with their parents. While Garifuna individuals desire the approval of consanguineal kin and peers, they will select the less socially acceptable course if they deem it appropriate to their situation. The fact that they are rarely if ever permanently ostracized by the community or their kin is simply one indication of the range of behaviors which is ultimately tolerated.

The respected elders of the community, both male and female, are referred to as the "old heads." Their influence, as Coehlo notes, "is pervasive, and extends to the private as well as to the public spheres of activity" (1955:59). As the "living interpreters of tradition, their opinions always carry weight...." (*Ibid.*). Yet, they have little political power beyond that exerted within their extended kin groupings. The Town Board functions as the officially sanctioned decision-making body within Punta Gorda. This board is made up primarily of Garinagu, and the two mayors who served during the time I lived in the town were both Garifuna. While the elders of the community are often participants in the Town Board, a number of younger Garinagu are involved as well. Despite the apparent control exerted over town politics by the Garinagu, it should be noted that the Town Board has little authority in most matters concerning citizens of the town and that the more important decisions are made at the District or national levels.

Perhaps the greatest control over behavior is exerted through gossip, rumor, ridicule and teasing. "... even [the 'old heads'] cannot escape castigation by ridicule, which is, among the Carib a powerful instrument of social control" (Coehlo 1955:59). Men often gather in the evenings in informal groups, during which time the behavior of both men and women is a major topic of discussion. Women may also gather in the evenings, separately or with the men, though it is more common to see groups of two to four sitting in the shade of a house during the hottest hours of the afternoon. Through such conversations is the status of individuals in the community established. Though these discussions may have little affect on the behavior of those being discussed, there emerges some guide to proper behavior which will likely influence those who are participants in these informal interactions.

Age is a significant determinant of an individual's status and role within the community and within the family or household, though perhaps less so now than in the past. The increase in numbers of those whose income is derived from wage labor, the decrease in number of men actively engaged in fishing, and the increased number of jobs available to women have somewhat altered traditional roles and relationships both between sexes and among age-groups. Within the family, relative age of siblings is still of considerable importance. Older siblings take on many of the responsibilities of an adult and thereby gain the same authorities and respect which accrue to parents. Older children, given the responsibility for the oversight of younger siblings, are often quick to use verbal threats or physical punishment in order to maintain control. Of the considerable respect accorded the father, Coehlo states:

> Overt manifestation of hostile feelings towards the father is seldom found, since he is the living link between the earthly world and that of the *gubída*, and to question this supremacy would wreck the foundations of Carib belief (1955:68).

Mothers and female relatives of the mother's and grandmother's generations are also due great respect, though children could hardly be described as obsequious. Adolescents and young adults who have gained some measure of freedom often avoid potential conflicts with older siblings, parents, and the male and female kin of ascending generations simply by taking actions without prior approval, presenting adults with a *fait accompli*.

A semi-secret fraternal order with approximately sixty members known as the Mechanics serves in certain respects to maintain order or control over individuals' behaviors. For example, secret codes are employed in public settings to signal fellow members whose behavior is considered inappropriate. Both men and women may join, though the two groups meet separately. The organization appears to be similar in several respects to the Masons in the United States with an overlay of Catholic ritual. I was told the organization originated in the U K. and that there are now chapters in many countries. According to one member, the top position within the organization is termed the "priesthood." Every Master Mechanic is said to know the actions of the Catholic priest "because he has learned them himself." Yet it also serves as a sickness and burial society. Such societies are common throughout the Caribbean. Members are recruited from all ethnic groups, however, and this is in no way a strictly Garifuna institution.

There is no one-to-one relationship between the role of the healer and the status and authority of such individuals. Recognition as a successful healer contributes to one's status, but healers are not automatically granted the rights and authority of a respected leader. Healers, however, may function to sanction socially acceptable behaviors, particularly in their role as diagnosticians. That is, they often serve to express and reinforce the cultural constraints placed on individual behavior. For example, a healer might suggest to a mother that her infant's "fresh" cold is the result of unnecessary exposure to a breeze, thus indirectly chastizing the mother for improperly caring for her child. Those healers who have the capacity to diagnose *obeah* or *idáhadu* or other spirit or man-caused illnesses, are in a position to confirm important assumptions regarding relations among individuals and relations between individuals and spirits. Certain diagnostic and therapeutic functions, however, are reserved to the *búiai*. Respected *búiai*s are accorded considerable prestige and authority and may well have played an important role in political decisions made within the community in the past. As no *búiai* has lived in Punta Gorda for several years, it was impossible to assess the local authority of the *búiai*. There is no indication from earlier published reports that the authorities and responsibilities of political or military leaders and those of the *búiai* coincided in any respect (see Gullick 1976a, de la Borde 1888 [orig. 1674]).

Of greatest importance to the discussion here is the role of illness as a tool of social control. More will be said on this subject in this and later chapters. For the time being, it is sufficient to note that the fear of illness, continuously reinforced by the appearance of illness in others, functions to assure some degree of conformity to the codes which guide behavior.

The Model of Health and Illness

Assumptions about illness are closely linked to assumptions about the world in which the Garinagu live. The Garifuna medical model thus cannot be said to be distinct from any general model of human-environment, human-human, and human-spirit interactions, or what is more commonly referred to as "world view."

According to Taylor (1951) every newborn possesses an *iuáni* (soul), which is said to be situated in the heart (*anígi*). The infant still lacks its spirit-double or *áfurugu*. For this reason, the child must receive special protection until it can obtain its *áfurugu*, which is to be acquired from the paternal ancestral dead. The child, says Coehlo, during this period must "depend on the spiritual substance of his father, having none of its own...." (1955:90). The *áfurugu* is described as composed of a "substance akin to that of supernatural entites." It is said to be the "other-of-a-pair", an astral body reproducing the material shape of the person in all its details (Coehlo 1955:138).

These distinctions between *iuáni* and *áfurugu* which were clearly documented during the fieldwork of Coehlo and Taylor seem to have been lost, at least in part, to the Garinagu of Punta Gorda. Characteristics attributed by some to *iuáni* are attributed to *áfurugu* by others, and vice versa. In some cases, *áfurugu* and *iuáni* are said to be identical and both terms are translated as "soul." Coehlo reported that with the proseletyzing of Catholic missionaries in Honduras, the term *iuáni* had increasingly taken on the identity of the world "soul." Though the Catholic notion of "soul" and those concepts expressed as *iuáni* and *áfurugu* are not identical, this coincidence or articulation of codes facilitates integration of belief systems.

According to several Garifuna individuals within the town of Punta Gorda, both *áfurugu* and *iuáni* are present at birth and both leave the body at death.

Death is defined as the asbsence of the *iuáni*. Death does not occur, despite other physical signs or the pronouncement of the doctor, until the *iuáni* has departed. When an individual is reported to be dying, it is said that his *iuáni* is traveling. The *iuáni* and *áfurugu* go to no particular place after death, but are said to wander. A wandering soul (whether *iuañi* or *áfurugu*) is referred to as *pantu*, which is translated by some as "ghost." Not all spirits or souls become *pantu*, only those which are said to be discontented or to have committed some crime or misdeed. *Pantu*, in any case, do not remain for long, though it is often necessary to use prayer to send them away. When a *pantu* is passing, it is said the body will feel heavy. Some claim to have seen *pantu*. One healer stated:

> Dead people have to arise again in three days. The *áfurugu* has to come back to the house. When my mother died, she came back plain and walked around the house for about half an hour. The soul returns during the wake. It has to keep close. The spirit of a person who has just died will come back and molest you if you don't have a wake.

Others said *pantu* could be seen moving quickly in the moonlight and that *pantu* appeared "like a bundle of fire." Whatever the form or the intention of *pantu*, they seem to cause no harm. It is only the *gubída*, the ancestral spirits of those who have been dead for many years, who return to bring illness.

Iuáni was described as "the spirit that is in the body" by one Garifuna man, a former school teacher. Coehlo said that his informants identified the locus of the *iuáni* as the head. He also stated that the *iuáni* was believed to be imperceptible to the senses, and, therefore, "incapable of making itself known to the living" (1955:137). The individual referred to above, however, reported that the *iuáni* was able to travel at night in dreams and possessed the ability to communicate with other individuals both through their dreams and in the daytime as well. A dream in which one individual dreams of another may be interpreted as communication between their *iúanis*. Such experiences do not generally appear to be regarded as threatening, but an evaluation of the dream by a healer or other person skilled in such interpretations may be required. An individual has no control over his *iúani* and may be unaware of extracorporeal experiences involving the *iúani*.

The *áfurugu* is, on the other hand, a spiritual icon which, according to Coehlo, possesses "faculties of discernment, even clairvoyance, which enables it to know of dangers threatening the individual to whom it is attached before he is aware of them" (1955:138). "In the face of unseen peril", he continues, "it may fly away, leaving the person plunged into a stupor, which is, according to the 'weight' of the *áfurugu*, more or less prolonged and seirous" (*Ibid.*). Taylor's informants located the *áfurugu* in the small of the back (1951:102), while Coehlo states simply that it is "indissolubly tied to [the physical body]" (138). Though he reports that the *áfurugu* may wander away from the body [a characteristic generally attributed by my informants to *iuáni* and only occasionally to *áfurugu*], "prolonged absences [entail] dire consequences for the person's health" (138). One bush doctor suggested an individual who had been engaged in strenuous physical labor and who had failed to feed or care for his *áfurugu* might die in his sleep. "Your soul" (*báfurugu*), he continued, "leaves you at night to drink water. If you leave a glass of water under your bed at night, you will find it reduced in the morning because your soul has taken some. You dream at night because your soul is traveling."

One of my principal informants stated that the *áfurugu* was distinct from *iuáni* and of a "lower concept than *iuáni*." *Áfurugu*, he explained, denoted a physical feelings, something "more related to the mind and the senses than to the spirit or soul." If an individual says, "I thought so", or "I felt so", it is his *afurugu* which has responded. "If you make a noise in the house, a child may shake because his *áfurugu* has been affected." When a child smiles, this individual stated, people will say, "He has a fine *áfurugu*." Another individual reported that when a newborn baby smiles or laughs in his sleep, it is because he is laughing with his *áfurugu*. One man suggested that while the *iuáni* can communicate with others, the *áfurugu* can communicate only with the person possessing it, suggesting the retention of certain aspects of the concept of "spirit-double", though *áfurugu* was never defined or described in those terms by my informants.

Every infant possesses an *iaua* which is variously defined as a shadow, reflection, or image. Taylor (1951) regards it as a component of the total person (*mutu*), but states that its role is a minor one and ill defined: "it leaves the body before death, and in life acts as a kind of general index to health" (102). Coehlo also gives little attention to the concept of *iaua*, suggesting "it was a moot point if the shadow, *Iaua*, is a direct projection of the body, *ugúbu*, or of the *anígi*" (135). Interestingly, among some of the Garinagu of Punta Gorda the term *iaua* has now taken on the additional meanings of "picture" and "photo", suggesting that the *iaua* is the iconic representation of the individual; that is, there is self and the appearance of self or the obvious physical characteristics by which we identify an individual. Alterations in appearance are indicators of illness or some abnormal state or some affect upon the 'true' self which is not visible except as *iaua*. Severity of illness is sometimes expressed in terms of the perception of relatedness to "self." For example, in discussing a serious illness, the individual may state that "I hardly even knew myself."

Coehlo defined the *anígi* as a separate spiritual component, "a kind of vital force or animal spirit" whose seat is the heart. The *anígi* was thus said to be one of three components of the soul. The Garinagu with whom I spoke, however, used the term *anígi* to refer to the heart itself and there is no indication the term refers to any component of the soul. The definition of *anígi* provided by Coehlo is similar to that of *iuáni* reported by Taylor, and Coehlo admits that "some elders... hold the *iuáni* to be synonymous with the *anígi*, the number of the parts of the soul thus reduced to two...." (*Ibid*.:137). If the term *anígi* ever carried a meaning other than "heart", it appears to have lost that meaning among the majority of the Garinagu of Punta Gorda.

Every adult is thus constituted of various separate but interdependent components: the physical body, *ugúbu*, the *iuáni*, or "vital force" (Coehlo 1955) or soul, the *áfurugu*, or spirit-double or guardian spirit or protector which is sometimes treated as equivalent to the "soul", the *iaua*, or shadow or reflection or appearance, and the personality which is, in part determined by the nature of the *áfurugu*.

The self (*nungua*)[5] arises out of the interaction of these components with one another, with the physical or natural environment, with other 'selves' and with the larger universe which includes all spiritual beings. That is, the self is not equated with the physical body (*ugúbu*), with the *iuañi*, the *áfurugu*, or *iaua*. The distinction between physical body and "self" is manifested in the following statement made by an elderly Garifuna women: "When your body don't give you to do nothing, then you can't do anything. Your body has to help you." Nor does the self (*nungua*) emerge except in interactions with other beings and with the various forces which constitute one's environment. The self, as psychiatrist and semiotician, Harley Shands often noted, is a "social invention, linguistically derived and normatively evaluated" (1970:26).

> ...the self appears to be a development, emerging in a particular culture at a particular epoch in time; within this cultural setting, the self becomes an object only by becoming susceptible to description in a series of human relationships in which self-description is a recognized goal. The eventual form of the self is that of a comprehensive symbol of the universe, reciprocally related to the universe as a computer program fed into the memory of a computer is reciprocally related to every subsequent action of the computer while under the influence of that program. The self appears as the master symbol reflecting and represting the complexity of the universe;.... (*Ibid*.:250)

This universe of social beings to which Shands refers is expanded by the Garinagu to encompass the spiritual beings with whom the Garinagu also interact. The most important of these, the *gubîda*, were once themselves actors in the world of living social 'selves.' Their power derives, in part, from their ambiguous status as persons who are both present and absent, distant yet threatening. They continue to command authority and respect. And they continue in death as they did in life to interfere in the affairs of living Garifuna people. Spiritual entities, whether the *gubída* or any of the many other spirits who inhabit the Garifuna universe, serve, in many respects, as the symbolic transformation of social realities; they are the "social facts" of Garifuna existence projected on a larger screen.

Self, then, emerges from a continuing set of interactions, and, in turn, influences or determines the nature of those interactions. It is the interaction of the physical body (*ugúbu*), the spiritual self (*áfurugu*, *iuáni*), and the social self – that is the individual located in a complex matrix of kin and non-kin relations – with the environment, both natural and cultural (or social, spiritual, and culturally modified) that is believed to be the source of illness.

But each individual self makes certain moral and behavioral decisions which may have consequences for the state of health as well. Thus, there is a moral component of self which is part of this set of interactions. Moreover, the physical body is itself the cause of some illnesses, that is, the physical body is imperfect and is said to possess inherent defects or characteristics which may be expressed as the signs and events which are constituents of the illness process or may affect the individual's response to physical and emotional stress. Multiple causation is not only a possibility, but a central feature of the Garifuna medical model.

Taylor, in his now classic ethnography of the Garinagu (1951), identified four categories of causal agents or factors recognized to result in illness. Sickness, he said,

> ...is attributable to: 1. neglect of the ancestral dead; 2. the maleficent attention of other spirits, probably–though not necessarily–brought about by the breaking of some taboo; 3. abįąragole, under which term are classed together both sorcery and poisoning; and 4. purely physical causes such as accidents or snake bite. However, many cases which would appear to belong to the fourth class are put down to the machination of ill-disposed persons, who may, for example, use sorcery to set a snake in one's path (1951:96).

This categorization, however, ignores those illnesses which are said to result from the individual's interactions with his natural environment – and it is to this category that most illnesses are now assigned. Garifuna people do not live in a world which they perceive as noticeably dangerous or unpredictable, provided one follows certain rules of behavior and moral precepts. The vast majority of illnesses are said to be *lisándi ubáo*, "sicknesses of the world" or "of the land."

Taylor's classification does not address the issue of personal responsibility; yet, the common assignment of responsibility for illness to the afflicted individual or to other members of the household, past and present, is, in my opinion, a striking feature of Garifuna beliefs concerning illness causation. In a society which historically appears to have had few overriding legal or political sanctions against inappropriate behavior, the models which govern interpretations of the signs of illness and the causes of death have functioned to assure the maintenance of proper relationships and correct personal actions. The *gubída* (ancestral spirits) institute clear sanctions against disrespectful behavior toward the dead. Certain spirits serve to provide temptations and test the strength of individuals, often with the most severe consequences for those who do not behave in socially and morally appropriate ways. Some spirits are regarded as exceedingly dangerous, but correct actions generally assure their impotence or temper any interactions. There are, as well, those spirits whose punishment is light, perhaps because the offending behavior is not regarded as serious. *Súsia*, for example, appears to drunken men in the form of a beautiful woman and leads them "into the bush" with the promise of love-making, where they will awake in the morning, often to find themselves sleeping on a grave in the cemetery.

There are, finally, the sanctions which men may impose upon one another through recourse to the supernatural. While individuals may direct *obeah* or *abiñariguile* against others because of jealousy or out of spite, and victims describe themselves as innocent of wrongdoing, *obeah* is often defined by the community as justifiable punishment instituted by a previous "victim" against the perpetrator of some anti-social action. The threat of *idáhadu* (the words of others, "mouth water") in theory functions to assure proper personal relationships and to inhibit careless talk. But these various spiritual and supernatural causes are, in fact, only infrequently mentioned as the cause of specific illness. That they appear often in the case studies (Chapter VII) is directly related to the nature of the cases chosen for study. These 'causal agents', dramatic as they are, exist largely as potential explanations, to be exploited when other interpretive solutions fail to create the desired result.

It is possible that with the increasing transferrence of responsibility for control over the behavior of individuals to various governmental institutions, the need to explain illness in terms of "uncommon" causes has diminished, with the subsequent movement of an increasing range of illnesses to the category of *lisándi ubáo*. However, it appears equally probable that the tendency to assign responsibility for illness to the afflicted person or to a member of the family is a practice of ancient origin which assured some degree of individual conformity to or acceptance of major cultural themes.

The focus in much of the discussion to follow is on concepts of causation rather than on the meanings assigned specific signs. The individual sign, in fact, remains largely 'meaningless', that is, devoid of useful information until linked with an interpretant. In the process of eliciting information from bush doctors, I found that Garifuna healers often disagreed on the signification of any given sign or syndrome. The diversity of opinion was, in part, the result of the fact that the signs which were presented were devoid of any personal or social context. It was also illustrative of the autonomy of individual healers. As shown in the case studies, context is critical in the determination of signification. Further, significations, once assigned, remain susceptible to negotiation. Meanings evolve; they are not inherent to the sign. Hence, the sign alone cannot be the center of our investigations.

NOTES

1. Island Carib males who migrated from South America took Igneri wives. The women maintained elements of the Igneri language which they passed on to their daughters. Today, there are few remnants of these linguistic distinctions, but in a few cases words utilized by females are different from those utilized by males to refer to the same thing, event, or person.
2. "Garifuna households" refers to households in which there was no evidence of inter-ethnic mating and no individuals in residence who did not define themselves as Garinagu.
3. Female headed households are those in which no adult male was present, excepting the son(s) of the woman. In all cases, it was evident that the residence was regarded as that of the woman and that the sons were not providing significant support to the household.
4. I utilize Gonzalez' definition of the household:
   ... the group of people who live under one roof, who eat and sleep together and who cooperate daily for the benefit of all. A household may derive nearly all its financial support from non-members, but economic cooperation of some sort is characteristic of the group (1979:45).
5. *Nungua* translates as "myself." The term *ugúbi* is also used.

CHAPTER 5

The Model of Cause and Effect Relationships

Each interpretant is, or provokes, a response; some (it might be argued that all) of these responses constitute the therapeutic process. The social and technological intervention in the chain of signs which constitute or imply an illness process follows from or is greatly influenced by the assignment of signs to a particular etiological domain. Since signs assume 'meaning' according to this assignment, which is, in turn, affected by the total context in which the signs occur, the concern here must be with defining and delimiting those domains. What Comaroff has said of the Tswana with regard to the 'meaning' of signs is equally true for the Garinagu:

> ...no fixed relationship existed between specific causes and symptoms, and explanatory principles, such as 'sorcery' could be applied to what appear to the observer to be a variety of physical signs, just as seemingly *similar* signs were attributable to a range of potential causes. Indeed, our own logical distinction between 'cause' and 'symptom' is not reflected in Tswana epistemology, where symptoms were perceived as the tangible dimensions of causes and were given meaning by the dominant metaphor of causality (1981:371).

Out of the total set of "diagnostic" or "etiologic" categories generated in discussions with Garifuna healers and patients, there emerge four broad categories of illness causation. Signs are, therefore, not necessarily indeterminant, but to be interpreted according to the category of causation to which they are assigned. Assignment to a category (or conceptual domain; see Dominick 1980; Staiano 1981) is determined only in part by the nature or characteristics of the sign. Each conceptual domain is derived from or dependent upon a specific set of self-object, self-self, self-other, or self-spirit interactions; at least two domains contain both natural and "uncommon" illness and each is affected by decisions made by both the moral and social selves.

The four sets of interactions which form the logical basis of the four domains of illness causation could be depicted schematically as an ever widening set of concentric circles, moving from the interaction of the various components of the body and self at the center, to the relationship between the individual or the social collectivity and spiritual beings at the periphery.

Causation is defined here in terms of the nature of the interactions, and the relationship of the body (*ugubu*) or self (*nungua*) to other elements or actors in the interaction. Organisms, persons, natural elements, spirits, and so on, are not causal agents per se. Rather, illness is seen as the result of *interactions* between these 'agents' and the body/self. The Garifuna medical model, in this respect, exceeds in sophistication the modern "scientific" model of illness causation.

The causal/conceptual domains appear to have little correspondence to a taxonomy of illness terms which might be generated from an analysis of Garifuna lexical items. Any taxonomy constructed on the basis of a lexicon alone would have produced an "explanatory model" (Kleinman 1981) composed of names for symptoms, syndromes or diagnostic labels, and causes, without regard for the logical distinctions among them. The taxonomic approach may be valid under certain conditions and useful in the generation of ethnomedical concepts, but it fails both to account for the dynamic nature of interpretation and to demonstrate the fact that the meanings of signs and symptoms are negotiable and context sensitive.

Each of these domains provides to the individual and to those who may participate in some manner in the social event of illness, an array of "cognitive resources" (Locker 1981) which permits sense to be made of suffering. Once signs are allocated to one particular domain, the therapeutic alternatives are limited, though not necessarily determined. Where signs are non-specific and conceivably referable to more that one domain, the therapy itself may become one method whereby the correct cause is determined. That is, a successful therapy utilized experimentally may point to the inclusion of signs within one domain rather than another when the therapy normally indicated by that domain is the "successful" therapy. Repeated failures to achieve a cure with what is, in theory, an appropriate therapy, may lead to the reassignment of signs to other domains or the search for a prior *object*.

Body-Self Interactions and Models of Organic Interdependence

The first of these conceptual domains is generally not described in the literature and is the most difficult to isolate. This causal domain evolves out of Garifuna notions concerning the nature of the human organism, the interaction of body systems or components, and the relationship of the moral and social self to the physical body. Several principles emerge from an analysis of all cause and effect relations which are assigned to this domain:

1. Individuals are believed to exhibit a range of variation in terms of biological and emotional or psychological characteristics. Such variation is normal. Individuals thus have different capacities and respond differently to various stresses.
2. In all individuals, internal regulatory mechanisms are susceptible to failure. The human body is imperfect and therefore unpredictable (though predictability is, in general, an important feature of Garifuna explanatory paradigms as we shall see). Closely related to this is the tenet that:

3. Some illnesses arise spontaneously, without prior or known cause. The body is thus the source and cause of some of its own disorders.
4. Individuals may be born with abnormal or limiting conditions. Some of these are attributable to actions of the mother and/or the father prior to the birth of the individual. Other illnesses are said to be inherited, though the genetic basis of inheritance is not understood. Certain illnesses, defined as "inherited" or "familial" further demonstrate the dependence of individuals on other 'selves' and the links between generations. These linkages, and especially the dependence of each generation on the one preceding, are further emphasized in prescribed and proscribed behaviors for the parents-to-be and the parents of newborn infants.
5. Some illnesses are present from birth, but generally manifested later in life. Such illnesses are sometimes referred to as "inborn." Inborn illnesses are not necessarily identified as inherited illnesses nor are they always traced to some failure on the part of the parents or to any other agent.
6. Some illnesses may arise as the result of 'mechanical' failures; these are generally explained in terms of pressures exerted by one organ upon another and the emphasis is thus on the integration and interdependence of organs or organic systems.
7. Human sexuality leads to a propensity to certain illnesses. Sexual roles are, therefore, emphasized in the interpretation of some illnesses. Males encounter few problems as a result of male sexuality though certain herbal 'remedies' are used to improve sexual performance which is occasionally said to suffer for any of several reasons. It is the females who endure the greatest suffering as a result of their sexuality. Such "illnesses" or dysfunctions as arise from sexual functions are granted less importance among the Garinagu than among the Spanish and East Indians among whom the maintenance of a nuclear family household and a monogamous sexual relationship (at least for the females) is given greater emphasis. That is, the suggestion here is that the more confining the female role, the greater the tendency for females to express illnesses or disorders in terms of their sexuality and the limits that places upon them.
8. The moral and social components of self may cause an individual to take actions which adversely affect the physical body. The Garinagu place greater emphasis on preventive behaviors and therapies than any other group and exhibit a greater tendency to place responsibility for illness with the afflicted individual. It is thus the failure of the "self", or rather, the controlling, conscious, decision-making component of the self, to properly manage various natural, social, and supernatural interactions, which results in much illness. The decision-making component of self may choose actions in direct contradition to basic bodily requirements for the maintenance of health.
9. Garifuna men and women rarely attribute illness to old age; they continue to work well into their seventies or eighties if work is available. When illness appears in the elderly, the reference is generally to overwork, previous injuries, or dissolute behavior rather than to old age.

Notions of cause and effect derived from the above principles are commonly expressed in discussions of illness. For example, several characteristics simply attributed to human variability were said to cause physical or emotional disorders or possess the potential to do so. Individuals were described by one bush doctor as born with one of two kinds of "flesh" (*huguru*; the same term is used to refer to "beef steak"; the term for skin is distinct: *urau*). Those with "thick" flesh are said to have more heat in their bodies. Individuals with "free" flesh, on the other hand, were said to be more likely to feel pain with the movement of the moon if they had previously undergone surgery.

Individuals are believed to differ in terms of the weight of their soul or *áfurugu*. According to one bush doctor, the weight of an infant's *áfurugu* is determined during the mother's pregancy. Poor nutrition and a failure to seek appropriate care could result in a light *áfurugu* in the newborn. Others simply attributed differences in the *áfurugu* to human variation. Men were said to be as likely as women to possess "light" souls. An individual whose soul or spirit is light is more likely to be affected by evil spirits or by the *gubída* and less likely to be able to resist *obeah*. "Persons with heavy souls", it was said, "can drive off spirits." Coehlo describes a similar belief for the Houduran Garinagu:

> Those gifted with a "heavy" *áfurugu* who are less exposed to spiritual danger, may abandon themselves to dream experiences, which are valued by the Black Carib as a source of prophetic knowledge and a means of communicating with the dead, through which the ancestors make their will known to their descendants, indicating processes of obtaining large catches of fish, or revealing the secret designs of enemies, or the perils that must be faced by those who embark upon long journeys (1955:139).

In what may be a related notion, it was said that "craziness" is more likely to occur in individuals whose "nerves" are "tender" or "weak."

Emotional stress which leads to psychotic reactions ("craziness" or "uncontrollable behavior") in some will not produce the same effect in others because it is believed individuals inherently possess different capacities to cope with such stress.

One bush doctor stated that a number of illnesses are "inborn." That is, whether they appear at birth or later in life, their appearance is inevitable. Inborn illnesses were sometimes equated with incurable illnesses and their failure "to cure" was explained in terms of their cause. Asthma, diabetes, and cancer were said by this healer to be "inborn", though in this assessment he differed from the majority of persons with whom I discussed illness. Certain illness events – heart attack and cancer among them – are relatively unknown in the Toledo District and clear and consistent explanations of cause have not yet evolved. Most claimed simply that they did not know the cause of cancer.

Fits (*attacki, adérihani, ówehani*) were also said by one informant to be "inborn." If the mother, this healer stated, is treated badly by the father, when the child is born, "it will get the worriedness of the mother" and this will cause the infant to suffer from fits or to become crazy. This same individual described venereal disease as a "disease inside you are born with" though he believed that it could be caused by "heat and cold" as well. He had rejected the more commonly held notion that venereal diseases is caused by contact between a man and a woman.

The majority of individuals hold the belief that asthma is the result of the infant's drinking of amniotic fluid at the time of birth, though one prominent healer stated that asthma was caused by the bites of mosquitoes and sandflies, but added that some believe it comes from using unclean water for bathing, drinking, and washing clothes. If not treated very early, asthma is said to be incurable. Another illness, *costipo* or *costipao* is believed by some to result from the failure to remove fluid from the infant's nose at birth. If it is not "fought" when the infant is young, *costipo* will cause death. It is also said to affect the brain and to make one "crazy." Such illness might well be referred to the domain of relations labeled "interactions with the environment" (See following section); yet, they are thought to result from the failure of the body to properly regulate such interactions. They are illustrative of the Garifuna emphasis on the susceptibility of the infant, on the responsibility of parents, on the importance of preventive therapies, and on concepts of multiple causation.

The term "inheritance" refers to processes which result from the trauma of birth, to the interaction between mother and infant prior to birth, and to physical, behavioral and physical characteristics possessed by a parent and passed on to a child. Illnesses which were reported by Garifuna informants to be inherited included "fits" ("I believe it to be from inheritance; foam comes up and chokes the baby" [reference is to the trauma of birth]); malaria (said to pass from parent to child); diabetes ("It runs in the family") syphilis ("It can be inherited and can leave children crippled or blind"); lack of development (see Lambey case study; the fetus may be small if the mother is small. "He takes after his mother; she is small"), and hernia.

Inherent characteristics manifested in a child or adult may be referred to a similar characteristic in one or both parents, but theories of recessive and dominant genes and the concept of a "genetic" illness are not known. The appearance of a hernia in a child, for example, "may come from the father." One woman stated that "something your mother or father do, you will do too. If your mother has a hernia, you will have a hernia; if your mother is a thief, you will be a thief too." A prominent bush doctor, when asked about the term "inborn", responded that "you are born with certain characteristics or habits which may result in drinking, smoking, stealing, killing, fighting, causing trouble, or many other unusual things."

The body according to one elderly midwife, who was described as "gifted" (i.e., assisted by spirits) is composed of three elements in varying proportions.

> Our body must have wind and water and blood. These three come together and form you. Some people have too much wind. It is mostly in the stomach. That's where the main pulse is.

The excess of wind may cause a variety of problems; the specific problem depends on the location of the wind. For example, excess wind in the head can cause headaches. This healer also stated that physical characteristics (or the lack of them) may make the individual susceptible to certain illnesses.

> The cause of tuberculosis is a cough. If you don't care for yourself, that cough will drop

lower to the area around the sternum. If you have no bump on the sternum you are prone to develp tuberculosis.

Statements concerning mechanical causes of disorders included: "Your own weight presses on you when you lie down at night" (said to be one cause of chest pain). "The air in your stomach walks around on your chest until it reaches your heart" (also said to be a cause of chest pain). "Blood leaves the womb as you get older and gets solid" (resulting in pain in the lower adomen, commonly referred to as the "stomach" [*uragai*]). "The bones in your chest may sink in and give you a cough." "The top of the baby's head falls in from straining while sucking" (said to be a cause of mole drop [sunken fontanelle which often accompanies severe dehydration in young infants]). "The heart doesn't pump properly" (one cause of "fits" and "fainting").

"Female sexuality" as a component in models of health and illness is pervasive; it is found in the medical models of every ethnic group in the community. Among the Garinagu, illnesses identified with female sexuality generally reference either pregnancy or menstruation. Women were said to have a "badness" inside of them after the birth of a child; it was thought to be necessary to utilize herbal teas to rid the new mother of this. Cold or wind in the ovaries resulted from "walking around after the birth of a baby." A midwife stated that a woman may develop a "sore" inside following the birth of an infant and that the sore may not heal without appropriate treatment. It was noted that women sometimes had convulsions or "fits" when they were pregnant. In some cases this was attributed to "trouble with the kidneys", but this "trouble" was not referred to any prior cause other than the woman's pregnancy. For the most part it was assumed that pregnancies would proceed in a normal manner, provided that the mother-to-be looked after herself properly.

Pain in the abdomen was said to occur when the womb was either too high or too low or when the ovaries became twisted. Pain in the legs was believed to result from the "poor condition of the vein which passes through the abdomen." This, in turn, was attributed to the position of the womb. A midwife told me that the "belly pulse" sometimes swells and prevents a woman having a baby. Pain in the lower abdomen was said to occur in women prior to their periods because the womb was stretched. It was also said to occur in women as the result of the change of life. The blood, in this case, was said to leave the womb and to "clot down" or become solid.

The period during birth and the days and weeks following are regarded as somewhat dangerous periods for both the mother and infant, though not all women adhered to any special practices or regarded this as a period of greater susceptibility. Proscribed and prescribed behaviors may govern the mother's activity following the birth (see Sentino case study, which reports an illness caused by the failure to observe these rules).

As stated earlier, men and women are generally expected to establish sexual relations relatively early in their lives and usually produce children shortly after. Men are rarely if ever criticized for "excessive" sexual behaviors, and assumed or proffered levels of performance are one determinant of a male's status. Virginity is not a highly valued trait among young Garifuna women, which is not to say that promiscuous behavior on their part is condoned. It is not. Yet it is expected that women will "want" or desire men and this is considered normal for all females. While Garifuna females are often extremely independent, Garifuna men seem not to believe that women can live happily without male companionship. A male healer stated that some young men and women are afflicted by a "double nature." "That nature run into the head and make them crazy." In women, this double nature was manifested in a desire both to engage in sexual intercourse and to maintain chastity. "Certain young ladies, they may want to hold themselves, but they want a man; this might drive her crazy."

In general, a decline in sexual performance, especially among men, was not considered normal. Some of the local Creole and Garifuna bars were said to keep on hand a supply of rum in which had been placed a certain amount of "medicine" known as *gangwao*. *Gangwao*, the name of the plant from which the medicine is obtained, was said to greatly increase sexual desire and sexual performance. Some women also admitted to its use (with similar results, I was told), though for the most part, jokes about use of *gangwao* made reference to men and not to women. Those who knew the location and proper procedure for harvesting *gangwao* were said to have a valuable skill indeed.

In general, illnesses are not thought to be a necessary part of the aging process, though a general decline in energy and strength is accepted. One Garifuna man of seventy-five with whom I often spoke was a teacher in one of the remote Kekchi villages. At an age when most individuals in the States have settled into the routines of retirement, he twice a year packed up his belongings and hiked some fifteen miles over jungle trails to the village where he taught. He returned to his home in Punta Gorda during school vacations in like manner. A Garifuna man of seventy-three, totally blind and almost deaf, reported that his physical state had been affected in recent years by his sexual excesses. In a consultation with a *búiai* located in Guatemala, he was advised by the *búiai's hiúruha* (spirit guides) that he should limit his sexual encounters to once a week if he expected his physical condition not to worsen. "This every other day stuff has got to stop" he was warned by the *hiúruha*. He was also told to send his female companion away. He claimed he could not bring himself to part with her. He believed the spirits had taken care of the matter because one day she left and never returned.

Illness is often attributed to personal failures and moral defects. Sickness was said by one individual to occur on occasion to stop actions which were "wrong." One healer reported that "when the patient is evil, his evilness works against him." The bush doctor stated that he instructed such patients in the ways in which they must change their behavior in order to help the cure. Another informant stated that an individual's sickness could result from treating someone else badly.

If a man treats his wife bad, he punishes himself too, and it reacts on him. I don't think God would cause illness as punishment. God made the good and the bad. If you want to do somebody bad you have the will to do it, but it will cause your own punishment.

Another expressed the same notion in somewhat different terms: "If you do anything wrong that hurts anyone it will turn against you." A second bush doctor reported that "when people wish bad to others, their own words will turn on them." When such persons come to him for treatment, he refuses to provide a cure. "They have to stop thinking that way before they can be cured", he explains.

There were sometimes conflicting views regarding the individual's responsibility for his own illness. However, most illnesses are ultimately attributed to carelessness or neglectful behavior which are recognized as contributing *objects* in the progressing triadic sign relationship. Even the illnesses of children were often said to be a result of the negligence of the parent(s). Nevertheless, "carelessness" was but one motivating event in an etiological chain containing causal factors from one or more of the four conceptual domains.

While unavoidable physical and emotional stress were also factors in illness (see below), individuals were often thought to abuse their bodies to the ultimate detriment of their physical (and moral) state (see Arzu case study). The section to follow focuses on the interaction of the individual and the natural and culturally modified environment, but personal responsibility often functions as an unstated cause in what are commonly multicausal explanations.

Interactions with the Natural and Culturally Modified Environment

The second set of cause-effect relations incorporates Garifuna beliefs concerning interactions between the physical body (*ugúbu*) and the natural or culturally modified world in which individuals live and act. The following principles define this domain.

1. 'Exposure' to a variety of natural stimuli is one of the chief threats to good health. The concept of 'exposure' implies some stressful contrast between the body in its particular state at a particular moment in time and the natural or culturally modified environment as encountered at that moment.
2. In like manner, the use and abuse of food and drink are thought to be a frequent source of illness. As is the case with illnesses which result from 'exposure , individuals

must often assume personal responsibility for their physical state.

3. In general, the notion of "intrusion" of a foreign or unnatural object into the body is not utilized to account for illness. Specifically, I refer to two beliefs which are common components of other medical models: (a) the belief that illnesses may be caused by the introduction of an object or organism or substance through supernatural means, as is common to the medical models of many North American Indian and West African populations, and (b) the germ theory of illness which is the basis of biomedical models. Two exceptions to this must be noted. First, as stated above, both food and drink if abused or inappropriate may lead to illness; these must obviously enter the body in order to have such an effect. Second, poisons or magical potions may be introduced into the body by someone who wishes harm to the individual or to control some aspect of the victim's behavior. Such intentional actions are assigned to the third conceptual domain.
4. Mechanical causes are assigned to this domain if the causal 'agent' is external to the body. Thus, injuries are placed within this domain and are regarded as a natural outcome of self-environment interactions, unless another cause such as *obeah* or *abiñaraguile* is suspected. In the great majority of cases, no such personal or supernatural causation is imputed.
5. Overwork or physical stress endured in youth may result in disorders in later years. Physical stress, including injuries, may result in disorders in which cause and effect are separated in time and in which the injured or affected organs may not be the organs which exhibit the effect.
6. Interactions with the enviroment expose one to a variety of potentially dangerous spirits. In certain respects, these are regarded as a part of the natural order of things. They are dangerous for the most part only if one does not take preventive actions or appropriately mediate the interaction. The illness in infants which is attributed to or referred to as *húmo* thus may sometimes be treated by 'natural' means. Cases which do not respond may be taken to the *buiái* who uses supernatural or spiritual means to diagnose and intervene. In some cases, *húmo* is defined as a natural or common illness (*lisándi ubáo*) and yet treated with both natural and spiritual therapies simultaneously. While certain 'spirit' caused illnesses may be regarded by the Garinagu as essentially 'natural' in origin, all 'spirit' caused illness have been referred to the fourth conceptual domain.

Examples of cause and effect relationships referrable to this domain are numerous and diverse. 'Exposure' is perhaps the most commonly employed of all explanations. "Walking at night without a hat", "getting out of bed suddenly in the morning and peeping out", getting wet without drying one's head, the accumulation of excessive heat in the head, "being caught in the rain when there is heat in the body", and general 'exposure' are all identified as causes of a "fresh cold." "Constant wetting of the feet or head" can result in an "inside cold"; exposure to heat or a build-up of heat in the body with subsequent exposure to cold may lead to "pain in the bones"; lengthy exposure to heat from a stove may causes sores on the body, the excess heat of the body being released through the lesions, or may otherwise affect the blood adversely. Sores were also said to result from too much heat and cold in the body simultaneously, in which case the blood "mixes with water" and sores develop. The bites of insects may also cause sores. "Traveling across a river or creek under a hot sun" may result in "pain when urinating"; taking off one's shoes and putting the feet on a damp floor may also cause pain during urination. Heat may cause a headache or make "the pressure" worse or lead to loose stools. Exposure to a "sudden dew" results in a "shock to the body" which may, in turn, cause a stroke. The contrast of heat and cold combined with "the wearing of dirty clothers" was said by one woman (a hospital nurse and midwife) to cause measles. To "take out the washing and then do the ironing" will result in "trembling in the body" if the individual is old. "Fever" may result from "heat and cold" during the rainy season. Baking bread can cause pain in the fingers if one submerges the hand in water while baking. Heat and cold in the blood simultaneously may lead to "pressure." The contrast of heat and cold are also said to cause backache, tuberculosis, venereal disease and *costipo*. The Maya are said to catch cold from the floor. "They don't eat well enough to assist the blood", explained one woman, "and they don't have enough blood." Cramps in females are associated with menstrual flow, but are also said to be affected "by the tide." Heat may develop in the *ariunun*, which was said to be located under the navel. It "sucks your blood", and "swells you." This is described as a "black thing" which can prevent women from having babies unless the body was rid of it, according to a local male healer "Bad air", such as was said to be found commonly in the States, is identified as an additional source of illness. Some illnesses were said to occur more frequently in either the dry or the wet season, though some additional environmental factor (e.g., dust, heat, wet) was often cited as the principal cause. Mumps is said to be a "seasonal" illness, while measles is more commonly attributed to "heat and cold." Food and drink, which occur both in a natural and culturally modified form, may cause illness, though, in general, such illnesses are preventable. "Eating contrary to one's stomach" was said to cause loose stools; eating tainted food or drinking bad water might result in vomiting, diarrhea and fever; food which contains insects such as roaches or ants may cause illness; drinking on an empty stomach will cause liver damage; eating too much cold food can result in an upset stomach or other sickness, especially in babies. Coca Cola was said to contain acid and to work adversely on the kidneys and liver. Poor blood may be caused by drinking too much, by eating dry bread and then drinking a beverage, but not eating sufficiently, or by eating mud which was said to "suck the blood." "Biliousness", described by one individual as "like a boil inside" was caused either by eating improperly or by consuming too much alcohol. Eating something "which doesn't agree with the blood" can lead to serious illness. "Not eating sufficiently can result in either "pain in the stomach" or "fainting." Eating beef, pork, oil, lard, greasy foods, or salt are all said to result in or exacerbate high blood pressure. "Too much fresh food" (defined as "starchy") was said to have the same effect. Eating too much sugar or too much salt or "liking sweets too much" was thought to lead to diabetes, though one healer protested that sugar dissolved itself in the bood and could not reconstitute itself as sugar. The cause of diabetes (sugar in the blood), he stated, must, therefore, lie elsewhere.

"Pain when urinating" could be caused by eating too much pepper. A nursing baby might suffer from *impacho* ("swelling of the belly") if the mother eats something which "doesn't agree with the baby." Medicine, logically enough, is given to the mother rather than to the infant. There were occasional food restrictions imposed on pregnant and nursing mothers for the sake of the baby's health. For example, several individuals stated that too much salt was not good for a pregnant woman while others expressed the belief that certain types of fish or shellfish were bad for expectant females. After a baby is born, some claimed, it was bad to eat after three P.M. If one eats after that hour the baby will develop "puff belly." One woman with a newborn infant said that some foods are too heavy for mothers of infants, but if beans and garlic are eaten by the mother, the child will not develop *impacho*.

Certain interactions with the environment result in injuries which are generally regarded as "natural." Only occasionally is supernatural or personal interference suspected. A friend who injured his leg playing soccer was told by a local healer that the pain and swelling was a result of the "veins being twisted against one another." A compress of leaves was applied and the leg wrapped with bandages. Injuries which initially appear inconsequential may lead to more serious problems at a later time, at which point the linkage between cause and effect may be unclear, at least to the biomedical practitioner. Some believe that cancer is caused by an injury which results in a bruise that fails to heal. A childhood fall or "knock", improperly treated, might manifest itself as cancer in adulthood. One woman attributed her heart trouble to a harpoon wound suffered many years earlier. The injury had been to her leg. Though she had apparently fully recovered from the wound, the doctor had warned her that "it would rest on my body some day." In the same manner, physical abuse of the body during youth was said to manifest itself in a variety of disorders in later years. Any type of physical stress might result in illness. Disorders attributed to physical stress included venereal disease ("your foot bucks something and it affects your whole body"), cancer (see above), inability to sleep ("body tense from too much work") headache across the temples ("from straining the eyes") hernia ("from hard work"), headache ("from bending over too much") and general debility ("I worked very hard when I was young and once I fell from a tree").

Insect bites are recognized to cause a localized reaction and occasionally to result in sores. Few take measures to prevent insect bites and for the most part insects are not regarded as dangerous. Many accept the biomedically generated notion that malaria is caused by the bite of a mosquito; however, if there is understanding of the disease organism-vector-human host relationship it was never mentioned. One woman expressed the idea that the mosquito caused malaria by "sucking the blood", while a bush doctor suggested that mosquitoes, botlass flies, or sandflies will leave a trace of blood from someone else or from a snake or other animal "and that is one cause of malaria."

No one at any time expressed concern about "germs." The idea of contagion (see below) does not involve the transfer of such foreign organisms. It was stated by two individuals that there might be "bugs" in your food if it was not properly prepared and the introduction of such "bugs" into the stomach might cause pain in the abdomen, but, otherwise, no reference to "bugs" or "germs" was made.

Interaction of the Body/Self with Other Selves

Every Garinfuna individual is a social being entwined in a complex matrix of social and kin relationships. He or she interacts on a daily basis with other social selves, most of whom are Garifuna. The nature of these interactions determines, in part, the health or absence of health of any Garifuna adult. Whilė the presence of a nuclear family is hardly critical to the survival of the Garinagu as a social collectivity, the presence of other Garinagu is essential to both the survival of the collectivity and the individual Garifuna "self."

> On a quiet, restful afternoon when few people are around, and hence little noise is to be heard, one is likely to hear the remark, *hirúgati*, which comes from the root *hiru* - meaning 'sad.' In other words, it is sad when there are not a lot of people around; to be alone, for the Carib, is tantamount to being sad (Hadel 1972:86).

"It is unthinkable for a Carib to be perfectly contented away from his family", Hadel continues. Yet trust of one's fellow Garinagu is not a given, and individuals often express suspicion of one another's actions and motives. "And so, we have the enigmatic situation of a people who are unable to work together and unwilling to work apart" (*Ibid.*:87). This ambiguous stance towards one's fellow man is illustrated in this verse:

> What am I going to do to please
> My fellow Caribs?
> Even when you are on good terms with them,
> They always have something to say against you.
> I will not envy a man for what he has got, my friends,
> I'll just try hard (*Ibid.*:199).

Thus, interaction with other Garifuna individuals, and, in particular with the members of one's extended family, is the *sine non qua* of Garifuna social existence. Yet, it is also the source of disorder and such disorder is often manifested as illness.

The principles which define this domain are as follows:

1. Illness may pass from one person to another as the result of physical contact or proximity, though proximity may not always be necessary.
2. Emotional stress, caused by failed or stressful interactions with other individuals, can affect physical and mental states.

3. Just as interactions with others are often the source of emotional and physical problems, so, too, is the lack of interaction a cause of such problems.
4. Actions of others may inadvertantly or unintentionally bring harm to someone.
5. Witchcraft (*obeah*, *abiñaraguile*) or magic may be used to influence the behavior of another individual or to bring misfortune, illness, and death. Such actions are always intentional. Concommitantly, *obeah* may be turned against the initial user.

Among those illnesses which were said to pass from one person to another as a result of proximity or physical contact were measles, mumps, chicken pox, *costipo*, and venereal disease, though each was assigned to other domains by different informants. One woman accounted for the apparent increase in cases of "high blood pressure" through reference to contagion. "They say it isn't catching", she explained, "but everybody is getting it." Another remarked that diabetes could be contracted by "sleeping with someone who has it", or by being close to that individual. Malaria was also said by some to pass from one individual to another, as was tuberculosis. One healer noted "when you talk to someone and a breeze passes between you, tuberculosis passes in the wind." It can travel long distances, he explained further. "When a volcano erupted in Guatemala, many people here developed tuberculosis." Another healer stated that when individuals develop cancer they must be isolated from the rest of their family because it can pass to other members of the household.

Of an entirely different order, but, nevertheless, the outcome of social interactions, are those misfortunes which come about as the result of contact with someone who has "bearsy-bugs." "Bearsy-bugs", the term used by several individuals in Punta Gorda, are the 'Belzing-bugs' or *ogoreu*[1] referred to by Taylor (1951) and Coehlo (1955). Individuals in Punta Gorda also used the term *uguri*. Bearsy-bugs or *uguri* are not insects, but animals which are "attached" to and travel with certain individuals. Only women are afflicted and, according to Coehlo, they are transmitted matrilineally. They may change form, but always appear (when they are visible) as animals. Coehlo notes that among the Honduran Garinagu their most common form is said to be that of a blue lizard. They may bring sickness and death to those with whom their owner associates and no woman wishes to gain the reputation of having acquired an *uguri*. They may also harm their owners, but often function as 'protecters', though their protection may be undesired. One healer explained that all *uguri* are male and may easily be provoked into jealousy. "If a man is a lover of a woman who has a *bearsy-bug* his belly may swell if the *bearsy-bug* doesn't like him", I was told by another. The *uguri* may drive away possible lovers or fetch one back if the woman desires. Two brief stories serve to illustrate the power of the *uguri* in matters of love.

A woman with a *bearsy-bug* was going with a Creole man. The man left her and did not intend to return, but the *bearsy-bug* went and brought him back.

One individual offered the name of a woman said to have a *bearsy-bug*. Another woman interjected that this particular woman had had the same lover for some time. "Well, that's because the *bearsy-bug* likes him," the first woman explained.

Another woman told me she knew of two women who had *uguri*. She reported she was always polite but never stopped to engage in conversation with them. "You can hail them, but don't accept food from them." It was said to be best to avoid them altogether.

Coehlo's account of *ogoreu* describes them as "malignant supernatural beings" more feared tham *umeu* [*húmo*] (1955:152).

When neglected, they provoke domestic accidents and "connect themselves" with girls just like *gubída* do at a *dogo* [*dugu*] ceremony; moreover, one of them may kill the first born of a family, and, if not "restrained" by the *búiai*, will go on provoking stillbirths and death of infants until the extinction of the line. One of the reasons given for breaking a union is when a man discovers that his mate has an *ogoreu* attached to her (1955:152).

One healer described *uguri* as "evil wandering spirits which work on the shadow" or *iaua*. "Once it works on the *iaua*, you are gone. You can't get over that. The belly grows until you die. You can't sleep when one is around." A Garifuna female stated that "possession by animals" was "more common in Stann Creek." The Garinagu of Stann Creek are thought by many Garinagu to be more traditional in their beliefs and practices than those of Punta Gorda. This woman also said that her sister had been "possessed" by such an animal (*uguri*) and had died as a result. "These animals can kill you or they can kill others. They possess you and may kill you then leave." The "cure", according to this woman, was relatively simply. "You can get rid of them by taking off your old clothes, walking some distance naked, then putting on new clothes." Other individuals in Punta Gorda stated that the lover of a woman afflicted by an *uguri* could escape its influence by leaving behind all his clothes and walking away from the woman's house naked, essentially the same treatment suggested by the individual mentioned above for riding the "possessed" woman. Only by leaving naked is the *uguri* denied any means of tracking the unfortunate lover.

Coehlo suggests the process of riding oneself of an *uguri* (*ogoreu*) is more difficult:

The case is not always desperate, however, for an experienced religious practitioner knows how to drag the pernicious spirit to a place far away, and keep it permanetly there so that it cannot come back to the afflicted woman (*Ibid* :152-3).

A bush doctor with whom I spoke told me he had rid a house of an *uguri* and that the process was very difficult and very costly because of the time involved.

It is unclear what specific function, in anthropological terms, the *bearsy-bug* serves. It may, on the one hand, provide an explanation of sterility or stillbirths, a relatively serious occurrence in a society in which the perpetuation of the family and the production of children is so highly valued. It should be noted that such a cause- effect relationship places the responsibility for sterility or lack of fecundity on the female. One woman stated that women with *bearsy-bugs* were identifiable by their behavior. Thus, attributions of possession by a *bearsy-bug* may serve to explain socially inappropriate behavior or communicative techniques and permit individuals to reduce, limit, or avoid interactions with these women.

Garifuna individuals believe that interactions with other individuals are a common source of emotional stress and that emotional stress is one cause or contributing etiological event in physical and psychological disorders. Illness or disorders which were said to result included "fits", "craziness", "heart trouble", "palpitations", "stroke", "hemorrhage", "pain in the stomach", and "headache." Most recognized that stress can adversely affect already existing conditions. Specific emotional states that result in illness were described as follows. The term "vexation" (*higániti*) implies anger, worry, and anxiety. Statements specifying the relation between "vexation" and illness included:

When the mind is vexed, you start to feel bad. Maybe you don't live a good life at home. You are going to worry about why your life isn't happy. Your mind is not contented. If you put if to your heart and soul it can lead to craziness and many other things.

What is unpleasing to the sight or ears will affect the nerves. The nervous system gets irritated. Many sicknesses will descend from this and from ill feelings. I had a female companion in the States. I believe she was driving me into psychological insanity with her actions. I started trembling, got nervous, and suffered from loose bowels and palpitations.

A man I knew found his wife in bed with another man. It caused the man to strain his brain and he went crazy and is still crazy.

The heart is bothered when you get vexed. It beats faster when you get into a temper because of children and for other reasons.

Iuanimati was said to mean "out of heart" or "discouraged in your mind." Taylor (1951) says that it also refers to loss of blood. "*Miúanihadina nadaguni le nabusuerbai*", translates. "I can't do what I want because I am discouraged." Both terms (*iuanimati* and *miúanihadina*) are derived from the word *iuani* or spirit or soul. *Miúani* was said to mean, "I have no spirit", while the term *mánigi* (*anígi* = heart) connotes a lack of heart or courage. "Sometime a child might be injured in front of you and you don't have the heart to see that. That's *mánigi*", one woman explained.

"Worriness" was also identified as a cause of or a contributing factor in illness. The word may be the English translation of either *higániti* (vexation, anger) or *miúani* (lack of spirit). In Garifuna, the words *arítaguni* and *sámina* are closely related and often used interchangeably. Both denote the activity of thinking, but may be used to denote "worry" as well. "*Arítaguni nuágubi*" translates as "I have worries", while "*nasáminaruan*" means "I am worried"or "I am thinking deeply." On several occasions I tried to elicit a separate term for the concept "to think" which did not imply to notion of "to worry" as well, but was unsuccessful. "Thinking too much" was identified by more than one individual as a source of stress and hence a possible contributing factor in illness.

Worries get you upset, frighten you and can cause a hemorrhage.

Worry can cause illness. When you are worried you can't do nothing good to yourself. It affects your mind and nerves. You get nervous and don't eat right. Your mind is in your brain.

The sickness ("craziness", *lelúluau*) comes out when you are worried. It turns you upside down and acts on your mind. Sometimes it can be cured.

Other statements in which emotional stress was referenced included:

Sudden fright can make you sick.

Your body is worked up from too much tenseness.

If you have heart disease and get annoyed, it takes affect on you. It also affects the pressure.

A past event (the infidelity of a wife, desertion of a wife, and the death of parents were offered as examples) stays with you and rests on your nerves.

You have something on your mind and it works on you.

The failure or inability to interact with other Garinagu is a source of emotional stress as well and can lead to or exacerbate physical conditions. "You have a disturbance with someone and you don't have anyone to talk with", one healer stated in describing one source of emotional stress. "Some people, maybe they have something on their mind and don't want to tell and it works on them", another suggested. Thus, appropriate interaction with other Garinagu may be a requisite component of therapy. One noted midwife was asked if "vexation" could cause illness. "Yes", she replied, "it can cause pain in the stomach and pain in the head." I then asked her if it was to be treated in the same way as other illnesses.

No, as long as that person is vexed, she will keep the pain. You must comfort and advise her. I sit down with two or three other women and talk with her, find out what her problem is. One begins to make jokes and when the lady begins to laugh, then you give her holy water to drink. I keep joking with her.

A category of cause-effect relationships which I have characterized as "non-directive actions of others" includes both natural (*lisándi ubáo*) and "uncommon" (*wamálisian*) illnesses. Whether the illness is regarded as "of the world" or of some other origin, disorders in this category are thought to be the result of an action performed by some individual who intended no harm to the "victim." A father, for example, may cause the navel of his newborn infant to bleed by engaging in sexual relations with a woman other than his *umári*. This is regarded as a "natural" disorder and it is unnecessary to request the services of a *búiai* or to utilize spiritual therapies of any sort. Similarly, a baby may lose its hair if a nursing mother who "has not yet seen her period" or who, according to another woman, has not waited a full three months since the birth of her child, eats barracuda or striped fish. "Evil eye" or *mal ojo*, a commonly reported affliction among Spanish-speaking

Garinagu, was mentioned infrequently in Punta Gorda. However, informants did suggest that an infant might become ill "if a neighbor or friend looks upon the child in a certain way", the classic etiology for *mal ojo*. Gonzalez reported that the concept of the evil eye, "which is believed to be an inborn trait in some persons – particularly women" was frequently mentioned as an explanation for children's illnesses among the Garinagu of Guatemala (1970: 97). In Honduras, according to Coehlo, "strong sight" or *uburagudina* (also *lérei agu, heriti agu*) was said to be a characteristic possessed by the father during the first month of a child's life. "If he looks fixedly at any infant, including his own, during this period, it is believed that the child will become afflicted with muscular tension and persistent constipation" (211). In Punta Gorda individuals referred to two separate but related concepts. If a woman is pregnant and possesses *heritau agu* (strong eyes) it is said her gaze will "kill every chicken or duck or other animal." "Oh, when I was pregnant", one woman said, "my neighbor wouldn't led me walk among her chickens." "Stay away from my chickens", she said, "I don't want them to die." If an individual is sweating heavily and comes into proximity with an infant, the mother of the child may pass the child over into the hands of the individual who is sweating. "If a person is sweating, his shadow is too heavy and may sicken the child if he doesn't hold the child."

The concept of illness caused by envy and the bad feelings of others was pervasive, though I encountered few who would attribute specific instances of illness to this phenomenon. "If people grudge you and speak badly of you", I was told, "their words alone may harm you." This is referred to as *idáhadu*, which one informant translated as "mouth water" and another as "the words of the people." *Idáhadu* was said to cause an illness known as *fiáfia* which is characterized as "a swelling of the body", though others said *fiáfia* resulted from *obeah*. Coehlo stated that "concealed hate is supposed to materialize as a kind of fluid, called *idáhadu*, which of itself has harmful effects" (1955:68). It is clear, however, that *idáhadu* may manifest itself in other ways as well. "You will feel heavy, nervous, and sick", one healer stated, while another offered the opinion that "when people talk about you, you can't sleep. Their words are hot, like fire." *Idáhadu*, he explained, makes you sick because it drives your soul away. Because the soul (*áfurugu*) is essential to life itself, *idáhadu* was described as "worse than *obeah*." No direct contact is necessary for *idáhadu* to have such effects, nor does the afflicted individual need to know of the envy or hostility of others to be affected, for words were said to "travel in the wind." Coehlo found that *idáhadu* appeared only "when anger and envy are denied outward expression" (1955:210fn). Initially, he stated, its effects are slight and, if detected early, are manifested only as fever or symptoms of nervousness or migraine, "but with the passage of time [*idáhadu*] may produce grave illness or even death" (*Ibid.*:211).

Such illnesses or symtoms as produced by *idáhadu* are said to be "uncommon" or unnatural and, in the later stages of illness, extremely difficult to treat. One healer described certain preventive treatments, but stated that *idáhadu* could be cured with the assistance of certain Biblical psalms. Another Garifuna elder stated that some "herbalists" could treat the physical and emotional manifestations of *idáhadu*, but such illnesses or afflictions were generally said to be "under the *búiai's* control." Some equated *idáhadu* with *obeah*, but the intent of the speaker to harm another is not explicit in *idáhadu*. *Obeah*, on the other hand, always involves such intent.

The term *obeah* is of West African (Ashanti) origin, but is ubiquitous throughout Belize and most of the Caribbean. Every ethnic group has some understanding of the term, though the connotations attached vary. In general, the term can most easily be translated as sorcery. Sorcery, which is always used to bring misfortune to another, is distinguished by the Garinagu from magic or love potions which are used for other purposes. Among the Garinagu, the word is used almost interchangeably with the Garifuna term *abiñaraguile*. *Obeah* or *abiñariguile* may be performed in a number of ways. One may make *obeah* without the assistance of an *obeah man* bush doctor, *búiai*, or *gabiarahaditi* (though all are said to be able to make *obeah*) if the appropriate techniques are known. Or one may "hire" someone knowledgeable in *obeah* to perform a service. A variety of methods and materials were described. One may obtain soil from the tomb of a dead man, mix it with *guinea pepper* and put it in the fire. The bone of a dead man sewn into an intended victim's pillow will lead to "craziness." One can "talk to a dead man" or bury the picture or clothing of the individual one intends to harm in the hearth. "You must return every Tuesday and Friday [the days which evil spirits work] to say prayers. As the picture withers, so will you wither." The most commonly mentioned method involved the use of the image of San Antonio del Fuego or prayers said to this "saint" along with the use of candles. The Maya were said to turn to San Antonio del Fuego most frequently to work *obeah*. Gullick (1976) states that "St. Anthony is nowadays considered by Caribs to be the patron saint of sorcerers" (45). Prayers are often said to be utilized in *obeah* and Evans reports that on Roatan Biblical psalms are memorized for use in *obeah* (1970:117). Gonzalez refers to the use of a variety of materials, inculding "plant materials, tiger's claws, alligator's teeth, various unidentified 'chemicals' and... hair and nail clippings, blood, or excreta of the intended victim" (1970:100). In general, *abiñaraguile* or *obeah* is said to require an appeal to evil spirits. Individuals were ambivalent on the question of the involvement of the Christian Devil in such actions. It should be noted that it is uncommon for Garinagu to make reference to either God or the Devil in explaining either natural or "uncommon" illnesses or other misfortunes, though both were otherwise acknowledged to be powerful. In general, the

Catholic spirits (with the occasional exception of certain saints) are thought to do little to influence or "interfere" in the day-to-day affairs of Garifuna people.

While at least one individual suggested that *obeah* was used less frequently now than in the past, there are times when an illness or misfortune is attributed by members of the community to *obeah*. The victim, whatever the consensus of the community, may reject such a diagnosis, for among the Garinagu *obeah* is often thought to result indirectly from the wrong doing of the person who is afflicted. Several individuals described *obeah* as punishment inflicted on a guilty party. In addition, a knowledgeable *búiài* or bush doctor, detecting evidence of *obeah* in a victim's illness, will possess the techniques to turn *obeah* back on the initial perpetrator. Stories such as those that follow were fairly common.

> This woman, she took some money from the man she was living with. He didn't know she was the one who took it and when he asked her she denied that she had taken the money. So he made *obeah* against the person who took his money. He didn't know it would hurt her. She got this sore on her leg that won't cure. That was many years ago. Now there isn't anything anybody can do because the man is dead now. He came to her once in a dream and said, "Why didn't you tell me you took the money? I would never have done this if I had known it would hurt you."

> One man here went to Guatemala [to the temple of the *buiáis*] to report something stolen from him. He told the *búiai* to use *obeah* against the thief. He didn't know it was his own cousin and she died. She got a chop on her hand and then got tetanus.

Sanford (1976MS) reports the story of a woman who tried to steal the plantain of another. She entered the woman's yard and was bitten by a snake which had been "set" for her. She subsequently died since the family was unwilling to explain the circumstances surrounding the incident to local medical authorities. As the cause was thought to be *obeah*, it is unlikely the family believed a physician could have helped in any case. As these and many other such stories indicate, to accept a diagnosis of *obeah* may be equivalent to acceptance of personal responsibility for the afflication.

The incautious or uninformed use of *obeah* may result in misfortune befalling the perpetrator or his family. A Maya girl of fourteen, afflicted by a "tropical disease of unknown origin" was admitted on several occasions to the hospital in Punta Gorda. She was treated without much success and was eventually transferred to the hospital in Belize City where she died. It was rumored that her illness was the result of *obeah* attempted by the girls' father which turned back on the family because of his lack of skill in its use. The Mennonite nurse who transported her by horseback from her isolated village to the hospital, after repeated attempts to treat the child in her village, said she was now prepared to accept the villagers' assessment.

Self-Spirit Interactions

The final conceptual category of cause-effect relationships incorporates all those physical and emotional or behavioral disorders which result from interactions between living 'selves' and spiritual beings, unmediated or unprovoked by human intent. The basic principles of this domain are as follows:

1. In the course of everyday actions and interactions the potential for attack by a wide range of malevolent spirits exists.
2. Control over, or mediation or avoidance of such interactions with spirits, both good and evil, can generally be accomplished through adherence to well-known principles governing moral and ritual behavior and through the individual acquisition and expression of the qualities of wisdom, respect, maturity, and prudence.
3. The apparently distinct domains of the living and the dead are, in reality, a single universe in which the interests of both are intertwined. The spirits of the deceased are dependent upon their living descendants as the living are dependent upon the spirits of their ancestors.

The Garinagu recognize many spirits; some are regarded as inherently evil, while others are benevolent, though all are to be feared under certain conditions, and any spirit is capable of causing illness, death or other misfortune.

The spirits identified in the sections to follow do not constitute the total pantheon of spirits known to the Garinagu. They are, however, the spirits most commonly mentioned in discussions about illness. If they are accorded relatively little importance here, it is largely because few illnesses or disorders are now attributed to them.

Upon superficial inspection, they appear a 'motley crew', adopted into the pantheon of supernatural beings over an extended period of time, the acculturative legacy of the Spanish, the French, the West Africans, the Caribs, and the Miskito Indians. There are, first of all, the various spirits who seem always to have inhabited this universe, that is, who can be traced to the Carib and Arawak ancestors: *húmo* [*umeo*], the seaside spirits who cause sickness and death in children (an illness identified as *kwashiorkor* by researchers [see Gonzalez (1963) and Jenkins (1980)]), *uináni*, who is most commonly identified as the "Chief of Devils" (Taylor 1951:104) or the leader of *mafia* (Coehlo 1955:153), the *mafia*, or *mapoya* (see Taylor 1951: 103, Gullick 1976:14, Coehlo 1955:153), often identified as bush or evil spirits or referred to as devils; *ogoreu*, or *uguri*, *ulasa*, *Bearsy-bug*, and *belzing bug*, described previously, and *agáuima*, an evil spirit found near rivers who is said to capture men's souls. *Ulasa,* the name given a particular *ogoreu,* is said to be derived from Miskito (Taylor 1951:105) while Coehlo suggests that the "significance that the *ogoreu* came to have in the Black Carib belief system is also due to their Africal cultural inheritance" (1955:257).

There are the spirits introduced as a result of contact with the Spanish, French, and English: *duénde* or *duéndu*, *súsia*, and *faialandia*. Interestingly, these spirits, which were apparently incorporated into the Garifuna pantheon at a later date, are, excepting *duénde*, relatively innocuous by comparison with those mentioned above. *Faialandia* or *faialanda* or *fialanta*, described by Taylor as a "supernatural light at sea" (1964), may throw canoes off course or cause boats to sit immobilized. I was told by one individual that *fialanta* was the "spirits of the baymen." One woman reported that when she was a child her mother had received a message that another of her children was ill. She set out in a small boat at night to reach the sick child, taking with her her other children. On two occassions, a mysterious light passed them. Finally, her mother pulled the boat into shore where they remained hidden until daylight. The mother never explained the source of the light, but the girl was later told it was *fialanta*.

Súsia is said by Taylor to be a spirit or demon of "relatively harmless character", and was so identified by the Garinagu of Punta Gorda. Coehlo's Honduran informants, however, attributed to her considerably greater evil intent and powers. In Punta Gorda, *súsia* is generally described as a female spirit who plays "pranks" on drunken men and causes them to lose their senses.

If a man is a habitual drunkard, he sees someone who he believes to be his wife or girlfriend. He follows her and she goes to the cemetery. There they start to make love, but he awakens to find himself in the cemetery alone or in some similar place.

A Garifuna elder told me he had been haunted by *súsia* at one time. "However, my *nafurugu* is very strong and I avoided her." This same individual reported that *súsia* had once appeared to a friend of his. "But my friend was a wise man. He said to *súsia*, "You are not my wife. My wife does not walk about at night." And he went straight home."[2]

Duénde (*duéndu* in Spanish = goblin or gnome) was identified by one healer as the "devil of the coast", though others stated that he inhabited the interior Pine Ridge area of Belize. *Duénde* is said, like other *gnomos*, to be a short, stocky man who wears a "big hat, like a Mexican and short red pants." He is considered by some to be far more dangerous than *súsia* or *faialandia* or other *gnomos*, capable of possessing an individual or driving his *áfurugu* away. It was said that children who are suddenly exposed to him may die. Great wealth is attributed to *duénde* and he may be appealed to for money "if one knows the correct prayers [*lagásurui*]." According to Coehlo and individuals with whom I spoke, *duénde* will demand the soul or life of a family member or a friend in return for the granting of such requests, though one local healer stated he could turn *duénde* back with other prayers.

Agáiuma is described by Taylor as a "nymph" who inhabits particular cascades or pools. She may, according to Taylor, assume many forms but in her encounters with men, she is always seen as a naked woman with beautiful long hair" (1951:104). Both Coehlo and Taylor state that *agáiuma* may bring sickness or death to her victims. In Punta Gorda, stories of *agáiuma* and her powers vary. One Garifuna male, a man in his sixties, stated he had once seen *agáiuma*. "She appears like a young lady, possessing a golden comb. She is shy and very sensitive to noise. She resembles the East Indians in her appearence." *Agáiuma* may appear, according to this individual, between 11:30 and 12:30 during the day when there is a "calmness" and quiet.

When I saw her, I was quite young. She dashed herself into the bush backwards when she became aware of our presence. There were a group of us going to the river bank to do some fishing. When I saw her, I turned back at speed. The others, having become alarmed, followed me. Four days later, one of my youngest brothers died. He was only five at the time. On the second day after we returned he had fits. He had been well until then. *Agàiuma* may be harmful to the human body and may cause death. I believe it was the effects of the haunting which caused him to die.

A Garifuna woman described *agáiuma* as a female who is Spanish in appearance.

She can make you sick. Your illness may start with a fever or chills. She appears to a sick person in their dreams. If it is a woman who is ill, she will come to her like her husband. This is an illness which must be treated by a *búiai*.

A male healer stated that *agáiuma* was "worse than the devil. The *buiái* got to work hard if she causes illness."

The Garinagu of Punta Gorda recognize two additional evil spirits known as *uinани* and *mafia*. The term *mafia* is generally translanted as devil. In some instances, the term Lucifer and Satan are given as glosses of *mafia*. Yet Taylor identifies *mafia* as a "malevolent bush spirit", while Coehlo reports:

The spirits called *mafia*, who wander through the streets at night, sometimes entering the house, are responsible for domestic accidents, and may strangle people in their sleep. They also attact women coming from the gardens in the hills, especially if aroused by the odor of menstrual blood. The chief is named *Uinани*, often identified with Satan (1955: 153).

The term *mafia* is clearly of ancient origin. Gullick states that the belief in *mafia, maboya, mapwiya* or *mapoya* can be traced to pre-contact Island Carib beliefs (1976a:14, 44), and that *mafia* were bush spirits. The current practice of describing *mafia* in terms reasonably consistent with Catholic dogma represents a gradual articulation of codes. The distinctions between *uinани* and *mafia* are not always clear. The confusion occurs when one identifies *mafia* as devil or satan, which is inconsistent with the earlier position that *mafia* were bush spirits, one of whom was *uinани*. In one case, I was told that *duénde* is a type of *uinани*, suggesting that with the passage of time all evil spirits are classified as *uinани* or *mafia*. The phrase "*Uiñani nuágubi*" translates as "I have an evil spirit on me." *Uinани* was said by one individual to be a spirit who causes illness, but another stated simply: "*Uiñani*'s illness is death. He lives on blood." Like *duènde*, he was reported by one bush doctor to offer wealth, but to demand a high price. "I could have been wealthy, but *uinани* would have taken my oldest son." Another healer described *uinани* as the "chief of the devils", an interpretation consistent with that of Coehlo's informants. In general, the Garinagu of Punta Gorda defined *mafía* as the devil, but stated that *uinàni* is also a *mafía*. The descriptions of *uinàni* were often explicit.

Uinàni is a monster seen by the soul or spirit alone. It is a terrible being, a demon or dragon. It may appear as an alligator. It is dangerous to the body and terrible to the sight. He jumps on you physically. Some people go to the plantation or go fishing at certain times to avoid being attacked by *uinàni*. His hours are eleven in the evening to three or four in the morning. However, *uinàni* is very rare in our time.

Uinàni is a devil. Sometimes you will dream it like an animal. It is an ugly sight. It can make you ill and give you all different feelings. *Búiai* must work against *uinàni*. You may have a dream, maybe dream an animal is chasing you, like a snake or like a dog. You may have been to the doctor and got no relief from doctor medicine. Then you have to go to a *búiai* and relay your feelings to her. She will know what to do and maybe by tomorrow you will feel plenty better. *Uinàni* only appears to you in your dreams.

Pantu was defined as the spirit that lingers after death, or in Catholic terminology, as a ghost. In general, individuals believe that the *iuàni* leaves the body at death but may remain in the area for days or, in some cases, weeks. The spirit or *iuàni* may become a *pantu* only if at death it was discontented or had committed some crime or misdeed (see Taylor 1951 on *ahári*), there is no mention of *pantu* in the writings of either Taylor or Coehlo, though both make reference to *ufię* ["ghosts" or "spectres"]. Coehlo identifies them as the ghosts of those recently dead, but Taylor states they are, as a rule, not connected with the spirit of a dead person. *Ahári* are described by both as the "spirits of one recently dead." The *pantu* seem to cause no particular harm, though their appearance may be disturbing. If the *pantu* is present for too long "someone complains and everyone starts to go into prayer and the *pantu* leaves."

Of far greater importance in any discussion of illness are the *gubída*, or the spirits of those who have been dead for many years. The *gubída* are described as the souls or spirits of parents, grandparents, or great grandparents who may return after a period of fifteen to twenty years to make demands upon their descendants. They cause or permit illness or death if their requests are not met or if they feel they have been ignored or offended in some manner. More will be said of the *gubída* and their powers and the therapeutic response to *hasándigubída* (the illness of *gubída*) in the following chapter.

Almost all Garinagu describe themselves as Catholic. As Kerns notes, they often explain even the most traditional Garifuna beliefs in terms of orthodox Christian theology (1977:264). Coehlo's statement continues to serve as an accurate depiction of the relation between Garifuna and orthodox Catholic beliefs.

The ancestral cult, therefore, when considered in terms of its practical implications, and its role in preserving the traditions of the group, must be regarded as the core of the Black Carib system of belief. The typical Carib virtues of flexibility and versatility enabled them to incorporate this non-Christian tradition into their Catholicism, thus achieving despite the vigorous denunciations of the official representatives of the Church, a synthesis that comprised a coherent and unified body of doctrine (1955:135).

When questioned specifically about the role of God, healers are generally consistent in their statements that their healing power comes from God. Many utilize Biblical psalms and passages to assist in curing or to ward off evil. The "blessed Virgin Mary" is appealed to by the *búiai* in his treatment of *hasándigubída*. Several bush doctors utilize holy water obtained from the church in the preparation of medicines.

Nevertheless, discussions of illness and its treatment rarely invoke references of God, to Satan (except as *mafía* or *uináni*), or to any of the Catholic pantheon of deities or saints. Satan possesses the power to cause sickness, but references are generally to *uináni* or *mafía* or other evil spirits as the source of certain unnatural illnesses. Some expressed the belief that God might occasionally cause illness, generally as punishment for misbehavior, while others insisted God never inflicted illness on individuals, but allowed them the freedom to undertake actions or indulge in behavior which might bring about illness. One bush doctor said God might cause illness as proof of his power, but added that this would be rare indeed, while another stated that "causing sickness is God's power. He allows the *gubída* to wander about and he allows *idáhadu* or *obeah* as well." Nevertheless, among the Garinagu, illnesses are never referred to as "illnesses of God", but as *lisándi ubáo*, or illnesses of the world. These 'grander' spirits are, perhaps, too distant to be frequently and directly involved in the day-to-day affairs of Garifuna people. The most obvious exception to this attitude is seen in the increasing emphasis on the healings of Señor Esquipulas.

NOTES

1. Most likely derived from "Beelzebub" or Baal-zebub, god of the Philistine city of Ekron.
2. On my last visit, while drinking in a local bar, I was informed that there are male *súsia* as well.

CHAPTER 6

Therapies, Therapists, and Therapeutic Resources

Garifuna herbalists, bush doctors, midwives, and *búiais* operate autonomously. There are no "social, jural, or economic arrangements" which provide for the coordination of practitioners' activities or restrict competition (see Young, 1982, on structural relationships between and among practitioners and their clients). The absence of collective action or the corporate legitimation of individual actions diminishes the potential control of healers and restricts access to resources which might otherwise be more effectively exploited by a corporate group, but, at the same time, makes it more difficult for the state to legislate against an amorphous 'body' of healers or to enforce existing legislation. In additon, since each healer controls specific information, his power in relation to that particular resource is increased. 'Traditional' systems survive because they exploit econiches which state medicine cannot exploit or fails to recognize.

In contrast, state biomedicine succeeds not only because its therapies are often successful, but because it is based upon universally legitimized paradigms, professional and legal support of actions and interpretive decisions, effective access to financial, material, and illness resources, and standards for training and practice which result in quasi-corporate structures.

The authority and position of the Garifuna healer are derived from his or her effective control over certain therapeutic resources, including knowledge concerning appropriate therapies, technical information regarding the proper preparation and utilization of therapeutic materials, control over diagnostic techniques which produce signs which are not or cannot be generated by biomedical personnel, acknowledged relationships with spiritual intermediaries or assistants, and access to the paradigms which justify diagnostic, therapeutic, and prognostic pronouncements. The Garifuna healer has access to and control over a range of etiological and diagnostic interpretations which are appropriate to the individual client, in general conformity with the broad parameters permitted by the medical model, and which validate and provide meaning to Garifuna social, economic, and historic realities. The absence of corporate healing institutions is totally consistent with Garifuna values regarding automomy and the expression of individuality, and provides for greater flexibility in the search for appropriate solutions to problems manifested as physical or behavioral disorders.

Healers differ in several respects, any of which may affect their authority within the community and their right to successfully impose diagnostic and etiological interpretations. They vary in terms of their recruitment to the role of healer and the manner in which the knowledge they possess has been produced. They are diversified with regard to the range of illnesses they treat, the diagnostic techniques they employ, the therapeutic methods utilized, and the object-representamen-interpretant relationships offered. Finally, they differ in terms of their personal status within the community and their right to assign 'meaning' to the signs of illness.

Healers, herbalists, and midwives may learn their therapeutic (and preventive) techniques and the justifications for their diagnostic, etiologic, and interpretive declarations from another healer. Most commonly, this individual is an older healer, usually a relative one or two generations removed, who wishes to see his or her knowledge preserved. Training may begin when the 'initiate' is quite young, and may proceed over a period of weeks or years. Most healers supplement this learning with experimentation, personal experience, and information gathered from other healers, though there is no systematic or concerted attempt among healers to share information.

Certain healers are referred to as "gifted", that is, they are said to be assisted in some manner by spirits who often appear to them in dreams, direct them to the correct "bush", and instruct them in its preparation and use. Even healers who do not claim to be "gifted" may dream therapies and the distinction between "gifted" healers and others is not always well defined. Of seven Garifuna healers interviewed, five claimed dreams as a continuing source of knowledge.

Individuals who have learned their medicines from another healer may still have such dream experiences. A healer who treated only one sort of affliction reported she had dreamed the therapies for this affliction when she was young and apparently continued to have such dreams. She had stopped practicing at the time of our interview, however, because she felt her clients had failed to properly acknowledge the source of their cure and often refused to pay. She had asked that she not dream the medicines any more and claimed to have forgotten most. Those who are not healers may occasionally dream medicines as well. One woman who had never practiced as either herbalist or healer and claimed no special skills reported she had twice dreamed the medicines (*árana*) necessary to treat a family member who was ill. The cure was effected in both instances and no further dreams of this sort occurred. A second woman related a similar story to me.

The *búiai* is a "gifted" healer of a special sort who serves in a special capacity within Garifuna communities. The role of the *búiai* (*bóye*, *búye*, *búiei, búwiye*) was described in mid-seventeenth century European reports of the Caribs of the Antilles. While descriptions of the practices of the *piaye bóye* differ from those offered today, there are sufficient resemblances to suggest that the *bóye* of pre-contact Caribs and the *búiai* of the Garinagu are essentially the same.

They consult the Devil through their Conjurors or *Piaye* Doctors as to their recovery from sickness, as to their where-abouts at sea in bad weather, as to the issue of their wars, or to learn the names of those that have bewitched them. Each *Piaye* has his particular *Chęmeen* (spirit), or familiar devil, and they are governed by the evil counsel of these detestable socrerers....

To know the cause of their illness they send for a *Piaye Boye*, or sorcerer, at night, who orders all the lights in the house to be put out and turns the suspected persons out: he then retires into a corner, where the sick person is brought to him, and, after smoking a piece of tobacco, he mashes it in his hands, and blows it in the air, shaking and flipping his fingers. They say that the *Chemeen* always comes on scenting the odour of this incense, and, being interrogated, he answers with a clear voice, but sounding as from a distance. The sorcerer then approaches the sick person repeatedly, feels, presses, and manipulates the suffering part, aways blowing on it, and extracts sometimes from it, or rather appears to extract some thorns or small pieces of cassava, wood, or bones, making the sick person believe that this was the sole cause of the pain. (De La Borde 1888:234, original 1674).

The degree to which the role of the *búiai* was altered by exposure to West African beliefs and Spanish or French Catholicism cannot be fully ascertained, though there appears to be considerable syncretism. The "cult of the ancestors", in which the *buiái* plays a critical role, seems to have been present among pre-contact Caribs, but the emphasis on the importance of the ancestors in all matters was likely reinforced by the introduction of West African beliefs. The recruitment to the role of the *búiai*, which is not described by De La Borde, bears certain similarities to the recruitment of healers to the "cults of affliction" documented by Turner among the Ndembu (Turner 1968). However, there is no evidence of such cults among the Garinagu now or in the past. The healer referred to above who treated only one affliction had suffered, prior to her recruitment to the role of healer, from the same affliction which she treated, but she did not claim to be a *búiai*, nor did she work in association with any other healers.

The *búiai* achieves his or her status only after a long and arduous journey. Generally, though not always, he is directly aided in the transformation to a full-fledged *búiai* by another living *búiai*. In cases in which no living *búiai* is present or accessible, the candidate must progress at a slower rate and with the assistance of his *hiúruha*. There was said to be a young man in a village to the south who had received the call to become a *búiai*. Because there was no *búiai* present in the village, he was having a difficult time of it. He was described as "only a messenger" (*onaglí*), though he had five or six *hiúruha* and did some curing. He reportedly received some assistance from a *búiai* living in Los Angeles.

The signs that one is destined to become a *búiai* generally appear early in the individual's life. An elderly Garifuna man related the following:

The *búiai* is born. There are symptoms from the time he is an infant which tell the parents. They often know very early that a child will be a *búiai*. The child acts abnormally. He can't eat certain things. The child appears haunted in his sleep and will awake suddenly. From the first week he behaves this way. When he begins to creep, he may act as though he is aware of something others aren't. He is never healthy, but he is not sick. He suffers from "allergies." He is born with spirits. These spirits are astral spirits from an astral spirit world. After death, spirits live in a world like the world we live in.

From the time they are little children they can start to foretell things. They know the spirits already. They may sometimes go behind a door and be heard to be carrying on a conversation. They may giggle and talk as though with someone else.

To reject the signs that indicate one is to become a *búiai* is to jeopardize one's health and life (though see interview with Mr. Avilez).

The *búiai* has no choice. He has to dedicate himself. The spirits force him to be a *búiai*.

No single set of signs indicate that one is destined to become a *búiai*. The child may have been said to have cried out in his mother's womb or to have been possessed by the spirit of a former *búiai*, to have spoken with the voice of a deceased *búiai*, or to have known the cure for what was thought to be an incurable illness. One local healer stated that he was a *búiai*, but chose not to function as a *búiai* at this stage in his life. He added the following:

My mother knew I was going to be a *búiai*, that I had a special gift. When I was born, the house was filled with butterflies [a form which certain spirits are sometimes said to take]. They are still here. They follow me.

Commonly, the future *búiai* suffers from a series of illnesses or from a poor state of health as a child or young adult. Only acceptance of the call to become a *búiai* will alter permanently the individual's physical condition.

The *búiai* possesses several spirits (*hiúruha*) who communicate with him and through him. Each *búiai* has a principal *hiúruha* who takes charge over the others; more than one *búiai*, however, may be aided by the same *hiúruha*. One famous, now deceased *búiai*, Balthazar or Din, now serves as chief *hiúruha* to a *búiai* in New York and to one in Stann Creek (Dangriga) as well.

There are many *hiúruhas*. Any astral spirit may become a *hiúruha* Many are known to have been living people, but they only become *hiúruha* at least twenty-five years after their death. Not all astral spirits act as *hiúruha*. They can give explanations about things way back. Some astral spirits and *hiúruha* may only be spirit world dwellers and not people who lived before.

The *hiuruha* can 'see' many things which remain invisible to others. This gives them the power to detect uncommon illnesses, that is, illnesses which are caused by evil spirits, the maleficent intentions or actions of living persons, and the disappointment of the *gubída*. But the *búiai* can inform of many other things as well.

In the States, there was a *búiai*, Bando, who visited me one evening. After he left, I had a dream in which a man appeared with a calf lying by his side. I also had a bottle of gin with me and the man asked for some. I refused and offered him holy water instead. I got frightened and went downstairs where I met a man leading a cow. I hid the bottle. Early in the morning, the *búiai* called me and asked me how I had gotten along with my visitor. He related the entire dream to me. Years later a *búiai* in Livingstone did the same and told me the man was the spirit of my maternal great grandfather. The man who first settled Punta Gorda was a man by the name of Phillip Zuniga. I was in Livingston at an *arairaguag* [usually referred to as *arairaguni* or "calling down of the spirit"], a spiritual consultation. The foreman of the *hiúruha* asked me for my name and I said I was here to ask about a dream I had in New York. The foreman said that spirit was annoyed with me now. I had denied him a drink. The *gubída* of this man's wife was brought to me and I explained the situation and apologized and she went back to her husband and reluctantly he came forward. He only asked for a mass to be said for him and his wife.

While the *búiai* himself may be knowledgeable about medicines, his principal function is as a medium, as illustrated by the above story. It is, in fact, the *hiúruha* who direct the therapeutic process.

The *búiai* can foretell sickness or disease. The doctors cannot cure such sicknesses. You must go to the *búiai*. After incantations, the spirits arrive and communicate directly with the sick person through the mediumship of the *búiai*. The spirits will walk around the house and shake hands with you; you will feel someone hold your hand, and they will tell you surprising things about yourself.

There was a woman who was a spiritist [*búiai*] who visited here recently during a *chugu*. She sat down and almost immediately the spirits arrived and began a conversation with the others. If you have relatives in the States they can tell you all about them. If your mother has just gone shopping, they can tell you. They know many things.

After the spirits enter the *búiai*, the *búiai* will give no account of anything. Someone will have to tell him what has happened. He needs a competent person to tell him what has happened. If there is not a competent person present, the spirits will come again and tell him what has happened and what the person is to do. The *búiai* can't see spirits; he can only hear them. You will see the *búiai* make a shake when the *hiúruha* enter him. The *búiai* won't know what is happening around him.

The *búiai* will have an invocation of spirits. These *hiuruha* are the ones who give instructions on what to do, what herbs to use. The *búiai* is not an able person, he is nothing without the *hiúruha*. The *hiúruha* will make the diagnosis. They will make a diagnosis according to the sickness. The *búiai* must look for herbs, but the *hiúruha* give all the instructions. It could be a natural sickness, They can cure that, but may tell you "It is not for us" and send you to see a doctor, a *grisanu* [white man].

A *búiai* may not be a *búiai* for life, but must work to maintain his relationship with the spirits.

If the *búiai* do contrary to orders of the *hiúruha*, the *hiúruha* will leave him. The youngest person ever to become a *búiai* was a man by the name of Thomas. He became a true *búiai* around twelve to fifteen years of age, but it was long known that he would be a *búiai*. But he lost his spirits. He was a brilliant *búiai*, but began to make all sorts of claims for himself. He did things contrary to the spirits.

As stated above, the *hiúruha* are frequently the spirits of former *búiais*, but there are other spirits who serve as *hiúruha*.

The *hiúruha* are not ancestral spirits. According to traditon they are Garifuna; but there are those astral spirits who may speak many languages. They will speak to you in your language. After death, any spirit can respond. Now they respond much earlier than in the past. It may be only four years now before they can be invoked, but it is twenty-five years at least before they become *hiúruha*. Nobody knows why the spirits appear so early now.

One healer had been taught his medicines by his father, who was a *búiai*. He stated that his father had spirits as guides "which came to him through illness."

My father's *hiúruha* included the spirit of a past *búiai*, the spirits of some who have lived, and the spirits of some who have never lived.

This individual claimed that he has a special ability to tell what is bothering someone, but he added that he had no spirit guides and knew the treatments for only a few illnesses. While therapeutic means and materials may be passed from one generation to the next, the role of the *búiai* is not.

Even *búiais* may not be able to cure all illnesses. If you are far beyond a cure, they will tell you that. I am blind because of a weakened optic nerve. I went to a specialist in the States and to a doctor in Belize City. They both told me no one could cure me because the optic nerve was very weakened. I went to Sarah and she cured me of several minor illnesses, like loose bowels. She used baths for seven days. Din spoke to me and told me what I knew was true. He said, "When you go to work on the train I see you. When you ride the train and get out of the subway to go to work, you stand deep in the snow. When you work in the bakery or kitchen, you get hot and it affects you from top to bottom. If affects you from the brains to the feet. Waste no more money on cures." I went to Livingstone to the spirit center and the *hiúruha* there said the same thing. The spirits at the spirit centers know about all sorts of things. They know all about our conversation right now.

Garifuna therapeutic specialists treat a wide range of illnesses, each provides somewhat different therapies, and each prepares his or her medicines in different ways. Some restrict themselves to the evaluation and treatment of *lisándi ubaó*; others may treat only a single affliction. Even those therapists who treat a wider range of illnesses will frequently recognize an illness as "beyond their competence" and refer the afflicted individual to a *búiai* or to the local biomedical practitioner.

Hasándigubîda, or the illnesses which are brought by the *gubída*, often necessitate a mass at the Catholic church or a special "offering to the *gubída*." If neither suffices to send away or placate the *gubída*, then the services of a *búiai* are required. Healers who claim no special relationship with *hiúruha* or other spirits may be able to treat *wamálisian* (uncommon) illnesses if they have learned the correct procedures or receive guidance from a spirit in a dream. *Obeah, idáhadu* and illnesses brought by the variety of malicious spirits known to the Garinagu, can be treated by healers who are neither "gifted" nor *búiai*s, though it is generally acknowledged that *búiai*s will have greater success in treating uncommon illnesses, that only *búiai*s can perform the *dugu* and *chugu* ceremonies, that not all those who know herbal and other treatments for illness are skilled in the treatment of uncommon illnesses as well, and that biomedical physicians successfully recognize and treat only illnesses which are classified as *lisándi ubaó*. Nevertheless, there is no consistent one-to-one relationship between the recruitment of the healer to his role, the existence and nature of spiritual intermediaries or assistance, the ability to dream medicines, and the range of illnesses which can be treated. The following chart shows the sources of healing knowledge, the type of illnesses treated,

	Healer A (male)	Healer B (male)	Healer C (male)	Healer D (female)	Healer E (female)	Healer F (male)
Occurrence of Dreams Revealing Medical Information	Once	Sometimes	Frequent	Frequent	Frequent	Never
Individual from whom training was/is recevied	Old *búiai* who was close relative	Grandmo., Spirits in dreams occasionally	Relative, *Hiúruha* or guides	Mo. and Gr. Mo. and others	Spirits, Doctor	Father who was *búiai*
Spirits who direct or offer assistance	None	Black man in white, Angels	*Hiúruha* - two kinds of small men	Mo. and Gr.Mo. and other black people	White nurse	None
Materials used in preparation and/ or treatments						
1. Use of Prayers	Treatment and Prep.	Treatment and Prep. (Carib prayers)	Treatment Preparation	Treatment? and Prep. (Spanish & Catholic prayers)	Treatment and Prep.	Treatment and Prep.

To be Cont'd.

	Healer A (male)	Healer B (male)	Healer C (male)	Healer D (female)	Healer E (female)	Healer F (male)
Materials Used (cont.)						
2. Candles	Diagnoses Preparation of medicines	No	Diagnoses	Preparation of medicines	No?	Preparation of medicines
3. Use of Holy Water	No	Only once	Yes	Yes	Only as treatment	Yes
Types of illnesses treated						
1. Natural	Yes	Yes	Yes	Yes	Yes	Yes
2. Uncommon	Yes	Yes	Yes	No	No	Yes
3. Hasandigubida	No	No	No	No	No	No

To be Cont'd.

	Healer A (male)	Healer B (male)	Healer C (male)	Healer D (female)	Healer E (female)	Healer F (male)
Major therapies employed						
1. Massage or "nointing"	Not major component	Not major component	Not major component	Yes	Yes	Not major component
2. Use of incense or 'smoking'	Yes	Yes	Yes	No	No	?
3. Bathing	Yes	Yes	Yes	No	No	Yes
Functions as:						
Midwife	No	No	No	Yes	Yes	No
Healer	Yes	Yes	Yes	Yes	Yes	Yes
Búiai	No	No but says he is a *búiai*	No	No	No	No

the material utilized in preparation of medicines, the presence and nature of spiritual assistants, and the role of dreams in determination of therapies among six local Garifuna healers.

The functions of the many individuals who claim some knowledge of healing therapies vary. Those who are mere herbalists, preparing medicines for simple afflictions, are not usually called upon to diagnose illness or to offer elaborate etiologies, and, therefore, do not serve to reinforce moral and social values in any significant way. Nor do they treat 'uncommon' illnesses. The better known and more respected healers, on the other hand, are in a position to serve as "moral agents" to the community, to provide interpretations which are consistent with and reinforce basic behavioral and philosophical principles. All of the healers interviewed had either been trained by a *búiai* or were guided in dreams by spirits. Only two claimed not to treat uncommon illnesses. Both were midwives, but treated other illnesses as well. The function of treating illnesses which have been brought by the *gubída* is reserved solely to the *búiai*, though on one occasion when I was privileged to attend an "offering to the *gubída*" ceremony, the highly respected healer I had accompanied to the ceremony was asked for advice on the proper procedure to be followed, though he was not a *búiai*.

Presentation of Signs

As in any medical "system", the first task of the healer is to determine the nature of the patient's complaint. In some cases, a family member may approach the healer and ask that he attend to the afflicted individual. In others, the patient may come to the healer's home or send someone to "fetch" him. Only a brief description of the patient's state may be provided or sought at this point in the encounter. It is generally sufficient that the healer knows that his services are required.

The healer proceeds. once with the patient, by obtaining a brief history of the patient's current illness or soliciting signs from the individual or his family. The healer will commonly ask, "What is your problem?" or "How does your body feel?" or "What caused the pain in your stomach?" He (or she) may ask whether the person has been eating properly, whether he or she has been resting well, and whether there have been any unusual dreams. The diagnostician may examine the patient physically, depending on the nature of the individual's complaint. The eyes, mouth, ears, tongue, abdomen, back, fingernails, gums, and so on may be probed for additional signs. The patient may be asked whether he has received an injury or a "sudden twist", whether he has dreamed of enemies, whether he has noticed mucus in his stool, and so on, depending on the signs which have already been presented or generated.

Patients and their families rarely attempt to apply diagnostic labels to signs or to a series of signs, but rather describe an illness in terms of the affective and visible alterations. The tendency to discuss illness in terms of the manifestation of specific signs is reflected in and reinforced by the Garifuna language which contains relatively few explicit terms for "diseases" or "syndromes", but possesses many lexical items which describe objective and subjective signs of disorder.

While there are terms which refer to various body products, such as blood, urine, and mucus, the range of terms for body organs or parts is limited. The term, *uragairugu*, for example, refers to the stomach, gallbladder, intestines, and other internal organs collectively, though there are separate lexical items for the liver, intestines, and womb. Notions of the interdependence of body components or systems are not highly developed. In response to a question asking whether all parts of the body work together, one healer offered the following:

I guess so. I'm not certain. Once the heart, liver, spleen, and guts are in the body, they work together. But if there is some defect or disease of the liver it affects the whole body. Then the heart. When the heart is not beating right, it affects the whole body. When the brain is not working right, it affects the whole body. The kidney is the most essential part of the body along with the heart and liver. The kidney causes backache, stoppage of water, especially when inflammated. It affects the whole body. It may also affect the circulation of the blood. The blood depends on the heart. The heart is the fountain. Poor blood is caused by malnutrition, lack of exercise, and hard work.

There is, as well, a tendency to express or describe symptoms in terms of alterations in sensation, for example, "I feel my skin like broke up...." "I feel my hand numb", "I felt cold on my stomach", and to express severity in terms of alterations in "self" ("I hardly even knew myself").

The range of complaints generated in discussions with Garifuna individuals included the following as well:

- pain (*gariti*) (e.g., "pain across belly", "pain in umbilical area", "heart pain", "striking pain", "pain when urine in all of belly", "pain like blunt needles")
- fever (*abirauha*) (e.g., "fever", "fever in the night"; *nabiruahani nuragairugunian*, "I have fever inside"; "I have fever in my bones" [often interpreted as sign of malaria].
- headache (*ligári nichug*, "I have pain in my head"; "I have pain all over my head")
- sneezing (*nachuhani*, "I am sneezing") ("I have a cold" = *nachuhani*)
- coughing (*natunahani*, "I am coughing"; *anéhain latunuhana hítu luágu*, "He is coughing up blood")
- chills (*anéhain lediligiti nuágu*, "I have cold on me"; "I have chills", "chills give me cramps inside", "chill comes on me"; *Dilígiti nuhn laduga abiruaha*, "I feel cold because of the fever" = chills).
- bleeding (*hítu*, blood) (note: bleeding post vaginally is *nichigutidan*, the same word is used to refer to menstrual flow; the word *hítu* is not used).
- vomiting (*anéhain areruhani nuágu* "I am vomiting")
- vomiting blood
- loose stools, diarrhea (*anéhain luburu uragairugu nuágu* [*uragairugu* refers to abdomen]; *anéhain hítu lidan namúru*, "I have blood in my stool").
- nausea (*ligiri buao*; same expression is used to indicate dizziness, giddiness)

- loose stools, diarrhea (*anéhain luburu uragairugu nuágu* [*uragairugu* refers to abdomen]; *anèhain hitu lidan namuru*, "I have blood in my stool").
- thirst (*busientina natun duna*, "I want water")
- digestive distress ("gas in my stomach", "my food won't digest", "my stomach feels full", "I have gas around my heart")
- excessive urination (*nasísihani*, "I urine")
- pain when urinating (*garíti nasisihani*, "I have pain when urinating")
- can't pass urine (*ligári asísihani*)
- blood in urine (*hìtu lidan asísihani*)
- distress in breathing (*dúnti nawaragu*, "I have shortness of breath", "I couldn't breathe", "I have short wind", "It's hard to breathe"; *mawáragutina buída*, "I can't breathe good")
- trembling (*adadaguruni*; "I have trembling in my body", "I feel my body nervous [shaking]"
- nervousness (*anéhain adádagaruni lidan nugurugu*, "I have nervousness on me" Note: word for nervousness is also used to refer to trembling or shaking; nervousness is described by its symptoms or physical manifestations)
- giddiness, dizziness (*ligiri buao*, "I suffer from giddiness", "I feel my head heavy", "My head is swinging when I get up", "I see darkness if I get up quickly")
- tingling ("I have tingling in the hands")
- numbness ("I feel my hand numb", "I feel my leg like asleep")
- loss of appetite (*negini*; also term for anorexia; "I don't have no appetite"; "This sickness takes my appetite")
- wind, gas
- dryness of the eyes (*lumabe agu*)
- dryness of the mouth (*lumabe iumolugu*)
- swelling (*laludunburuo, aluduni*)
- poor blood (term anemia is not used) (blood = *hítu* or *hítau* "I don't have any blood", "I have poor blood", "My blood is weak", etc; see Chapter VII).
- inability to sleep (*siénti narumugun*, "I can't sleep; also *marumuguni*)
- sores (*gumáin*)
- wound (*chuñti*; terms for wounds suffered during chopping and cutting differ).
- rash (*anéhain luágu urau tuágu*, "She has an itch on her")
- burn (*churadina*)
- cut (*bèti, ibaguni*, also refers to wound)
- abcess (*gahuguwani*)
- ulcer (*yága*; *anèhain yága tuágu luágu tugudi*, "She has an ulcer on her foot")
- loss of speech (*maragalihali siñanti ladumerahan*)
- weakness or general debility (*debiliti; anehain debili nuágu*, "I have a weakness on me" "He is sickly from the time he is born", "He isn't sound from inside", "I'm not so strong"; *debiliti nadaragun nugúbu*, "I feel weak in my body; also *tuátuadina*)
- paralysis (*fadagua*)
- cramps, menstrual
- cramps, non-menstrual; "I have cramps in the legs", "chills have given me cramps inside", "cramps catch me" "I get cramps over my legs, stomach, and arms")
- palpitations (*heriti tafaru nanigi;* "My heart is beating hard", "I have palpitations"; also *tafarahani anigi*, "pounding of the heart")
- stiff-eyed look (*adérihani*, also refers to "fits")
- staring (*mamalisiaga*)
- worry (*anehain sámina nuágu*, "I have worries on me"; note: *samina* denotes "mind"; also *aritaguni nuágubi*)
- sweating (*harougati nuhn*, "I am hot")
- fits (*attacki, aderihani, ówehani*, Note: some ethnographers report *ówehani* is used to describe the trance-like state of the *dugu*, however, one informant used the term *ówehani* to refer to fits, paralysis from polio, and convulsions as well)
- paleness (*anéhain páleruni tuágu*, "She is pale" *anéhain lilougua hítu tuágu*, "She is short of blood")

- trouble with vision ("I suffer from blindness", "My eyes are blurred", "I can't see")
- discharge (term varies according to whether discharge is from a wound, from the ears, or from the genital area; in the case of discharge due to gonorrhea, an individual might describe his symptoms by stating that he has a cold (*iadu*) in his privates.
- injury (*beléseti*)
- profuse bleeding (*seinenti*)

The following terms are diagnostic labels known to many through exposure to a western or bio-medical model of illness. In some cases, these 'illnesses' or syndromes were recognized and labeled by the Garinagu prior to contact. In others, Garifuna terms were created to label, usually in descriptive terms, an illness which was previously unrecognized until 'diagnosed' and described by the biomedical model, or, as many Garinagu argue, did not exist prior to the introduction of "civilization."

- tuberculosis (*tuna*, "cough"; *hatuna hatina*, "I have a bad cough."
- tetanus (*hederahani*, "He is stiffened")
- dysentery (*denési*)
- polio, epilepsy (*ówehani*, the term also refers to "fits", "actions before death", and possession by spirits during the *dugu*)
- scarlet fever (*abírauha*, "fever")
- malaria (*abírauha*)
- chicken pox (*pox*)
- measles (*chagayanbeh*; *minsula*)
- bronchitis
- pneumonia
- asthma
- whooping cough (*terentene*)
- rheumatism
- appendicitis
- hernia
- cataracts (smoke in the eyes from old age)
- diabetes (*sugáru hítu*, literally, sugar blood)
- stroke
- high blood pressure (*inuiti hítu*, literally, high blood)
- syphilis
- club foot
- glaucoma
- flu
- tumor

Terms which were employed only by the Garinagu, that is, diagnostic terms which were not recognized by biomedical personnel, included the following:

- *impacho* - an illness in which the baby's belly swells; it is considered to be *lisándi ubaó*
- *costipo* - a sickness which is more or less serious depending on the individual with whom illness is being discussed. In general, it refers to a "head cold"
- *húmo* - an illness in small children caused by the smell of certain fish. It is sometimes referred to as a natural illness and on other occasions treated as a sickness caused by spirits.

- *hasándigubida* - an illness (symptoms may vary considerably) which is brought by the *gubida* or ancestors
- *fiáfia* - an illness characterized by swelling of the body, caused by *obeah* or *idáhadu*
- *alima alu tuagubi* ("She has a sickness of the spirit) - refers to any spirit-caused sickness. Spirits may be "of the water" or "of the land." The phrase "*Nuagubi uinani*" translates as "I have a devil on me" and refers to a sickness caused by an evil spirit.
- *labuhanuanbadi*, or mole drop - an illness of infants characterized by vomiting, diarrhea, and sunken fontanelle. Generally diagnosed by biomedical personnel as gastroenteritis.
- *obeah* - in many cases where it was suspected that an illness was caused by intentional actions of another, the term *obeah* was used to refer to the ultimate cause of the illness but was used as the diagnostic label as well. The same was true for illnesses thought to be caused by *idáhadu*.

This is not meant to serve as a complete list of all complaints which may be presented to the healer or to other concerned individuals. It serves as a general indicator of the broad range of signs which may be presented and illustrates that illnesses are almost always described in terms of their symptoms and signs, that is the objective and subjective representamens, rather than through use of a diagnostic label. Additional comments offered during the course of discussions about illness will be found in Appendix A.

Generating Signs

The subjective signs presented by the patient may provide the healer with sufficient information to offer both diagnosis and therapy, but the healer makes his own observations and, where necessary, generates his own signs, that is, produces signs which otherwise would have remained 'invisible.' It is important to note that the word used to describe uncommon illnesses, *wamálisian*, also means "things which are not visible." While both common and uncommon illnesses may produce objective signs, it is up to the knowledgeable healer to generate the signs which indicate the true nature of the illness.

If you think someone has been *obeahed* you can burn wild garlic and ask the individual to stand in the middle of the smoke; he will feel a reaction like something loose off of him. You can tell who caused the *obeah* with a deck of cards.

(The midwife may check her patient's condition by "feeling inside" called sounding or pressing; the technique calls for external examination only). I can tell from this whether it is womb business or ovaries.

The main pulse is in the stomach and it can be felt through external examination. Feel the main pulse and the pulse in the wrist. If the pulse in the stomach is normal, the wrist pulse will be normal. Sometimes the pulse in the stomach is too high and inflamed.

The inside pulse must work with the main pulse. There is a third pulse next to the eyes, along the bridge of the nose. If that pulse is fast, you will have a headache. Sometimes the belly pulse swells and a woman can't have a baby. When it is examined, it beats harder than the pulse in the arm. The woman can't eat.

Sounding will also tell if someone has an inside cold. Feel something in abdomen, but it isn't hard. Ask the patient if he or she has a discharge.

If the bone at the joint of the ribs is bent down (determined by sounding), it will cause coughing, vomiting, pain, and other feelings.

The vein that runs through the body can be examined by sounding the abdomen. If the vein passes through the womb, the vein is not in condition and your whole body hurt you. Can also feel knots like grains of corn in the veins. Sometimes the patient says she feels the vein in the knee biting. Vein is not correct, but the vein in the abdomen is the cause.

Sometimes people are troubled by evil spirits. People may say they are troubled or worried, but they don't know why. I can tell certain things through dreams. If someone who cannot sleep dreams of snakes it is an omen of evil spirits. I give medicine and tell the patient to return in one week. I can't give him an answer right away. I need time to think about it. The answer will come to me later.

You can tell if a bad spirit is on someone. You get one candle and rum. Put the rum in the person's hair. Rub the candle in the left hand. Make the sign of Christ. The noise made by the flame of the candle is the sign of the enemy. The direction of the flame tells who the enemy is.

You have to bring rum, a candle, and holy water to diagnose. You swear to the candle three times. You have to mention the name of the protector. If the candle comes down three times, it means the person has a bad spirit. An animal is following her.

People only have to tell me how they feel. I will know what's wrong. I can tell them I will use herbs to cure them. No physical exam is necessary. I was born with this power. If the illness is there for a long time, I can't treat it.

You touch the head or neck to feel for fever or pulsation.

If a man suspects a woman may have V.D., he can put lime juice on his penis and as he enters her, she will cry out in pain.

You can burn candles and look at the flame of the candle to see how it behaves. When the wind is not blowing it should keep steady. Sometimes when it is calm the flame will move. When it moves, there is an enemy or someone trying to harm you.

To diagnose *idáhadu* you must use two candles, one red and one white. The red one is from Guatemala. Sometimes the white candle cannot tell; the red candle is more powerful. If both move, you have an enemy who is working against you.

Diagnosis and the Assignment of Meaning to Signs

In some cases, the sign-interpretant relationship is determinant; that is, the objective and subjective representamens which are produced are clearly linked to an interpretant. This relationship further specifies or is specified by an object or objects, thus completing the triadic relationship which constituted the sign. More commonly, however, the healer must search for additional information. In the absence of other signs or when it is not possible to produce all the necessary signs, the therapist may attempt a therapy. A successful resolution to the case will indicate to the therapist that his assumptions were correct and will allow him to establish an etiology for the illness. The object, once determined, generally specifies an etiology, though it may be necessary to move regressively in order to identify additional objects, often from other cause-effect domains. That is, there may, on the one hand, be an immediate cause, or what I will refer to as an immediate object, but there may as well be one or more additional objects, any of which may be, in Peirce's terminology, the dynamical object, or, in anthropological terms, the ultimate cause. The interpretant which is produced by the healer may serve as diagnostic label. The entire triadic relationship comes to possess 'meaning' which is consistent with the broader paradigms of the society and is appropriate in a social, cultural, political, personal, and historic sense.

As seen previously, dreams play an important role in the therapist's determination of treatment. The dreams of patients may be analyzed as well in the search for additional signs which will allow for the completion of the triadic semiotic relationship. In many cases, the meaning assigned dreams may be fairly consistent across therapists. For example, to dream of someone who is attempting to harm you implies that you have an enemy. The appearance of an ancestor generally indicates that the ancestor is dissatisfied and wishes to make a request. Other dreams may refer to coming wealth, success, failure, death, and so on. The following interpretations of dreams were offered by Garifuna healers:

If they say they dream of a man running after me it is a sign of an enemy. I say to them, "let me see if I can help you by boiling bush." The enemy acts on the nerves. This is not a common illness. It is *wámalisian*.

Dreams about a snake biting your foot - means you have an enemy. I use *waiúri*, *lamúru*, *garlic titíe*, *cow foot leaf*, garlic.

Dreams about fighting means you have an enemy or somebody is talking about you - *idáhadu*. I treat them for *idáhadu*. I use cedar bark, take it off the tree, boil with garlic, *garlic títle, waiuri, cow foot, lamúru* and use it to bathe them.

If you dream of traveling in a boat, it means death is coming closer. The boat is a coffin. It means sickness will be on you or death is coming. Not necessary to bathe with the bush. I tell the patient to be careful.

Climbing a hill. This means you are a success in life if it is a clear bush. If it is a thick bush, it means something wrong is coming to you.

Dream of catching a big fish. It means somebody is going to die. I advise that there will be a death in the family or it will be a good friend.

Falling into a hole and cannot get back. This is a sure grave. Sooner or later you will be down there.

Running in your sleep means success in life.

Lose one of your teeth means a death in the family. There is no remedy or prevention.

Kissing. This means that an enemy is talking about you.

Bathing in unclean water. This means you will meet with bad luck. There is no protection from this.

Bathing in clear water means success in life.

Picking up money means failure in life. Nothing can be done.

Sometimes people are troubled by evil spirits. People may say they are troubled or worried but they don't know why. I can tell certain things through dreams. If someone who cannot sleep dreams of snakes it is an omen of evil spirits. I give medicine and tell the patient to return in one week. I can't give him an answer right away. I need time to think about it. The answer will come to me later (see page 141).

If your illness results from *idáhadu* you will dream of fire coming towards you. The direction of the flames will tell you where the words are coming from.

Sometimes you will dream that a relative is advising you to stay off the streets. Carib women are taught as soon as they have menstruation, they should stay home after five P.M. The blood draws spirits. These women don't always pay attention.

If you dream of happiness it means you will have a good job or a happy marriage. You will be successful in life.

You may dream that you have an enemy. If this happens, you should go to your enemy and find out what you did to him. Most of the time that solves the problem.

Sometimes people dream a spirit is attacking them. I give them a little medicine. The medicine I give is to ease the tension of their nerves.

Some of the most significant dreams are of deceased ancestors.

If my father wants something I will dream dreams beyond expectation and if I do not pay any attention I will feel the symptoms of an illness. You go to the doctor and the doctor can't cure you. You see an herbalist and don't get better. You must go to a *búiai*. He makes incantations and his chief messenger makes contact with the spirit world. He may say your father wants to have communication with you. In five minutes or so, your father's spirit will arrive if you agree to speak with him. If you have never met him he will introduce himself. If you know him you will recognize his voice. He will say what he wants. Perhaps all he wants is a mass.

I may dream of my sister with a towel and a calabash and a comb going to the river. It is clear that she wants a bath (the "bathing of a dead person's spirit").

If you dream of a dead relative, it means he wants a sacrifice, a mass or food offering.

Some illnesses are defined clearly by a constellation of signs (representamens) which appear simultaneously or sequentially. The therapist must know precisely what to look for in these cases. However, more commonly, signs are indeterminate. Different healers may provide different interpretations of identical signs. Context, as always, is an important variable. Among those linkages between representamen(s) and interpretants offered by healers were the following:

If the patient has biliousness, he will vomit out yellow stuff or pass it in his stool. Biliousness can also be seen in the eyes; the eyes turn yellow.

A yellow rim at the lower edge of the eyeball indicates a woman has venereal disease.

Too much blood will cause a headache over the whole head and a feeling of discomfort. The patient may also hemorrhage through his nose.

When the blood is low, the patient will complain of being tired, of being short of breath, of feeling weak and light in the head. An examination reveals that the tongue is white and the rims of the eyes are white. The fingernails will be pale.

Pimples inside the rim of the eye indicate the patient has been working in too much heat.

A baby with asthma will have a whistling in his stomach from the age of seven to eight months.

The signs of diabetes show on the body. You may get a scratch and it grows. You will want to eat sugar. Then the body begins to reduce.

The signs of high blood pressure are pain in the back of the head and neck and all over the shoulder.

Typhoid fever comes from other countries. You will have a strong, high fever and a headache. Then you will develop dysentery and diarrhea.

Sometimes when a child has worms, he will have fits (*ówehani*) and a stiff-eye look (*adéirahani*).

Biliousness will lead to giddiness. You will vomit yellow stuff. In the stool you will see brownish mucus with a little white. The eyes will turn yellow. Bilousness is from too much drinking.

Worms. The signs are a finger in the nose scratching, during sleep the teeth will be grinding, the belly may show.

Inside cold. Yellow lumps of mucus in the stool.

Inside cold. You will find something by sounding in the lower abdomen. It is not hard. You will ask if she has a discharge and how it looks and how she feels.

Tuberculosis causes a dry cough.

Pregnancy can be diagnosed in the early weeks by complaints of the patient: vomiting, a bad feeling, the loss of appetite, and the absence of a period.

An *ariunun* will cause your belly to swell. A woman with an *ariunun* won't be able to have a baby. You will know you had an *ariunun* if you pass a black thing in the stool.

Costipo is a certain disease in the head. There is mucus in the head and in the brain. When you blow you nose, the mucus smells bad.

You can tell an ulcer in the stomach because you will feel the pain and then the pain will disappear and then it will come back again.

If a child has a big belly, you must ask for his age. If he has passed one year, it is likely that it is worms. Condensed milk causes worms, as does meat.

With *húmo*, the signs are a slight fever, then it goes to a high fever, then you will notice the skin – the outer part of the body broke out with little bumps. Then the child begins to tremble (*adádaguruni*), has no appetite or will not take the breast, then you notice the mouth which begins to show red signs, then the stool turns green and waterish; then the crotch turns red. Then the stomach will be hard and the baby will feel discomfort and begin to bawl during the day and night. This is the order in which the signs of *húmo* appear.

In the illness caused by *idáhadu*, the hair falls out gradually, and the victim gets paler and paler. He can't sleep at night, he dreams a person has been throwing stones at him, running after him, wrestle and throw him down on the ground. You may dream that the person who is behind you will prepare food for you and set is on the table for you. If you eat the food you are in her hands. You will dream that there is smoke in your house.

In the illness called *fiáfia*, the belly begins to swell; in three days it will affect your heart. You will have diarrhea, vomiting, and sometimes you will go crazy.

Hasándigubída is the sickness of the dead spirit. The person who is affected may say words like a crazy person; he begins to laugh, talk alone, rock in the hammock, and use songs he has heard from the *gubída*. They say he is out of his senses.

The woman fell on the way to the well and she was unconscious when she fell. That is also a sign of the *gubída*.

In illnesses caused by *uináni*, the body is not active. All kinds of sickness comes in, like fever and pain, headache, and sometimes the victim is unable to move about. The doctor at the hospital may say, "We have no remedy for you, you had better look for another doctor."

In many of the cases encountered by the healer, the signs presented or produced may be referrable to more than one process and the healer must gather additional information regarding the context in which these signs appeared or must generate additional signs. As stated previously, the therapy itself may possess the potential to generate the representamens which allow for the production of one or more objects. The biomedical therapist thus often serves, in his very failure to "cure", to produce the signs or representamens which cause the therapy managing group to consider moving the illness to a different domain of cause-effect relationships and to move the patient to a different practitioner (see, for example, the Cowo case study in the following chapter).

If the healer is to continue in his service as "moral agent" and perpetuator of the basic medical paradigm, the interpretive decisions which are ultimately rendered must conform to those explanatory principles available within the four domains of illness causation. They must, moreover, be supportive of the socially constructed reality which is the Garifuna universe. They must function to regulate social and spiritual relationships. And they must serve to legitimate the role of the healer and to provide the authority for future decisions. The 'meanings' assigned to signs, that is, the full triadic relationship, are generated by what Coehlo calls "implicit principles" (1955:259) and what Hadel describes not as a world view, but an "event-orientation toward reality" (1972:81). Such an orientation includes a belief in the general orderliness of the world, an order which is ultimately determined by God but much affected by other spirits, the gradualness of processes, the concept of reciprocity, or, as Coehlo puts it, a "balance in the relations between the members of society and in those that are established between the group and the supernatural powers" (260) and an emphasis on the development of the characteristics of wisdom, caution, consideration, respect, and optimism. The world is dangerous only if one does not know and abide by certain behavioral rules. These rules or "codes" include the maintenance of a respectful attitude towards those who are the senior members of society, in particular deceased ancestors, care in one's relationships with other Garifuna people, and avoidance of extremes in work, in pleasure, and in interactions with the natural environment.

Though orderliness, wisdom, circumspection, and respect are emphasized as positive characteristics, the Garinagu cannot be described as significantly inhibited in their personal actions by the requirement that they exhibit these qualities. "In some respects", says Hadel, they "do not just live life, they attack it" (1972:87).

For them – as I suspect for any people who must devote the greater part of their lives to filling subsistence needs – life is not something to be contemplated in repose; there is no time for that. Rather, life is to be fought for, it is to be won. Reality is not static; it is dynamic, always moving like the sea which has traditionally fronted every Carib village and town. And so a Carib does not, he cannot, merely view the world; he must take a stance, a posture toward it. He must act and react (79).

Coehlo stresses the

...practical character of their morals...their abhorence of everything that depresses vital processes, and conversely, their appreciation of all that enhances the plentitude of living, [and] their belief that to be joyful is not only the natural state of man, but constitutes a kind of obligation.... (258).

The "moral value of suffering", Coehlo adds, is a concept not to be found among the Garinagu. The acceptance of responsibility for illness serves as a guide to future behaviors, not as a significant source of guilt for past actions.

Coehlo continues:

Melancholy... is distrusted, since, according to a generalized belief, it is conducive to antisocial feelings and acts....

And later, he states:

It should not be presumed...that the Black Carib deny themselves any outward emotional expression; on the contrary, their whole life is tinged by affect. Emotion is not given unbridled license, but neither is it suppressed; rather it is channeled... From the moment of his birth, the Black Carib finds himself in a culturally well-defined position, and in the course of his life, he moves to a successive series of well-defined sets of rights and obligations. But the culture provides a number of alternatives for him to choose from, so that his adjustment is not achieved through partial psychic self-destruction (263-64).

The basic tenets of the Garifuna medical model both derive from and give validity to this general understanding of the universe and relationships among all things which inhabit it.

Therapeutic Interventions

The patient or afflicted individual or therapy managing group is not without resources in the attempt to control interpretive decisions. The fulfullment of the sign relationship may be influenced through presentation of signs, reporting of context, and the choice of therapist.

...clients, by choosing practitioners and specialities, pre-determine the technical course of sickness episodes, that is, the technophenomenological events that are subsequently materialized, the etiological arguments that are raised and the moral claims that are eventually examined and negotiated (Young 1982:28-29).

The afflicted individual or responsible family member may serve as both diagnostician and therapist. The vast majority of Garinagu utilize both bush and patent medicines or prepared ingredients purchased at the local pharmacy or from one of the many dry goods stores in their search for 'health' or relief from suffering. Both are utilized to prevent illnesses as well as to treat them. During the course of interviews with healers, herbalists, patients, and household members I obtained the names of one-hundred and seventy-eight patent or herbal medicines or components of *arana* (medicines) used by the Garinagu. Of these, ninety-nine or fifty-nine percent are the names of herbs, roots, or some portion or product of a plant; sixteen or ten percent are 'natural' products or are used principally in conjunction with other bush medicines, and fifty-three or thirty-one percent are patent medicines or medicines which are largely justified by a biomedical model. Of the items in the latter category, the uses to which they were put is as follows:[1]

18 Tonic, to give strength, for nutrition
10 External use only; massage, localized pain, heat in body, sores, bruises, wounds
6 Purge
6 Pain, generalized
5 Fever
4 Internal or external use; soothing, healing, pain, cold, fever
3 Upset stomach, pain in stomach
2 Worms
2 Pressure
1 Cough
1 Loose stools
1 Heart, palpitations, gas around the heart
1 "Women's problems"
1 Undetermined

These 'medications', unlike most "bush", generally are thought to have a single use. They are normally not combined with other medicines, though any may be used simultaneously with either doctor or bush medicines. Approximately forty-five percent are used for prevention of illness, if both tonics and purges are included in this category. The remainder are most commonly used for the relief of symptoms and are not, with some exceptions, regarded as a cure. Of these fifty-three items, only two were mentioned by healers as components of their medicines (See Appendix B for list of preparations.) In general, they are regarded as neither especially powerful nor dangerous. Some are utilized for the relief of symptoms in chronic illnesses which have not been effectively or satisfactorily dealt with by either the physician or healer. Most are regarded as effective for the purposes to which they are put, but none are utilized to treat illnesses which are regarded as serious. For that, one generally turns to a professional – either the bush doctor or the physician.

Of the one-hundred and eight herbs, roots, and other components of what is commonly referred to as "bush medicine", forty-six were mentioned by healers alone. This list, lengthy though it may appear, constitutes only a partial list of all "bush" medicines. Cosminsky, during her fieldwork in 1965 and 1975, collected the names of approximately eighty botanical items. Of these eighty, only thirty-three appear on my list, while, in turn, approximately sixty names of botanical items which I collected do not appear on Cosminsky's list, indicating that there may well be several hundred herbs, roots, and other plant products known to and used by the Garinagu of Punta Gorda. Appendix C contains a list of the various bush utilized by healers and laymen in Punta Gorda and some of the uses to which they are put.

The following methods of administering medicines and therapeutic techniques are utilized:

– Ingestion of medicines
  Give the baby a chupon to suck on. Put in garlic, oil, cloves and other medicines.
  Cow foot leaf tea helps the heart because it helps the blood to flow freely.
  Use *fever grass* for tea. It helps the system. Foreign tea may cause constipation.
  Pepper is good for high blood pressure.
  Red Lavinda is for the heart.
  Use *trumpet leaf* with *garlic titie* for cough.
  Give *pasote* for fever and pain in the stomach.
– Ingested, emetic
  Gahela leaf with *guava* is taken to make you vomit
– Inhalation of vapors
  Inhale hot vapors for a head cold
– Inhalation of liquids
  Breathe in salt water to dry out the sinuses
– External application
  Put *maliba* on your head for a headache.
  Mash *ganabise* and apply to the skin for itch.
  Siwapat leaf in warm water is applied for pain in joints
  Vinegar with warm water and salt. Soak and it takes the heat out of the body.
– External massage/manipulation
  For a fresh cold, noint the neck and chest so they pass the cold.
  For tonsils, give coconut oil or pomade, along with massage.
  For sprain, massage with pomade or soft candle wax.
  Low uterus or twisted uterus; use olive oil for nointing. Move it back into place with nointing.
– Insertion of medications
  For an earache, use sweet oil inserted into the ear.
  If a baby is in the wrong position, you pour olive oil into her [the mother] and then you turn her. When you turn her back again, the baby will be turned as well.
– Suction
  When a baby has a lot of mucus from a cold, someone will suck it out and then spit out the mucus.
  If a baby has a sunken mole, you can suck on the mole and push on the palate until it comes up.
– Gargling/washing out the mouth
  Wash mouth with honey, salt and water for pimples in the mouth.
  Wash mouth with alum and gargle with it. This heals sores in the mouth.
– Bathing (for both common and uncommon illnesses)
  For sores, bathe in the sea. Use *makakao leaf*. This makes your skin smooth.
  Sores on body caused by *obeah*. Bathe in certain bush medicines in hot water in the middle of a room on Tuesday and Fridays.
  Obeah/evil spirits. Bathe in water which has been prepared with *wild garlic*, *flor de muerte*, and *essence root*.
  For *idahadu*, bathe with water prepared from *cedar bark*, *garlic titie*, *wariuri*, *cow foot leaf*, *lamuru*.
– Prayers
  Idahadu can be cured with the right prayers.
  When there are evil spirits, I bathe the patient with herbs, but I tell them to read the Bible more often.

- Dialogue

  Heart trouble can come from vexation. You must talk with the patient, advise them. Vexation can cause fainting away if you don't speak your mind to someone.
- Smoking with incense and other natural materials

  For *humo* you apply medicines to body for a few days. Then burn incense to make sure all of the sickness is gone.

  Oudlice is burned to keep the spirits away

  Conch shell - it stinks and gets rid of evil spirits.
- Use of objects without contact with the body.

  Tie a black thread to a white candle and mention the name of the person who is harming you. She or he will have to stop.
- Bleeding

  I prefer to let myself bleed sometimes. That way the body makes new blood which is better than the old blood.

The techniques which are most commonly employed by healers, in order of their frequency, are: ingestion of medicines, external application of medicines, massage or nointing, and bathing. Certain administrative modes and diagnostic techniques employed by the hospital, most specifically the use of intravenous fluids, injections, diagnostic tests which involve drawing off blood, and X-rays, represent control over resources not available within the Garifuna medical model.

Principles of Intervention

Beyond the principles or codes which govern the assignment of signs of illness to a category of cause-effect relationships and determine or partially determine the therapy to be employed, there are certain principles which all healers appear to accept in their therapeutic interventions.

1. Healers almost always caution against the use of bush and doctor medicines simultaneously. One healer explained that one is raw and the other processed and for this reason they may act against one another. Several healers felt that bush medicine was better than doctor medicine and if the appropriate bush were known and could be otained, it should be utilized first. Only lack of knowledge and access thus prohibited healers from treating a wider range of illnesses. On the other hand, other healers believed there were times when doctor medicine was superior and all advised their patients to consult the doctor for certain illnesses. Some expressed the belief that much knowledge about bush had been lost.

2. More than one method of intervention/mode of administration may be utilized at the same time for the same illness. For example, several healers reported giving oral medications and utilizing massage or 'nointing' simultaneously. The use of both baths and 'smoking' of patients is employed in cases of certain natural (i.e., *húmo*) and unnatural illnesses.

3. The weakest medicine may be used first, if not effective a stronger medicine may be employed. One healer stated, for example, "If there is an enemy trying to harm you, I will treat with *waiúri*, *lamúru*, and cedar bark. If this doesn't work, then I will apply *mangrove* or *crabu*.

4. One medicine may be thought of as more powerful than others or one may assist the others to work. For example:

You can use *gánabis root* and *gánabis leaf* with *sorasee* and epsom salts for cold in the stomach and also for dysentery. Certain herbs are stronger, but products like epsom salts and *senna* are *used as helpers*.

Garlic titie helps other bush to cure the sick. Without that it cannot help. *Garlic titie* is the *king of all plants*. It is used *to help all the plants develop a scent*

If you use three medicines, don't use four. You can use five. If you have eight medicines, you must add a ninth. You must always have an odd number because the *referee must be there to keep medicines from working against one another. The medicines work according to how they work with a partner or partners.*

5. Amounts of medication are adjusted to suit the needs of the patient. One woman, for example, stated she had tried *hammond's leaf* because she had heard it was good for high blood pressure. She fainted and was hospitalized for low blood pressure. She stated that one had to know how much of a medicine to take. The healers, she added, knew how much to give. A bush doctor/midwife added this comment.

If you drink too much *sorasee* you will get a hemorrhage from the nose from too much blood. Sorasee increases the amount of blood. You must know how much to use.

6. The techniques of preparation are important. As can be seem from the following, however, these techniques vary across healers.

When I prepare medicines, I use Carib prayers. They aren't prayers from the church. Still, I pray to the Good Lord. Once I used holy water from the church, but the important thing is the faith in the way you do it. The Lord knows you are trying to help someone (E).

Garlic titie must be boiled in a particular way if you are trying to drive away evil. But I can't tell you that (E).

It is essential to use holy water from the church when you make certain medicines. You can get that on Good Fridays. You can use it yourself to keep spirits away (A).

I prepare the medicines according to the sickness. If a person come today to be treated, I have to pick the herbs today. The person can come the following day. The medicine got to sleep overnight. It can't cure on the same day (A).

I use prayers and candles. The prayers are Spanish prayers and prayers from the Catholic Church. I may use Hail Marys. I also use Holy Water (I).

You get a can to boil. Before you light your candle, you put a broad leaf in the bottom of the can. You ask the patient for a nickle or a dime. If they don't have a dime you use a nickle. You put that as an offering for the spirit of the bush. After that you go slowly and pull leaves off the vine of *garlic titie*. Put the leaves in the can. Save the vine without the leaves. Put this aside. Then bring *lamúru* on top as second one. Then *waiúri* on top as third one. *Cow foot* is the bed, then money, then *garlic titie*, then *lamúru*, then *waiúri*. Then at the end, take a few leaves of *cow foot*, break them into small pieces and add them to the can. Then get a wider leaf of *cow foot* as a cover. Take two pieces of *garlic titie* vine and place them on top in the form of a cross. Then use water from the well or pipe but not water from the roof. Master says roof water won't work. Put in the water, then out your candle. Proceed to the fire hut. Boil until the scent of it spreads. Five minutes before bathing, put the water into a pail. Sit down and look at your shadow in the pail. [Direction is to patient]. This brings up the picture [iaua] and helps the patient by driving part of the sickness away (B).

You have to dry the medicines well or they will turn black. Sometimes I pray to the Blessed Virgin Mother to help in making medicines. I don't use holy water. I use one "our father", one "hail Mary" and make the sign of the cross (C).

Wash the root, cut it to proper size and split it. Tie down and leave until you get nine bundles. Then boil it. When it is boiled down by half, strain it on a piece of clean cloth (C).

7. Both the body and the medicines, being natural phenomena, may work in conjunction with other natural phenomena.

Medicines should be picked at certain times; you must watch the tide. You must know the correct hour. The medicine shrinks back if cut at the wrong time.

There is a medicine to ease cramps till the flow starts, but all this has to do with the tide.

Worm medicine should be taken when the moon is three days old. I have read in science that creeping insects and insects inside move together with the moon. There is no treatment for worms during a full moon.

The position of the moon is important when you pull *gánabis* root. You pull it the day after a new moon appears. You start from the north side of the tree and pull it until you get to the last point. There is just a little medicine in the point at the end of the tree. Get all you want till maybe next year.

You may get pregnant by the moon. If you have your period at the time of the new moon, then you have contact with a man five to six days later, you will become pregnant.

Some sicknesses you are born with, like when you are crippled or can't sleep. Some say that the moon affects them depending on when they are brought forth.[2]

8. One medicine may be effective in the treatment of a number of illnesses or symptoms. Conversely, an illness may be treated with more than one medicine.

9. As a general rule, illnesses which are classified as *lisándi ubaó* and which are 'internal' are treated with ingested medicines; natural illnesses which are manifested externally may be treated with ingested medicines or external applications of medicines, depending on the assigned cause. If possible, the affected part of the body is treated directly in most cases. Injuries, "twisted veins", etc. are most commonly treated through massage and external applications of medicines. Bathing may be employed in either natural or uncommon illnesses. If the illness is worldly, then only the affected part may be bathed, whereas if the illness is uncommon the entire body is bathed. "Smoking" is used almost exclusively for uncommon illnesses or illnesses in which it is thought spirits may 'linger about' and perhaps inhibit full recovery. Common illnesses almost always require treatments which act directly upon the body, that is, the body or some affected part or some component is the focus of the treatment. In uncommon illnesses, the healer may take no action which has a direct effect upon the body (see, for example, section on *dugu* which follows). This is not to say that such treatments do not alter the patient's

physiology, but, rather, the cause-effect relationship (therapy-alteration in physiology) is less obvious.

10. One sign may have several interpretations and the physician must differentiate among several possible diagnoses. For example, one healer said that a complaint of "cold in the private parts" might be either V.D. or an inside cold.

I get a white cloth or piece of paper and let it [the discharge] drip on it. If it is white it is an inside cold. If it is yellow it is V.D.

11. Etiological and diagnostic shifting are possible responses of the healer in cases where the individual fails to cure. However, it is more likely that other explanations will be sought which justify the healer's original diagnosis or diagnostic techniques.

Q. What would you do if you gave medicine to someone and they returned to say they hadn't been helped.

A. I would tell them they hadn't described their symptoms to me correctly, so we would have to find the real symptoms.

Where a cure is not effected, a common therapeutic technique is to repeat the entire treatment.

In cases of *húmo*, you apply the medicines for a few days and burn incense to make sure all of the sickness is gone. Then you pay them a visit and see if they are feeling better. If they are not, you repeat the bath once more.

Give 1/2 to 1 glass each day until two bottles are finished. Then check the eyes again. If the eyes are still pale, she need one to two more bottles.

But it is also not unusual for the healer to change the therapy. This does not necessitate a 'diagnostic' or 'etiological shift.' Rather, it requires only the recognition that one medicine may not be as effective as another in the treatment of the same illness and the medicine's effectiveness may vary according to the patient's constitution.

I may use one medicine. If that doesn't work, then I try another, just like the doctor.

Most healers qualify their initial statement of competence and control over the signs of illness by saying "I think I can help you."

12. Healers will frequently advise patients to see a physician.

You may feel a tumor in a woman in the stomach entirely. Lots of women suffer from that here. I tell them to see the doctor.

If they say they have a fever, I send them to the doctor for an injection. In most cases, I recommend to the mother of a baby that she take the baby to the doctor first.

If it is tonsils, I have medicine for it, but I send them to the doctor first.

The treatment for hernia is to have an operation.

When a woman is pregnant, sometimes all the body swell. When she gets into labor, she gets fits. The kidney causes this. This is bad trouble. You must take her to the doctor.

13. Prevention of illness is a major function of healers. Healers often provide advice on ways in which sickness can be prevented. They counsel care in relationships with other living people and care in relationships with deceased ancestors. They may advise that you speak with an enemy or suggest, on the

basis of the interpretation of a dream, that an ancestor wishes to have a mass or a bath (*amuiadahani*, "dead man's bath"). In general, only *búiai*s can advise on the need for a *chugu* or *dugu*, but the healer may suggest that the patient seek assistance from a *búiai*. They may suggest that individuals avoid hard work and practice habits of cleanliness and "tidiness." They may encourage individuals to get their rest and "to eat properly" (see Palacio 1982 on notions of what constitutes a proper diet) and to avoid certain foods. Establishment of an etiology which involves carelessness itself constitutes a recommendation to engage in, or not engage in, certain behaviors. Healers believe that one's bad or evil thoughts can come to rest on the individual himself and that failure to express one's self or to discuss problems with others can also cause illness. They caution against such attitudes. Finally, healers offer a wide range of medicines or treatments which are directed to preventing *obeah* (*abiñariguile*) or misfortune caused by evil spirits. Such techniques or medicines are reported in previous sections and in the interviews with healers to follow.

14. Healers do not offer explicit theories concerning the manner in which medicines work or the reasons for their effectiveness. Other researchers have stated that Garifuna healers believe each bush to have its own spirit (see Cosminsky 1976MS). However, of the seven Garifuna healers I interviewed, only one made reference to the "spirit of the bush" (see above). When another healer was asked why the "liquid" in some plants is effective in healing while in others it is not, he replied:"Well, that's nature's work." And when asked why the boiling of one component of a bush medicine gave it efficacy, he said: "I don't know. Perhaps the boiling brings the scent from it." A healer trained by a *búiai* stated that he did not understand why his medicines worked.

Some unstated principles emerge, however, from further examination of the medicines and the uses to which they are put.

a. Some medicines are efficacious because they have desirable characteristics, characteristics which are assumed by or transmitted to the patient during therapy. For example, cabbage bark is said to be good for poor blood because it turns red when boiled. It may be the same principle which governs the use of "bitters" for diabetes which is diagnosed by tasting the urine for sugar.
b. At the same time, certain medicines are believed to work because spirits are assumed to have certain human characteristics. Thus a variety of things which have an unpleasant odor (conch shell, *garlic titíe*, *essence root*, *flor de muerte*, and others) or which cause irritation (*haliwaya*) can be used to drive evil spirits away. In like manner, the *gubída* are placated by offering them things which they most desired as living persons.
c. Some medicines work because they alter the 'temperature' of the body, resulting in an appropriate balance between heat and cold. The medicine for dysentery is said to work like rum by "heating the blood." *Ganábis* or *caro* can be used in cases of high blood pressure to remove the heat in the blood. "Getting into a temper" was said to lead to heat in the head; *skagineal* was used to "draw out the heat." Herbs are recommended to "cool off the brain" when there is "heat in the head." Corn water

acts as a "coolant for the system." And so on. There were also medicines which acted directly on a lesion or growth because of their temperature. Thus salt was said to "cook up sores" and pepper was reported to "burn the root of appendicitis" and to work on cancer in a like manner.

d. Certain medicines or therapies were thought to work on the body in a mechanical way. For example, purging was used to "cut loose boils and worms", herbs were used in dropsy to "scrape the bag of the sickness" and there was said to be "something like lime" in the young pineapple which "cuts through cold."
e. To control body fluids, secretions or products was equivalent to controlling or curing sickness. Hence, many medicines were thought to work because they altered these body components. Several patent and bush medicines were said to clean or purify the blood; *cow foot leaf* was thought to keep the blood flowing freely; certain medicines strengthened the blood, an action which appears to be equivalent to increasing the amount of blood; herbs were used to cause the body to pass an "inside cold", emetics were used to cause vomiting of "biliousness", chupons to allow the baby to pass "black" stool, bleeding to allow the body to replace old blood with new, and so on.
f. A few medicines appear to be utilized because they exacerbate existing symptoms and thus 'cure' the illness. For example, certain medicines were used as emetics in cases of nausea or biliousness, and herbs like *flor de muerte* were said to cure fever by causing the patient to sweat a lot.

Interviews with Four Healers

In this section I present information obtained from four Garifuna healers on recruitment to the role of healer, the importance of dreams in the production of knowledge about curing, and certain underlying assumptions or experiences which govern their therapeutic interventions and interpretive decisions.

Mrs. Castro

Mrs. Castro is an elderly midwife and healer whose brother describes her as "gifted." She no longer delivers babies because of her advancing age and government laws which prohibit deliveries by unlicensed midwives. Pregnant women and women with small children still seek her out, however, for pre-natal and post-natal care. Mrs. Castro says she can remember the days when there was no doctor and no hospital.

In the old days, before there was a hospital, Rosa Zuniga had a big house near the front. The front has eroded away since that time. There used to be houses toward the sea where the sea is now. Rosa Zuniga set up her house as a hospital. Babies were delivered there and people were treated for illnesses there. In those days we didn't know about this illness called diabetes. Only nowadays when doctors tell us about it and show us these things. It might have been there, but we don't know it. Then we only have our own people as doctors.

I asked how she had learned her medicines and how she had learned to deliver babies.

I learned some things from my parents. I learned some things about midwifery from a doctor, but I can't go with the doctor [because of the law]. I was delivering babies in town privately but the government wanted me to go to Belize for training to get a license. But I couldn't go because I would have to leave my children. My husband was dead, so I couldn't go for studies.

But much of her knowledge has been obtained through dreams.

When a patient would come to me with a difficult case, I would dream all the herbs to use. I would mix them up and they got well, even when hospital cure didn't work. A white nurse appears to me sometimes in dreams. The nurse would ask "Well, what have you found?" I would answer: "I don't know." Then the nurse would answer, "Yes, you do", and would show me which herbs to use and how to prepare them.

She emphasized the importance of the 'veins' and 'pulses' of the body in both diagnosis and therapy.

There are three pulses in the body. The true pulse is at the heart. There is one in the arm and one in the belly. You must check all of them.

If a woman complains of pain in the legs it is the veins which run through the foot or leg or body. You must examine this vein through the abdomen. If the vein passes through the womb it is not in condition. Your whole body will hurt you. The cause is in the womb. I start nointing from the big toe, along the foot. Then I lift up the womb. I can feel knots like grains of corn in the veins. Others try nointing, but it looks like they don't know how to do it properly. Sometimes you will feel the vein in the knee biting you. The vein is not correct. But up here [the abdomen] is the cause.

The technique of 'nointing' or massage plays an important role in many of her therapeutic interventions.

Sometimes gas from the stomach goes under the heart and stirs the heart. I treat gas in the stomach. A lady came to me pregnant, and said she felt like her heart would come out, that the baby had gone up to her chest. She felt weak and had vomited. I began to massage on her toes, work up on her foot and leg. I massage her head, over the top of her head, and hold the veins[3] on either side of the spinal cord. Then I massage down her back, push up her ribs on the side and around to the front. I find the wind under her ribs. I hold it and worry with it. Then she belch, belch, and then she feel good(see also p. 107 for additional comments on wind and relationship to water and blood).

Sometimes if someone have pain in the stomach, I must check the bone at the joint of the ribs. It might be bent down. This would cause coughing, vomiting, pain, and other feelings. I have the person lie on her belly. Then I massage on the back up to the neck. Then I put her to her side and noint to the side. Then I take my knee and noint her tailbone way to the neck. but not touching the main joint of the spine, only along the sides. I get to the ribs and lift the ribs up until you can put a finger on the part that's under. I try to feel under it. One or two times and pain is gone if person knows what they're doing.

If a woman has pain in the lower abdomen, it is her ovaries. The ovaries are low, out of place. They get twisted and give you trouble, pain. I start from the back, from the waist, the tailbone and left side. I noint her, all the veins from the foot right up to the body. I hold her up by her pelvic bone and haul her up. I put my fingers under the pelvic bone and lift it up.

But 'nointing' was not the technique used in all cases. She had a variety of treatments for other disorders as well. For example, she described the treatment for dropsy as follows:

With dropsy, you get swelled, your whole body. In the hospital they draw off the water. That water is specific to that illness. When they drink my medicine, they urine water and sweat water. I use Christ's Cane (*Cano Christo*). Peel it, cut it at the joint, put it in a mortar and beat. Then put in a clay pot or soak in the mortar. Strain and get lime or sour orange and cut and boil with cream of tartar and magnesia and mix it up. Make about a gallon. The patient drinks the whole gallon, which leads to sweating. Before they couldn't pass stool. Now he begins to pass stool. The medicine scrapes the bag of the sickness. The sickness is in the bag inside. Water causes the sickness, but I don't know what causes the water. They pass a black substance. Black continues to pass till the black done. Then pass coal. Part of sickness is still in the body. Then yellow. Then green. By then, all the sickness is gone. Sometimes they get better and sometimes they kill selves with diet. They eat lard of different kinds. The only lard should be coconut oil. They eat poor food. When the medicine is done, you test to see what he can eat. Boil meat and serve with rice and give him a nice dinner. If that don't do him bad, he can eat that. No soda, no lard, little salt. Use to make tortillas. Make tea with dried *pia leaf*. Then, time for testing with salt water. If no feel nothing bad, can go back to salt. The last thing is, I tell the man he can't fool around, not even with his wife, until he is better.

While she treats many illnesses, her primary work was as a midwife. I asked her what questions she asked when a patient first came to her.

Well, I ask "How do you feel?" She will say, "I feel bad." Then I ask, "Do you vomit?" and she will say, "Yes." Then I ask, "Do you see your period?", and she will say, "No." Then I ask how long since she see her period and she will answer me. I will say "You must be pregnant." She will answer, "I don't know." You can see it in her eyes too. There is some sign in the eyes, but I can't describe it. I feel her abdomen. At one and one-half months I can feel the baby through [external] massage. I don't report it to anyone if it is first baby because the girl may deny it. I wait until three months to report. I will know if the baby is in good condition. I check the mother from the back and check from both ovaries and lower abdomen. I can feel the position of the baby's head. If the baby is in the wrong position, I will move it around with [external] massage till the baby is in the proper position. Sometimes, when I change the baby's position, I would call the doctor to see what I was doing. I worked with a doctor, but I couldn't get a license. The doctor liked my work very much. Even now all kinds of women come to me to be checked.

From three months you can be sure she is pregnant. I feel her lower abdomen because the uterus is in the middle and her ovaries to the side. *Taga hiñáru*, that's her womb inside, the uterus and the ovaries. You can feel the baby when it is young yet; it is growing until at three months it gets to the navel. Some children in some families only grow to seven months, then they born. But by treating him [the baby] within three months, you will see him good size. As she gets bigger her breasts will develop. At five months her breasts will have water. You look to see if the baby is normal when she comes to see you. You can tell how the body of the baby is. Sometimes it is transverse or breech and then I will try to move the baby. If she is in pain from labor and the baby is in the wrong position, I can move the baby. I have always been able to move the baby to the right position.

Some deliveries present special problems.

Once, a family called on me. A woman was in labor, but the baby was in a transverse position. It was a dangerous position. By the time I reached her, the baby's hand had appeared. I took a needle and put it in the flame. Then I stuck the baby's hand until she drew it back. Every time the baby's hand would emerge, I would stick it again. Once the hand was back inside. I did massage until a normal delivery was completed.

Both mother and baby must be cared for following the delivery.

After the baby is born, he sometimes have water inside. I have to put my hand in his mouth and make him vomit to bring out the water. Sometimes they are half drowned when they come out because they travel far to reach the earth. I wash their eyes with holy water and cotton. Put the cotton in holy water and clean it, then squeeze it into the eyes.

For the mother, you must boil bush to get her to clean inside. Boil *sorasee*, *Santa Maria leaf*, *cow foot leaf*. Put in hot water and boil. Then put it in a basin and make her stoop over it. If there are any clots, they will come out. This can clean out everthing. She drinks some of the medicine too. Then you put a binder on her. This holds her back strong. Examine her to see if any clots are retained inside the womb. Give her medicines to drink to pass it. Given her Spanish medicine.

You give the baby chupon with *mansinilla*. Rub garlic, put garlic under ashes. When the garlic is roasted, put chupon with oil to clean inside of baby. When baby is born, he passes black stool. The chupon cleans out the black stool.

Some babies have a low mole. I don't know the cause. The mole is deep and gives them vomiting. I noint them from the neck, also the cheeks and forehead. I push the finger on the palate and suck on the top. This will bring it up good. Otherwise, it will kill them. Mole gets low and gives them vomiting to death and loose stool too.

Sometimes a woman may develop a sore inside after the birth of a baby. This sore won't heal without special treatment.

If she gets a sore she can't have more babies if the sore doesn't heal. I had it happen to me. I could feel the sore opening up each time I walked. Go the bush to get *gombo limbo* (*tura heurunai*) tree bark. Peel the bark and cut it open. Scrape it clean to get the salve from it. Use *romero*, Spanish medicine from the store, and another bush. I don't remember its name. Boil it and strain in a clean cloth all together. Drink it for your water until you feel the sore close. Then take *balsalm copayba* and mix with castor oil and take a purge. Notice your stool and you will see a scab from the sore inside. Use a warm cloth on the area after you are cured. Sometimes women with a sore won't do this and she will pass matter and clots.

Mrs. Castro recognized that vexation and worries could lead to illness. "Many people are vexed around here. Vexation stays with you." Vexation was said to lead to pain in the stomach and pain in the head. But no simple medicine could treat this pain; rather the woman must be advised and comforted and must talk with others about her problem (see p. 118). I asked if there were illnesses which affected the mind. "Craziness come out of nerves. The nerves are tender", she responded.

Q. Are people like that from birth?

A. I cannot say. Nerves work on them. I don't know the cause. I see them walking about, talking, talking to themselves. That is bad illness. With some people it is in the family. With some people, maybe they have something on their mind and don't want to tell and it work on them.

She attributed illness to natural causes.

Illness is normal. Anybody can get sick. But you can call upon God to help you in getting well. Most people would say illness is normal. It is not punishment from God for anything.

I asked specifically about certain uncommon illnesses.

Fiáfia. I don't know about that. I've heard the name of the sickness, but I don't know what kind it is.
Mal Ojo. I've heard that Spanish people have it, but not Garifuna.
Bearsy-bugs. I hear about that, but don't see or feel that.
Strong sight. I have heard that some people have eyes that affect babies, but nothing like that happened to my babies.

Evil Spirits. I don't worry about evil spirits. I know there are some people who use incense and garlic, but I never do it.
Obeah. I never had anyone suggest that illness was *obeah*. There is no treatment for it because poison is put in your water or rum or food.

Only with *húmo* did she mention spirits, though her statements on the subject were contradictory.

Húmo is caused by shark and sting ray. The parents shouldn't eat this because the baby may have an allergy to the smell. It's not good for babies to smell the scent of fish. You must use bush to treat. *Surúsia* [doctor] cannot treat *húmo* because he can't treat spirits, but Garifuna doctor knows how to treat it. A *búiai* can treat it.

And on the role of the *gubída* in illness she offered this statement:

I don't know how *gubída* cause illness because I don't dream or see them. I dream my dead mother and dead father. I see them just like when they were alive. But they don't do nothing. I have heard others say *gubída* bring sickness, but I don't see that.

Estephan

Estephan is a relatively young Garifuna healer who has lived all his life in Punta Gorda. He is related to many people in the town and is well known. He serves as a healer only part of the time and otherwise is employed intermittingly at a variety of jobs. He was taught his medicines by his grandmother. He is occasionally assisted by spirits who appear in dreams.

Yes, I have dreams. A person comes to me in a dream in the form of an angel. Once a black man, an East Indian, dressed in full white appeared. This was when I was tending to a girl who was crossing a creek and they found her near a bush without marks on her body. Her brother came to me and I said, after looking at her, that it was an evil spirit. The black man said it was an accident, something hit her, but didn't show no marks on her body. The black man showed me the right bush and said to give one to the girl to smell and to soak the other in the water. She was bathed in the herb for two weeks every day at 12 o'clook. He told me when she should bathe with it. I didn't even know the name of the bush. The girl recovered. I told the brother not to take her to the hospital. When she started coming back, I knew from her frightened look that she had seen something awful.

Though dreams sometimes play an important role, he attributes his cures to God.

I pray with the patient, asking the Lord for healing touch. I work through the good Lord. You can know all the medicines in the world, but if you don't have faith, they won't work. Through the Lord all things are possible.

Estephan believes that most illnesses are natural.

Many people say to me that sometimes they feel like their illness is a curse, that God is punishing them. But I feel as long as you're a human body, you are entitled to sickness.

The emphasis in the treatments he offers are on bush preparations ingested or applied externally.

If you have heart pain, you must drink a mild medicine which cools the heart and slows the blood down because it is flowing too fast.

If you have fever and chills, don't go to bed. You sweat it out with bitters which are available in the bar. Rum with lime is also good.

Siwápat leaf in warm water is good for pain in the joints. This is applied externally. It is also good for twisted vein and swelling. The heat of the body draws the liquid out of the plant. Something in the leaf gets in the body and helps.

Cabbage bark is boiled for poor blood. This is good for the blood, it purifies it.

A cold in the penis can be treated with pineapple and salt and vinegar.

Corn water is a coolant for the entire system. It gets to the root of chicken pox and the outside starts scabbing and falls off.

Pepper burns to the root of appendictis. Pepper is also good for certain kinds of cancer.

Sorasee purifies the blood. The juice works on the blood.

Salt and water with *guava leaf* are good for an upset stomach or vomiting. The salt is used to cook up the sores. The *guava leaf* stops the vomiting.

For asthma, the cure is simple. You drink the water from a boiled rat.

Cow foot is good for tea and for sprains. The tea helps the heart because it keeps the heart on a cool system. It helps the blood flow freely. It is also good for pain. The liquid helps the pain.

He also places considerable emphasis on preventive therapies, and in particular, on the value of purging.

If someone says they have a pain in the belly I ask, "What causes your stomach to hurt you?", and maybe they answer, "I feel like it is something I eat." I tell them to observe their stools. If it is cold inside it will come out in a hunk like when you blow your nose. Biliousness may also come out. Biliousness leads to giddiness. You will vomit out yellow stuff. It is like a boil and you will vomit it. The stool will appear brownish with a little white. If either occurs, I will continue to give them bitters which are good for cold inside. When the cold or biliousness is getting thinner then I will lessen the amount of medicine. The cause of biliousness is too much drinking. You have to purge the body twice a month or biliousness can build up in the body. Biliousness can be seen in the eyes. The eyes turn yellow.

Sometimes pain in the stomach may be due to wind. Then I give them epsom salts and *senna*. This purges them and gets rid of the wind. Garlic and aniseed together also get rid of wind.

Sorasee can be used to purge. Whenever you will drink it, you know it will purge because you have gripping. This keeps the kidney and liver clean and these are the two that extract the waste. If you can keep the kidney and liver clean, you can get rid of wastes. My children are now on vacation. I will purge them now. This cleans out the system, purifies the blood, cuts loose boils and worms. This is why my children have never been sick. They don't even know what a fever is.

I have no trace of nicotine in my lungs. That is because of pepper which purges it out. That's why the stools turn yellow sometimes or change color. Pepper burns the nicotine out.

When asked what people could do to prevent illness, he responded that they should bathe every day, change their underwear regularly, eat properly, and catch their rest. He attributed diabetes to eating too much salt or to 'the food you eat", and stated that high blood pressure was caused by lard and salt and eating too much fried food, which continuously replenishes the body with fresh starch. He asserted that Americans eat too much "cold stuff" and that Coca Cola has acid in it which works on the kidneys and liver.

He recognized that the signs of illness might have many interpretations and that further information might be required to make a diagnosis. If the patient complained of pain in the leg, the cause might be overweight or a sign of rheumatism; if the pain was in the stomach it might be wind or a cold inside or an ulcer. If the pain is in the arm, the cause might be a strain or the patient may have twisted a vein. A woman's period or liver or kidney problems can all cause a backache. If the patient says he feels his leg sleeping, it could be either appendicitis or a hernia. Pain in the joints might be rheumatism or sugar in the blood or too much weight.

Estephan explained to me that he did not believe in the *gubída* and quoted Biblical scripture on ancestral spirits in support of his statement. He did, however, believe in a number of evil spirits, among them *duénde* and *uináni.*

You can make a deal with *uináni.* You can call him up with certain prayers. But you have to promise something in return. The bargain might be that you would get a plantation but *uinańi* will ask for your first child if you are successful. *Uináni* will kill that child in a way which appears natural.

He also expressed the belief that illness and death might be caused by *obeah.*

You use candles with prayers and an item belonging to the person you wish to harm, like a photo or clothing. That's why I don't like my picture taken because someone might use it. You bury the picture in the hearth and return on Tuseday and Friday to say prayers. As the picture withers so will you wither. The Maya use the image of San Antonio del Fuego to do *obeah.* I learned of that from the Mayans, but I don't use any of this knowledge.

Both *obeah* and evil spirits can be warded off by the proper use of certain medicines.

If an individual takes *bisi nut* and somebody gives him poison he will automatically throw it up.

Garlic titíe is used mostly for getting rid of any kind of evil. You boil it and bathe in it and you can walk through a thousand enemies and they can't touch you.

Flor de muerto. You can rub it on a person with rum. Because it stinks it gets rid of evil things.

You smoke *essence root.* It look like wax. You get it off a tree. It works on evil because of the scent. They use it in church a lot and at funerals to get the spirit in check.

Conch shell stinks and gets rid of evil spirits.

You can see in their eyes a frightened look. Then you try to shift the conversation around to find out what they are frightened of. Give them a bath in wild garlic (*garlic titíe*), *flor de muerte*, and essence root. They all stink and that sends the evil spirit away. You tell them to read the Bible more often. That way the good Lord will help them.

Someone might say, "Well, I think someone is tampering with me." Burn wild garlic. The person stands in the middle of the smoke. He feels a reaction like something loose off of him. Bathe him on Tuseday and Fridays. You can tell who's causing the problem after the first two baths. Tell him to bring underwear or a handkerchief. Get ashes, herbs, and boil. He drinks the water. Treat the handkerchief with a special oil. Give it to him to keep. This protects him when he goes out.

Quicksilver inserted under the skin of the arm will protect you against enemies. It will fight poison. If you hold a glass with poison, the glass will break.

During one of our discussions, a young man approached Estephan for assistance. The boy's uncle had been murdered. A man had been arrested, but there were those who did not believe this man was responsible. Estephan told me that the boy had asked him to find out who the murderer was. Estephan explained to me that he sent the boy away. "People don't realize that when I do such a thing I must pay a high tuition."

Alejandro

Alejandro says he was born with "spiritism", that he has special powers to diagnose and treat. Because his gift is "inborn" he cannot charge for the services he provides, but can only take what he is offered. His mother knew he was gifted when he was born. Butterflies followed him from the time he was an infant and still are to be found in his house on many occasions. He can cure only certain sicknessess, but he can treat illnesses which others cannot treat because of his special abilities.

My brother in Livingstone treats sickness, but he can't always cure because he isn't gifted. I have treated people from my youth all over Guatemala. I treat everyone. Sometimes, when people can't get cure elsewhere, they come to me. If you are gifted, you can look at a man and ask what is wrong with him and you know right away what is his problem. Sometimes you must put a candle into his hand, but then you can tell what is wrong with him.

Certain spirits [guides] are given by God to some people. You have to be inborn with them. You can see them in the daytime. They will appear on Fridays and Wednesdays only. You need a candle and a small bottle of rum. They look like Spanish people. There are two kinds of guides. One wears red pants. They are called *yawaraguna*. The others wear blue pants, but I can't remember their names. They are both very short.[4]

Alejandro learned some of his herbs from other healers, as did his brother. But he was and remains dependent on his guides and his grandmother who died many years ago for assistance in healing.

The mother of my mother come and tell me what herb is good for what. She was Carib but dead a long time. It was my mother that told me that it was my grandmother who appeared to me. I was born knowing how to cure. But my grandmother still comes to me and shows me herbs. My guides will also appear to me when I am sleeping. They instruct me and teach me new medicines.

Because Alejandro possesses spirit guides he could work as a *búiai*, he states, but he has chosen not to do so.

*Búiai*s are born with spirits to aid the world. I am a *búiai*, but I don't want to work like a *búiai*. The only *búiai* left in Belize in Sarah in Stann Creek. Some people have people who died. They swear to that spirit to instruct them for things. But they not *búiai*. *Búiai* cures, but I don't want to work like that. Maybe when I am older. Right now, they want me to work as a *búiai* in Guatemala.

Alejandro believes there are those who try to cure uncommon illnesses but fail because they lack the necessary skills.

If you give certain baths, the spirit will come to the curer and advise him not to cure. Some people try to cure, but they aren't born with the gift. This spirit can harm them.

There are also those who would serve as *búiai*s, but do not succed in their work. Alejandro was expecially concerned about the results of a recent *dugu*.

The men who come from Guatemala for the *dugu* were not *búiai*. They were not spiritisms. They left the spirits at the *dabúiaba*. They can call in the spirits only. I believe the spirits are still there. They threw the food in the creek after the *dugu* was finished. That woke up and drove out the spirits from the creek. The devil of the creek is upset now. Nothing good come from the dugu. The *búiai* don't know how to call the dead spirit [*gubída*] of the family. When you enter the *dabúiaba* your body feel heavy because of the presence of the spirits. The *búiai* has to know how to make the *dabúiaba* light. The spirits come in a rush, all at once. The *búiai* has to know how to make them come in one at a time. He has to be able to control them. Those spirits are gone now [*gubída*] but there are other bad spirits there. The *búiai* wasn't really a *búiai* because he couldn't send all the spirits away.

Like Estephan, he attributes his power to God and refers to his work as a healer as "God's work." He says he once dreamt of God and describes the experience as follows:

God is spirit too, like San Isidro who protects all plants. I dream of God too. He was only four feet. He was a Jew man with blue eyes. He was white, white with a white gown. He was nursing the Holy Ghost. Christ appeared to me. He tell me, "My son, I don't want you to stay in this place. I want you to quit this place immediately. There are people trying to set bad men against you." God the Son was nursing God the Holy Ghost. He was just a little boy. That night in a dream a black man come. I said, "Are you looking for me to kill me?" He said, "No, my son. I am sent by Christ. My name is Joshua." I never know Christ have a black messenger. I dreamed all this about three years ago.

The world has many bad spirits and good spirits. The bad spirits were at one time evil people God saved but then turned out to wander as spirits. "It's in the scriptures", he adds. The bad spirits can attack you if your soul (*áfurugu*) is light.

Bad spirits can work on you according to your soul. When you have a light soul, the spirit will bother you. It will try to harm you at midnight. If you have a heavy spirit you can conquer them.

I asked if Satan sometimes caused illness.

Yes, that spirit sometimes tries to bother people with a light spirit; there are other spirits too. There is *Uinańi*. He has only one foot. He can turn into other forms. You can see him in the distance and as he gets closer, he grows larger. He comes like an animal or as a white stick or post. You will feel the magnet of the spirit as he gets closer. He will come to you in a dream first. If you conquer him in your dream he won't molest you, but if you lose he will trouble you because your spirit is light. Then there is *agáiuma*. She stays by the river. She is worse than devil. *Búiai* got to work hard if she causes illness. Anytime you go to the creek she throw herself in and follow you. Spirits of devil, *agâiuma*, *uinâni* get you sick and make you feverish. They come to you in your sleep. Anytime you sleep they are driving your soul further from your body until you die. *Mafia* is a black man who got a tail. *Caraho* is a white man. *Susia* is a woman's spirit who tempts drunken men. *Duénde* is the devil of the coast. *Bearsy-bugs* are the Prince of the Devil. If he don't like you, he will kill you immediately. *Búiai* can't kill them either.

Given the large number of malevolent spirits, it is not surprising that many of Alejandro's clients come seeking relief from spirits and the evil intentions of other humans.

People only have to come to me and tell me how they feel. I will know what is wrong. I don't have to examine them. But when sickness is there for a long time, I can't treat it. I will prepare medicine according to the sickness. If it is a spirit, it will come to me at night and tell me. If it's a sad spirit I must treat it differently.

I can tell if there is a bad spirit on them. I use candles and can tell from the direction of the flame. They can't sleep because of a bad spirit. They have to bathe in herbs two times. Then you get *oudlice* and you get essence and other things. Any bad thing can't harm you. You smoke them with that.

Sometimes people come to me with a certain sad spirits. Because someone hate you. Someone buy soil from a dead man [grave]. Mix it with guinea pepper, *koetch*. Put them all on the fire. This causes a sad spirit.

To make *obeah*, you can buy soil from the tomb of a dead man. You can talk to a dead man. Dead man can do all sort of things. The owner of the grave wants to leap on you. He comes to you plain. Makes you bawl in the night. You can also take the bone of a dead man and sew it in a pillow. This will turn someone crazy. Can treat with herbs, smoke with *oudlice*.

Lots want to learn *obeah*. I can cure any *obeah* and I can tell who did it. It can be turned back on the person with a candle and two pieces of paper, folded in half. You mention the name, put the candle with the head down. It will turn back.

Idáhadu is the words of the people. When people talk about you, you can't sleep. Their words are hot, like fire. You must use holy water from the church. You can get that on Good Friday.

Idáhadu is worse than *obeah*. You will dream of fire coming to you. The direction of the fire tells you where the words are coming from. It makes you sick because you can't sleep. It drives your soul away. It can be cured if you know certain Psalms. Psalm 63 can be used against it. There is a book in Spanish with prayers. You take a white candle and black thread. Tie the thread to the candle and mention the name of the person who is harming you. He will have to stop.

Indian people use San Antonio del Fuego to make *obeah*. You can get an image of San Antonio. Indian people use three kinds of candles – red, black and white. The red is the dangerous one.

Obeah man can kill you. *Obeah* can come as a secret thing. You get thinner. Can get killed easy. People scarcely do it now because not many people born with the gift now [*obeah* men]. I don't know why. I don't harm anyone, but I know people that do harm. I cured a girl of *obeah* once and people tried to harm me. People here don't know much about *obeah* now. They use words now. They turn to the devil. If you have a light soul, they can harm you. Some people may have stronger words though. People will mention *obeah* sometimes. When people wish bad to the next person, their own words will turn on them. When they come to me, I refuse to cure them. If they stop thinking that way they will cure. They must respect everyone.

Some Indians [Maya] have bigger plantations than others. A man came to me with a sore on his foot. I tell him everything. I wash the sore with herbs. Smoke come out of the man's foot. He feels his head coming bigger and bigger. I say to him that it is man's work. He has to say prayers to get it back. When the man come back his foot was alright. I wash it again, but he no feel it this time. The man knows who did it. It was caused by jealousy. The man didn't tell me much, but I know anyway. It's done cure now.

Like Estephan, he suggested a variety of techniques which could ward off the effects of evil spirits and the machinations of evil people.

Oudlice. That's the devil's enemy. *Oudlice* protects the body from the devil's path.

If you have a light spirit, you must look for protection. Quicksilver [inserted into the arm] is good protection against poison.

You can use holy water to keep the spirits away.

Titíe can be used for a bath and for protection. It keeps away *obeah* if you bathe in it. It can be drunk for protection too. You will vomit poison if anyone gives you poison.

Alejandro knows treatments for *lisándi ubaó* as well.

For pain in belly or rheumatism pain, take a hot bath.

Pain in the stomach can be from too much heat and cold turned into dysentery. When cold settles in the stomach, it is like cooked starch. You use a purge for that.

Heat in the blood can make you feel hot. The doctor may tell you this is high blood pressure, but it is not. High blood pressure makes your heart pound. Use *gánabis root* and *gánabis leaf, sorasee*, and *senna*. Boil for purge. Add three parts epsom salts and one-half spoon cream of tartar. Drink for three days. Take from four o'clock in the evening. This will take the heat out of the blood and also helps pain.

High blood pressure is also due to heat in the blood. You can use *ganabis root* or *caro* to remove the heat.

Diabetes is an inborn disease. You can use *sorasee* and *Billy Web*, but that will only keep it down. As you get older it will get worse.

Use tiger fat for treatment of asthma. That is inborn too.

Shark's oil is good for tuberculosis when it first start. Mix Red Lavinda with shark's oil. Red Lavinda is good for the heart too.

Ganabise leaf can be used for itch. Mash it and apply it to the skin. It can also be used for backache or purge.

Boil *gahela leaf* with *guava* skin. This is used for vomiting. If you got biliousness, pain in the chest, you will vomit it out.

Trumpet leaf is used for a sad cough, like T.B. or a sad cold. Use garlic with trumpet leaf for cough.

Ganapistola is good for when the body has plenty of heat.

Perhaps because of the many years he has lived among the Spanish, many of his explanation of cause-effect relationships were phrased in terms of the balance – or imbalance – between hot and cold.

A fresh cold comes when you have plenty of heat in the body and the rain catches you. Certain persons have more heat in the body because they have thick flesh.

Pain in the stomach can be caused by an *aruinun*. This soaks up heat and cold. If you eat something against it, it will work on you.

Stroke is caused by heat and cold in the blood which has reached the bones.

T.B. is caused by carelessness. After you work a day in the sun and take a bath. This starts a cough. If you don't have a bump on your sternum, you can get T.B. when you have a cough. The cough drops to the lower area around the sternum.

Nerves or trembling is caused by heat and cold. It travels over the whole body until it reaches the bones or veins. If it reaches the veins, it leads to trembling. It can affect the brains too.

Mr. Avilez

Mr. Avilez is a well-known elderly Garifuna healer who, despite his age, maintains an active practice. Like all of the healers described here, his 'fee' is based largely on what his clients can pay. He first learned his medicines when he was a young man. He was trained by an elderly *búiai* who was a close relative of his mother's.

He [the *búiai*] said he didn't want to die without handing over his medicines to someone he likes. He said to me "I like you. I would like you to learn." He invited me to walk around the ocean and see all the bush that work on the sick. I began to learn names and how to boil them and how to apply them.

Mr. Avilez says he has cured all his children but it was only subsequent to his retirement from teaching that he began to work actively as a healer.

The *búiai* came to me in a dream five years after his death. He came paddling to Barranco in my dream. He told me "I am coming to take you to a certain place on the Temash River. Come inside the dory; sit at the bow." He started to paddle. Then a few minutes after in my same dream he arrived to the spot. It was the bank. He said. "We'll go ashore", and he walked behind me and showed me the spot. "This high spot is where you will put a building for your people to come to you so you heal them." Then he showed me bush around. "You will see them. There is for *idáhadu* (*two-nine-tails vine*), *húmo*, and so on. Then he said, "let's go back and the same vines will be used for water spirits and land spirits." I told the *búiai*, "Grandpa, I am not in a position to take up this job because I am a teacher." But all that he had shown me I reserved so I could use them when I was no longer teaching. They call me doctor, but I am no *búiai*.

I asked about the role of God and Satan in illness and healing.

Causing sickness in God's power. God allows the *gubída* to wander about. God allows *idáhadu* or *obeah*. God can heal the sick as well. If you are a bush doctor, God can give you help to cure the sick. When you practice medicines, you call on God's help, light a candle, say a few prayers so the sick will he healed. Satan can cause illness. He can cause any kind of illness. Some talk on Satan with special words to cause harm. The devil is a spirit and can present itself as natural in the bush. Satan is the same thing. He can form like a snake or a human being.

And he related to me this story about a encounter with *Mafia* in a dream.

The devil, *mafia*, is a wandering spirit that can cause sickness. He is a master of languages. *Mafia* has a beautiful wife. She came to me in a dream when I was at Big River. I was sleeping and she came right in and opened the curtain and said "Oh, this is the place where you are." I asked her to sit, but she said she was going right back. She reported to her husband because he hates people who heal the sick. The *Mafia* came about a week later in a dream. He said, "Oh, I've been trying to find you. I didn't know this was the spot where you are", and I told him, "Come and sit by my bed." He said, "No, I won't be able to sit by your bed because you have something by your pillow." I sat up on my bed and I asked him to shake my hand. He said, "No, I won't be able to shake your hand because you have something under your pillow." I said I would like to talk, but *Mafia* wouldn't come closer and I am too deaf to hear him well.

Mr. Avilez has large clientele, many of whom he visits on a regular basis. I accompanied him as he went to see a number of his patients.

This lady, her problem was that she was shaking from lack of sleep. Her illness was nerves. I bathed her with bush – *flor de muerte*, *waiúri*, *lamúru*, *garlic titíe*, and *cow foot leaf*. I also used incense to smoke the house and the patient. Sometimes you have to bathe them every day for three weeks. At the end of the treatment, get a fire coal and get incense and smoke the patient. I get the incense from the Indians in the bush. It is a gum which comes from a tree. The incense drives spirits away. Another cause of her shaking was a lack of nutrition because she didn't get the proper food. I advised her not to eat pork while being treated, but when the treatment is finished I advised her to eat pork and fish. As you cure the nerves you bring back the rest. You see the change on the patient.

Mrs. Castillo's grandchildren were ill. They have eaten something against their body which acted on their nerve. When I first see them I look at the mouth and the gums and crotch. I ask, "What did they smell and what did they eat?" Then she remembered that she brought shark into the house. The scent of the shark is too strong for children. *Húmo* is from shark or ox-bill. This is a natural illness. It is just the scent which affects them. I bath the babies with the same bush [see above] and that drives out the scent. You will see their testicles red. That is the mark of *húmo*. The skin peels. I check the mouth and gums. They will have itch or pus. This cannot be cured with one bucket of water. It may take two weeks to cure. They must bathe at 9:00, 12:00, and 5:00. On Thursday and Friday and Sunday there is no bathing. That is prohibited by tradition. I must follow the custom. The *búiai* [his teacher] said don't bathe the patient on those days. He didn't say why. The children are cured now.

These good people, they had a snake in their kitchen. It built a house under the cassava baking place. I used bush to drive it out and it has never returned. I used *lamúru* and *Santa Maria* or *Cow foot leaf*, and *garlic titíe*. *Haliwalu* has a very bad smell, the sap is very irritating. I use that too to drive the snake out. It can be applied when spirits linger about the place.

This lady's daughter is eleven years old. She had an attack of the brain. She will look at you steadily, then return to a normal state. The cause was heat in the stomach and the head. The temperature was too strong for her. I bathed all of her body twice with *flor de muerte*, rum, and garlic. This cooled off her brain.

These twins were born with a chest cold. It came up again when they got loose stools. I bathed them with bush – *lamúru, cow foot, and garlic titíe*. They are fine now.

This woman suffered from *ligári ichugu*, that is, pain in the head. She had heat in her head. You call tell because the eyes will show a certain color like red. This shows something is wrong with the brain. I applied a plaster made out of egg, vinegar, flour, nutmeg, and alum. I put them on a clean piece of cloth and plastered the head. In a few minutes it is dry. I leave it on for one and a half hours and change up to four times a day for up to a week or more. She had pain in her head and in her eyes. She is a hard working woman on her farm [the Carib Block or Reserve] and the sun was hot. For six months she had a problem until she came to me.

An inflammation of the eye can be very painful. I have to plaster the forehead with egg, vinegar, flour, nutmeg, and alum. This got this lady's eye into a normal condition. For four years she had a problem. She went to Belize [City], more than one time. The doctor said it was a cataract. The medicine helped the inflammation, but she still can't see very well out of that eye. There is a treatment for cataract. You have to use eggshells and grind them very fine.

There was a child at the hospital. She could not talk, eat, or swallow. Her face was swollen. She had a slight fever. She was like that for three days before the family called me. How did it happen? The water spirit had control over her. The spirit overcome her. She slept for three days. The water spirit lives in the creek nearby. When the creek is full it floods and that's the time the water spirit will take shelter near the bridge and attack a child or an older person. The girl has to pass the creek to go to school. She arrived at school and it began to happen. They took her from the school to the hospital. Her eye is steady and doesn't move. Her mouth is open and water drips out of it. I squeeze her nose and it was several minutes before she responded. These are signs of the spirit. The doctor gave her up for dead and said there was nothing he could do. The family came for me and asked me to treat her. I bathed her [*flor de muerte*, strong rum, *garlic titíe*] and smoked her with incense and then smoked her again. In the morning the doctor arrived. He was expecting to find her dead. He walked into the room and the bed was empty and he said, "Where is my patient?" I answered, "Here is your patient, doctor." And he turned and there was a girl looking at him and she was laughing. The doctor said to me, "Well, Mr. Avilez, you can come here anytime." And he told them to give me permission to work there.

Once this man have a bearsy bug, an *ugúri*, in his house. These are bad spirits, wandering spirits. They change into different forms. It can be a crab and then a rabbit and then a snake. It works on the shadow (*iaua*). Once it works on the *iaua* you are gone. You can't get over that. It mostly affects babies and young children. An *ugúri* can live under a house. It digs a hole there and works in different form. You will find a big hole under the trees or under the house. The signs are that you will see an animal that changes form. The person who is attacked, his belly is swollen. His belly grows till he dies. You can't sleep when it is around. It always visits you, especially women. There are only male *ugúri*, you know. Strange things will happen when the *ugúri* is present. You will boil a crab and then you don't find it in the pot. In Stann Creek they are called Lucifer or Belzing-Bugs. It attaches itself to a woman. It loves woman. If a woman has a lover and the *ugúri* is jealous it will attack the man or drive him away or make him sick so he [the *ugúri*] can possess. I cured this man's house of the beasry-bug. I had to work at night when the bearsy-bug is out. I put sea eggs in a hole in the shape of a cross. I put four in each hole and in between I placed a piece of copal and garlic. I covered it with dirt and it will never come there forever.

There are many illnesses which he will not treat. A variety of common afflictions are referred to the local physician "out of respect." And illnesses which he believes are caused by *obeah* or the *gubída* are referred to a *búiai* in Stann Creek.

An invisible spirit, like *gubída*, cause sickness, like, for instance, they came to you in a dream begging for something to eat. In that dream, that spirit will show you a calabash or a plate with food which is a sign that you should make an offering. If you don't make the offering, it may become compulsory that you do it. Then you find that certain sickness come to you. For instance, a sore on your foot, a terrible headache, stomach trouble. It doesn't heal. You may have vomiting. These are signs of *gubída. The gubída* makes the illness. Then they cause you to be talking foolish talk, to be bawling, crying, or sometimes appear to you and other people can't see them. This happens while you are awake. People will say they dream of you and see them [*gubída*] running after you with sticks to club you. Once the *gubída* club you, that is a sign of death. You must go to Sarah for this.

Somebody may use alligator gall or the gall of mountain cow [tapir] and put that in your drink. Or they may use other poisonous things. The belly begins to swell. Sometimes in three days it affects your heart and you are gone. It depends on your constitution. A heavy *áfurugu* can resist *obeah*. But if they have a light *áfurugu*, they cannot. I send them to Sarah.

His understanding of the development of the *áfurugu* differs from that of other healers.

Whether you have a light or heavy *áfurugu* is determined during pregnancy. You may have a light *áfurugu* because of your mother's poor nutrition or because she didn't visit the clinic.

I asked about the distinction between *obeah* men, *gabiarahati*, and the *búiai*.

Gabiarahati and *obeah men* are the same, but the *obeah man* has more power. The *obeah man* can heal what the *gabiarahati* put on you. The *búiai* cannot make *obeah*, but can heal *obeah*. He can't turn *obeah* back on the person who made it. An *obeah man* can turn it back. There are *obeah men* in Guatemala who are Indians. There are no *obeah men* in Punta Gorda.

He mentioned many treatments for both common and uncommon afflictions.

For headache, wash the head with *flor de muerte*, *garlic titíe*, and strong rum. Put it all in a calabash and burn it before using.

For an enemy who is trying to harm you, use cedar bark boiled and mixed with *waiúri* and *lamúru*. Apply [bathe] for a week or two.

For *idahadu*, use *two-cat-tails* prepared as a bath. However, it is seldom that they heal.

Cedar bark boiled with pork fat and vinegar for inside injuries.

Use *worm plant* with garlic for worms; *pasote* is also used for worms.

If you have sores on the body, wash with alum, then apply some sulphur.

Use *contrebo, Billy Web bark, palo de hombre, cedar bark*, and some other bitter roots boiled in water for diabetes.

Like other healers, many of his medicines were recommended to prevent illness as well as to cure it. Certain illnesses could be avoided altogether.

Poor blood is caused by malnutrition, lack of exercise and hard work.

Drinking too much alcohol leads to sickness.

Hibiscus can be used as a tea for tonic. It purifies something inside.

From time to time you need a cleaning of the stomach when the stomach is hard.

Weakness in the body is often on account of carelessness, poor nutrition, like vitamins, not washing the body frequently. The body needs tonic sometimes and plenty of rest. Some people work too hard and get weak. I believe that working too hard when you are young causes paralysis, stroke, nervousness when old, and also frequent pains.

Propitiation of Ancestors and the Major Ceremonies Directed Toward Healing

When ancestors become dissatisfied, illness often follows. The "sickness of the ancestors", or *hásandigubída*, is not a "worldly" illness and must be treated by special means. Ceremonies performed at the time of death or subsequent to the burial are meant to get the spirits off on their journey and to prevent their lingering about (see Kerns 1977; Wells 1980, 1982a, 1982b; Coehlo 1955; Taylor 1951, Hadel 1972). They may be expected to reappear in dreams, however, and to make requests of their family from time to time. Most commonly, they wish only that a mass be said for them, a relatively inexpensive tribute costing a few dollars. The price of ignoring such a request may be high.

When parents and grandparents have died and they want something they may cause illness. Down the street, an ancestor wanted something. A girl of fourteen or fifteen became ill because her shadow was light, so the ancestor bothered her. Others in the family had already died because they didn't believe. The girl was in the hospital twice, but she didn't get well. They started leaving food out for an ancestor when the girl reported she saw a man with a guitar who had been dead since before she was born. When the girl saw the spirit, he wet her with rum and she recovered. He wanted a mass and they wouldn't give it. Now they will have to have a *dugu* next year.

Small offerings of food and drink may be made to indicate to the ancestors, who are never far distant, that they are remembered and respected. Such offerings are believed to postpone or negate altogether a request for a more costly and dramatic ceremony. Occasionally, an ancestor may appear in a dream holding a calabash or a comb. This may be interpreted as indicating that he or she wishes to be 'refreshed.' The ceremony required in this instance is referred to as *amuiadahani* (also *agowaduni*, see Wells 1982a), or the "bathing of a dead person's spirit." A prominent healer in P.G. used the term *lagounhelal;* the general intent and procedure appear the same. A low grave approximately one and one-half feet high is built of mud or sand within the house. Raw cassava is grated and soaked in water and a certain amount is put inside the grave or thrown on the grave. "If the deceased was a man, you bring a calabash, soap, and a face towel. If the deceased was a woman, you bring a comb, calabash, clothes, and soap. You light a candle." Religious songs are sung and a certain amount of food left near the 'grave' for the day. On the same day the grave will be leveled.

The ancestor may ask for an offering of food, which may be more or less elaborate depending, perhaps, on the seriousness of the illness.

I was ill in May and my family wanted to *búiai* me. I only agreed to certain things to please them. I had a mass said for my father who had been dead for exactly ten years. I put all the foods he used to like in a bowl and left it overnight. Friends said I was sick because he wanted this. In the middle of the night I got up and went into the other room where the food was and I felt strange as though someone were there. In the morning I felt much better. But I don't know why my father would want to hurt me as he liked me.

A woman fell on the way to the well and was unconscious. The doctor said it was not a stroke but did not know what was wrong with her. These were signs that it was the *gubida*. She had been in the hospital for several days without improvement when the family decided to have an "offering to the dead."[6] Many family members gathered. The women had been cooking all day. Much food had been prepared and was placed in a separate room where dishes and a lighted candle had been left as well. Each person entered the room and took some of the food in a dish, then put the dish on the floor. No food was consumed. Everything was left for the spirits. After approximately two hours all food and dishes were thrown into a hole and buried. The woman was much improved the following day and released from the hospital within two days.

The *chugu* or "feasting of the dead" is, according to Kerns (1977), rarely requested less than ten and more than fifty years after death. It is much like the ceremony described above, except that it is required a *búiai* be present. "If you don't have a *búiai*, the evil spirits will come and cause trouble." I witnessed no *chugu* and cannot report on the procedure followed in Punta Gorda.

The *dugu* (*dogo*, *adogorahani*) rite or ceremony is the most elaborate and expensive of all ceremonies, usually costing participants well over $1000 BZ. Despite the expense and the absence of a *búiai* in Punta Gorda at present, a number of *dugus* have been held in P.G. in recent years. Two more were reportedly planned for the coming months when I was last in Punta Gorda in 1984. This contrasts with the situation I encountered in 1979. No *dugu* had been held in the town for at least two years. Two were conducted during the seventeen months I was there and I was privileged to be able to attend portions of both. This increase in the number of *dugus* held in Punta Gorda may be the result of several factors. According to Wells (1982a), one explanation is that *dugu* frequency responds to resource flow. During the years 1978 to 1981, when the above mentioned *dugus* would have been planned, there is evidence that the flow of cash into the community had increased. Other researchers have implied that as psychological stress increases, the performance of the *dugu* can be expected to increase as well. Wells concludes, however, that the *dugu* serves primarily as an "identity symbol" which

> ...reflects individual and group strategies which are situationally directed toward identity maintenance or improved socio-economic status (1982a:76).

This interpretation is consistent with my own findings which suggest several parallel and related events: 1. the increasing dominance of state and private networks for the delivery of biomedicine; 2. the growing body of shared interpretations, justifications, and therapies which I have referred to as the "lay therapeutic system", and 3. the retention of ethnic specific markers of identity, specifically the performance of the *chugu* and *dugu* ceremonies.

The *dugu* is described by the Garinagu as a "thanksgiving ceremony" in which ancestors of living participants are honored. According to Kerns, it

> ...represents the pre-eminent cooperative activity, the maximal limits of exchange, the paramount demonstration of generosity and gratitude.... (1977:294).

The motivation for the *dugu* occurs when one or more family members fall ill with some sickness which does not respond to ordinary therapy. Both physicians and healers may state that they can find no cause for the sickness. The expansion of symptoms outward from a single individual to others in the family is a common occurrence and represents an instance of what Janzen refers to as *symptomatic proliferation*. Whether or not the afflicted individual(s) or another family member dream of the *gubída*, a decision may be made to engage in an *arairaguni* or "bringing down of the spirits." A *búiai* is consulted and the ceremony performed. If the *búiai*, though the assistance of his spirit helpers, determines that a *dugu* is required, the family will generally ask that they be given at least a year in which to gather the resources and consult with other family members.

The following explanation and description of activities and procedures which are part of the *dugu* and the preparations for the *dugu* were offered by several persons. For the sake of clarity, I have integrated their accounts into a single narrative. Where explanation seems required or discrepancies occur, I have inserted notes.

The *dugu* will begin this month. It is my father's father's father who wants the *dugu*. Each male member of the family will contribute $25 BZ; females will contribute $20. It is true that someone is ill. If they don't believe in the *dugu* they will die (G).

Sometimes the ancestors appear to someone in a dream. Sometimes somebody gets sick and can't cure. That is how you know they want a *dugu*. Sometimes the ancestor comes natural in a dream. He or she will warn of death in the family if a *dugu* is not held. This time [the reference is to the same *dugu* referred to above which her family sponsored], there weren't any ancestors in dreams, just sicknesses. The family gets together. Everyone in Livingston, Stann Creek, Hopkins, everywhere must be contacted. One family member sets out to visit them all. Sometimes the family has to pray to the ancestors to ask for a year because it takes time to grow the cassava for the bread. The one who is sick becomes the leader. The leader gives instructions to the family and sends round for help. Everybody is supposed to contribute money. If a person says he will have the *dugu* and changes his mind, he will get sick and nothing will cure him. The leader must work hard and collect money from the others to buy two pigs. They raise chickens and ducks for the ceremony too. Only male animals are used in the offering; female animals are used to feed the family and others. They will kill a female pig on the day of the *dugu* for the family to eat. They will have a meeting every Sunday for six months until the week of *dugu*. They take a little bit of money with them each time and wrap it in a calabash. The leader decides which *búiai* to use. There is one in Stann Creek and one in La Buga (Livingston). Those may be the only ones left. (F)

The last time there was a *dugu* it was a woman who had trouble with one of her eyes. She got cured after the *dugu*. This time there are three people ill with illness that won't cure. The *gubída* cause illness. It could be a parent, grandparent or great grandparent.(F)

The *búiai* won't work between Ash Wednesday and Easter [actually, it is his *hiúruha* who won't work during Lent, except, as one individual put it, "on a emergency basis."] The *búiai* comes in a few days before the *dugu* and starts to prepare the temple [*dabúiaba*; this building is specially constructed for the occasion. An existing *dabúiaba* may be used but will require rethatching]. The room in the back is called the stable [also *gule* or sanctuary] and no one but the *búiai* can go there. The candles are kept in there. The *búiai* sleeps there too. He prepares the whole place. He gives instructions to everyone. He tells people to get things. He prepares people for the trip to the cays. (F)

The *búiai* prepares the room in the back [*gule*]. The *búiai* consults the people about what things are required to be brought to the place. The *búiai* brings cotton. He puts cotton in place of the cork in a bottle of rum to allow the smell to get to the spirits. He brings his own incense [copal] and holy water. (Z)

On Tusday morning they [several family members] leave and he goes with them to the seaside. They leave for the cays from P.G. about 3 A.M. on Thursday morning and come in about 6 A.M. [This signals the 'official' start of the *dugu*. Most family members have gathered by now and hammocks are strung everywhere inside and outside the *dabuiaba*]. They look for fish, conch, hairy crab. Everything is cooked. They throw some in the sea on Saturday morning [at the end of the ceremony] and some is buried. Some may be thrown into the sea at midnight Firday night. The *gaiusa* [singers] come with the *búiai* too and they have to be fed. The drummers come with the *búiai* too, but there are also local drummers. The drums and the singing help to bring the spirits. The women are cooking [a separate kitchen has been built beside the *dabúiaba*] Everybody has a job. (F)

The statue of the Virgin Mary is present to show that the blessed virgin is present. The *búiai* got to beg through her to help the sick and to help his operation. He has calabash with seed [*sisira*] for dancing and for the singing of particular hymns. The *sisra* are place beside [on either side of] the Virgin Mary and are a sign of the blessed angels who brought gifts when they visited Mary. [There are supposed to be three calabash rattles, each symbolizing one of the Wise Men. I saw only two at the first ceremony I attended]. You are not to move those gifts unless the *búiai* give you the power or permission. (Z)

When the *dugu* starts the *búiai* looks for *copali* to be smoked. He smokes and blows smoke around. That's in case devils are around. Smoking gets rid of them. If *mafia* gets in maybe somebody loses his life. The drums must be there for dancing. The purpose of the dancing is to get the *gubída* satisfied because when they were here on earth they do all those things. (Z)

From 5:30 A.M. Thursday [when the boats return] they start dancing and singing almost continuously until Saturday morning. [According to Wells (1982a), an important part of the "work of the *dugu*" is performing sets of songs and dances bracketed by short rest breaks.]

> Four types of dance are used – the *abaimahani*, a semi- sacred song of the women; the *amalihani*, a song and dance of supplication; the *awangulani*, a dance of rejoicing; and the *hugulendi*...." (4)

The circular *hugulendi* dance, she continues,

> ...functions to 'gather, attract, and sooth the powerful ancestor spirits who are considered to be anxious to progress in their transition toward a pure state of existence. (6)

The *búiai*'s spirit helpers come and tell him if anything is wrong. Maybe somebody is taking the rum, for example. Or maybe some woman went there with her period. You can't enter the *dugu* with your period. You can't even remain outside. You must stay at home. (F)

The *gaiusa* are singing their songs. The singing brings the spirits in. But you must know the songs. The songs are to talk to the *gubída*. (B)

The ancestors, many of them, come back and cause fits [*ówehani*, the same word is used to refer to trance-like possession states of the *dugu*, to the 'fits' of epilepsy, to the seizures or convulsions accompanying eclampsia, to the rigidity resulting from polio and the actions preceding death; the Garifuna word for death is *owehni*. According to Taylor (1951) there are three stages of possession, each recognized terminologically: *adereha*[7] or "to stiffen" refers to the first stage; the second is called *agobuiha*[8] and indicates full possession; the third is called *aueha* amd means to "pass out." The term *ówehani* used by the individuals I interviewed is likely derived from the word *aueha*.] The ancestor comes to someone and they don't know what they do or say. The *búiai* brings the ancestors in and may bring them back again if that is necessary. The ancestors say things through the people they possess. They tell them what they want and what everybody should do and not do. Maybe they tell you're not doing something in a correct way like they want done. Maybe one family didn't believe in the *dugu* and the ancestor will say so, will point out which family didn't attend. Ancestors say they will teach them, they will reach into the home. The family or individual will lose a grandchild. If there is a family feuding and it isn't mended, then the *dugu* won't go through. The *búiai* will mention any family feuding. (F)

The *gubida* come on their family there, they fall down, can't talk, bawl, shout, and want to dance more. Sometimes they climb up [the rafters of the *dabúiaba*]. They act like crazy. It is the *gubída*. To get them eased down the *búiai* use rum. The possessed person is said to have *ówehani* from the *gubída*. (Z)

Some have fits and he [*búiai*] has to blow smoke [*buwe*, *bue*, tobacco smoke] on them until they recover. Many will be possessed. (G)

The *búiai* talks to the *gubída* and they obey. Your dead father comes when the *búiai* calls his name and joins in. [Any of these spirits may speak through the *buiái* who is, himself, possessed during these experiences]. (Z)

The *búiai* has spirits, but it is the same as though he is possessed by the spirit of your *gubída*. The spirit speaks through the *búiai*. [Many who have heard the *gubída* speak state that they speak with the voice of the ancestor and they recognize the voice; ethnographers have suggested that many *búiai* are highly skilled ventriloquists. This characteristic performance was reported as early as the mid-seventeenth century:

> Armand de la Paix (in Rennard 1929, p. 51) says: "Moreover, the devils enter even into men's bodies and speak by their mouth" and Rochefort (1658, p. 473): "These familiar spirits also enter into the bodies of females and speak through them" (Taylor 1951: 124fn).]

There are bad spirits too. The *búiai* is called to get rid of the evil spirits. The *hiúruha* are supposed to be there because there may be bad spirits there. You can have *gubída*, *hiúruha*, and evil spirits there at the same time. The *búiai* brings in *hiúruha* to assist in driving the spirit [land or water spirit] from the sick person. This spirit may be the cause of the illness. The *gubída* have the power to drive the evil spirit away. The *dugu* is held for either *lisándi wenani* [illness of devils] or *hasándigubída*. [In this he differs from all the others with whom I discussed the *dugu* and its functions. They stated that it was only the *gubída* who caused the illness. His statement that it may be evil spirits as well is, however, consistent with Coehlo's report that illness occurs because the *gubída* withdraw their protection (1955:147).] (Z)

The spirits [*gubída*] must be sent back after they are called. But certain spirits are hard to move. If there are family feuds, the spirits won't move until everything is settled. The *búiai* has to stand to settle matters and only then can he send the ancestors back. He may use prayers to send them back. Certain songs are used. He asks certain people to help him sing to send the spirits back and also to call them back. If the *búiai* knows the spirits are not contented he will call them back until they are satisfied. He calls people to make *mali* [Palacio, 1973, refers to *mali* as a placation ceremony; my informant said the famous *búiai*, Sarah, calls it a benedication]. (F)

The offerings [food, rum, and other items requested by the *gubída;* during one *dugu* I attended, the *gubída* asked for a special pair of pants which could only be obtained in Guatemala] placate the *gubída*. Then the *gubída* and the *hiúruha* get rid of the evil spirit through the power of the *búiai*. And the evil spirit goes never to return. If the illness is *hasandigubida*, the *gubída* leave the person alone and the person recovers. (Z)

They prepare the food and leave it on the table from early A.M. on Friday. [Among other things, large tubs of cassava bread are left up in the rafters of the *dabúiaba*]. They sprinkle *hiu* [a drink made of cassava] around the *dabúiaba*. At four P.M. on Friday, they bury the food away from the *dabúiaba*. They pour rum on the table. Then the spirits are satisfied. The flames [the rum is set on fire] will indicate the spirits are happy. (B)

At the end of the ceremony, the *búiai* informs the sick that everything is alright. *Agudahani*, that means the sprinkling of the rum in the hall or inside the temple to show the people that the *gubída* received the offering [Taylor refers to *agudahani* as a "burning" ceremony in which the *búiai* covers a table top with rum and sets it on fire (1951:127)]. Then they bury the food in any part of the compound where the operation took place. When it is buried, that is a sign that they are not coming back again to repeat. When it is not buried and they eat the food, the *gubida* are liable to repeat everything again. (Z)

On Friday, the food which has been in the *dabúiaba* is buried in back of the temple. Some of it is thrown into the sea. The spirits leave on Saturday. They are sent away by the *búiai*. As long as everyone cooperates with *búiai*, the *dugu* will be successful.

Sick people will get normal again. The *búiai* also leaves on Saturday. The leader must sleep in the *dabuiaba* for eight days to make sure the spirits don't come back. (F)

There are several aspects of the *dugu* which might be examined further (see, for example, Wells 1980, 1982b on color and spatial symbolism of the *dugu*). However, I have chosen to restrict additional discussion to the experience of *ówehani*. The occurrence of possession constitutes a transcendence of the body's boundaries, a movement of the 'self' from pragmatic considerations and constraints to a state in which the previously inexpressible may be expressed. It gives evidence that the distinction between life and death is illusory, that the social body is not defined by its living members alone. The cause of illness, and its consequent cure, can be found in a set of relations which have no boundaries in space and time. The *dugu* becomes a joyous occasion, a reunification and reconstitution of the social group. The *gubída* enter "in a rush" and their presence is physically felt. They have been called back by the *búiai*, assisted by the drums, and they have come to express their wishes and to startle the unbeliever into belief. They enter the bodies of participants who cannot, from that point on, be held accountable for their actions. Ironically, the unification of the corporeal being with the spirit of the deceased does not remove the possessed person from the social group which surrounds him, but rather brings together the entire social body, uniting it metaphorically in the actions and experiences of a single person.

NOTES

1. Total number exceeds fifty-three because of multiple uses.
2. Two women indicated that infants had died because of an eclipse of the moon. One stated that the child had "water head" due to an eclipse.
3. The Garinagu generally utilize a single term, *hilagulau*, to refer to the blood vessels, nerves, muscles, and tendons.
4. "Guides" wearing red pants and crossed shoulder straps are mentioned by other ethnographers as well.
5. Most believe any *búiai* can turn *obeah* back on the individual who caused or requested it.
6. This ceremony appears identical to the *chugu* described by Wells; yet the individuals with whom I spoke did not refer to this as a *chugu*. Further, several persons insisted that the *chugu* requires the presence of a *búiai*.
7. One healer referred to a child who had 'fits' and a 'stiff-eye look' as suffering from *adéirahani*. The cause, in this case, was said to be worms. The same word is used to refer to *tetanus*.
8. The state of possession by ancestors was also termed *hagubidahouna*.
9. See Wells 1982b on the use of *bue* or *buwe*.

CHAPTER 7

Case Studies, CultureTexts, and Culture Models

Illness episodes function as narratives, as stories of personal failures and successes, they display information about the moral and social order, about relationships as they are and as they should be; they derive from and speak of critical cultural concerns; they are built upon signs which incorporate "disparate significata" (Turner 1967:28); they provide models for and models of unique cultural realities. They serve as texts which both disguise and reveal through metaphor.

The illness episodes described in this chapter constitute, in the language of certain Soviet semioticians, "actual culture texts." They both interpret cultural models and are interpreted by them. Despite the obvious constraints imposed by the various medical paradigms upon the interpretive process, reality is negotiated according to the needs of the various actors. Signs acquire significance partially as a result of the contexts in which they emerge and in accordance with the requirements of participants, including the diagnostician, in the process.

In the case studies to be presented, several processes are evident. Individuals and their families engage in negotiation, in the reinterpretation of signs, and in the activation of a series of networks in the search for therapies, diagnoses, etiologies, and prognoses consistent with the patient's and the family's understanding of the case.

The primary goal of negotiation is the achievement of an interpretation or an alignment and stucturing of the relationships among signs which is acceptable within the parameters of the medical model and which leads to a therapy which is preceived as appropriate. Janzen (1973 MS) has identified two processes which are important to any discussion of negotiation. These are *symptomatic proliferation* and *etiological shifting*. *Symptomatic proliferation* refers to the change in perception of symptoms. For example, symptoms may suddenly be shifted outwards to the social group. Symptomatic proliferation thus relates several individuals' afflictions to one common cause. Symptomatic proliferation may also provide "an individual with a series of successive symptoms incorporated into a single case", that is, as the case progresses, new symptoms are incorporated into the illness. *Etiological shifting*, as Janzen employs the phrase, refers to a shift in diagnosis, where, for example, an illness may be moved from the category of "illness of God" to "illness of man." I have somewhat altered that definition for my purposes here. Etiology and diagnosis are closely related but not identical processes or phenomena. Diagnosis refers to the labeling process, even though that label may be so vague or broad as "an illness of the world" or "heart trouble." Diagnosis does not always occurs in illness episodes, nor, obviously, is it necessary to the recovery of the patient. One may proceed with symptomatic therapy without an understanding of either etiology or diagnosis. It is also possible to determine an etiology without determining, at the same time, a diagnosis, though a clearly stated etiology often specifies or implies a diagnosis as well. Diagnosis and etiology imply one another, but neither may be strictly determinate of the other. Further, diagnosis is more clearly linked to etiology (and vice versa) in biomedicine than in ethnomedical systems. At least this is true for the Garifuna medical model. Therefore, I have distinguished here between diagnostic shifts and etiologic shifts.

Etiologic shifts are of two types; 1. a change in the determination of the original event (sign) in the chain of events leading up to an illness, and 2. an alteration in the determination of the totality of events which are to be included in the sequence. There may occur, as the result of negotiation, a realignment of signs. That is, existing signs may be reordered in such a way that a sign previously incorporated into the syndrome may be excluded; one or more others may be added.

In some instances a diagnostic shift may involve an incorporation of new information into an existing diagnosis, rather than, strictly speaking, a shift to an entirely new diagnosis. It is likely that certain information, however, cannot be incorporated into previous diagnoses because of limitations in the flexibility of the medical model employed, and the patient or social group must select from among the acceptable range of diagnoses.

The utilization of a new model of illness may be expected to lead to an alteration in therapies. A Garifuna woman stated she had suffered for many years from asthma. She became a member of a Pentecostalist sect and took part in a healing ceremony in which her asthma was "cured." It seems probable, in this case, that only prior acceptance of the new interpretive model would have resulted in either the acceptance of the proffered therapy or the change in her physical state.

But, in general, individuals are slow or reluctant to accept entirely new models. Rather, the tendency is to incorporate bits and pieces of new paradigms into the old. The residents of Punta Gorda and surrounding communities very commonly seek out antibiotic therapies in the local clinics. Yet it is clear that this has not involved, in any notable way, the acceptance or incorporation of a new model or even some portion of it. "Man's interest in this world is largely practical", states Locker.

He is concerned with doing and achieving and not with acquiring a coherent understanding of the way in which it works. Rather, knowledge of the world is organized in terms of degrees of relevance to his actions and is only as systematic as it need be for the realization of his practical projects (Locker 1981:10).

It is likely, however, that new therapies will result in a slow change in models in which some elements from the biomedical model are incorporated into ethnically derived or lay models. The therapy, if deemed successful, may lead to a new model of illness causation and therapeutic intervention, or it may result in etiologic, diagnostic, or symptomatic shifts, or the incorporation of signs previously unheeded. The therapy which succeeds implies an etiology and a diagnosis.

The confrontation with biomedicine and its largely intractable codes may require that the ensuing interpretation incorporate, account for, or partially assimilate the diagnosis or interpretation of biomedical personnel. Such a resolution may result from the creation or utilization of new models based on an articulation but not an identification of two or more codes. A single sign may develop multiple interpretants, each consistent with or explained by one of the many available models of illness and health. These varying interpretants may exist simultaneously without inherent contradiction or threat to any given model. Even where contradictions are evident, consistency in interpretation may not be required for, as Locker remarks: "From within the natural attitude practical problem solving is of more relevance than matters of theoretical purity" (1981:171):

Both chronic and acute illnesses provide occasion for negotiation, though an acute illness which is of short duration and is satisfactorily resolved may provoke little. Chronic illnesses, especially those in which the diagnosis or etiology is non-specific, are most susceptible to negotiation.

Diagnosis and the assignment or determination of an etiology may be affected by the patient's manipulation of symptoms, that is, his or her reporting of signs. Signs, symptoms, past events and current problems are selectively incorporated into the presentation or altogether disregarded. Information is produced through the interaction of patient and healer, but the patient may manipulate this exchange in such a way as to avoid certain diagnoses or to predetermine a diagnosis and a therapy which is likely to be personally acceptable.

Several of the cases reported here began with the utilization of therapeutic resources outside the domain of biomedicine. All eventually utilized biomedicine – not necessarily because of its assumed superiority but, in part, because of its accessibility. Many were dissatisfied and turned again to other resources. Cases were often resolved by combining elements from various 'systems' and, to the extent possible, explaining the resolution in terms of the accepted cultural or medical model.

One critical issue not yet confronted has to do with the relation of such potentially esoteric sign systems as world view to the existance and exploitation of medical resources. Semiotics fails if it cannot provide a unified view of culture which demonstrates the interdependence of both.

Culture is described by Soviet semioticians as:

...a process and a mechanism characterized by the struggle for information which is received, decoded and translated from one system into another as well as exchanged.... (Winner 1979:106-107).

Culture, in this view, consists, in part, of information and the means whereby individuals or groups gain access and control over such information. The relationship between power and signs is thus made obvious.

Marx at once determined the necessity of the signs as intermediary in exchange and in the semiotization of the communicatory process (Lotman 1976:215).

Of the connections among signs, information, and power, Lotman declares:

The battle for survival – both the biological and the social one – is a struggle for information. An understanding of culture's essence as information explains the passionate involvement in this matter of both the bearers and the destroyers of culture, whose conflicts with each other constitute the history of mankind (Lotman 1976:215)

And further:

Culture, however, is not a storehouse of information. It is an extremely complex mechanism which preserves information while constantly working out the most efficient means to do this; it receives new information, encodes and decodes communications and *translates them from one sign system into another*. Culture is a versatile and highly organized mechanism of cognition. The sphere of culture is at once a sphere of constant struggle, of social, historical and class conflicts and confrontations. Various social and historical groups fighting for information strive to monopolize it. The means used toward this end vary between secret texts and codes (the secret languages of different age and social groups, religious, political and professional secrets, etc.) and the creation of misleading texts (*Ibid.*). [emphasis added]

Material resources and cultural models are unified through reference to the concept of the sign. The strategies which people employ in seeking relief from distress and in manipulation or exploitation of medical resources have to do with gaining access to and control over information. *Interpretation, from this perspective, is the manipulation and exploitation of signs for the purpose of effecting a desired biological and social state.*

My focus in the case studies to follow is not on the presence, absence, or nature of the signs which might indicate an actual alteration in physiological or psychological state, but on the individual's and the social group's perception or the response to such signs. Just as physiological changes may occur but not manifest themselves in signs available for interpretation, so may an individual define himself as ill and yet regard the signs as indicating no necessary and/or appropriate behavioral response. While instances of non-action may be found in these case studies, the emphasis is on the strategies utilized to effect the maintenance of or return to a 'normal' state. The notion of normality, it should be noted, must be defined anew with each case and in relation to the prior physical state of the afflicted individual.

The first five case studies presented are of Garifuna individuals and their families. The seven which follow are studies of illness episodes occurring among members of other ethnic groups. They are included here because they illustrate further a variety of negotiating strategies, the confrontation with biomedical personnel and beliefs, and some of the similarities and dissimilarities between the Garifuna medical model and those of other ethnic sections.

Case Study One: Peter Lambey

Peter is a Garifuna male child who was ten months old in May of 1979 when his case came to my attention. He was then a patient in the local hospital having been admitted with a "history of vomiting." My initial interview was conducted with an elderly woman in her seventies who described herself to me as Peter's grandmother. She was, in fact, Peter's father's mother's mother's sister. Peter, at that time, lived with this woman, whom I shall refer to as Ventura, and Emiliano, her *umári*.

I noted that Peter was many pounds underweight by comparison with other infants of his age, he was lethargic, and there appeared to be considerable muscular wasting. His hair was light in color and sparse; his skin color suggested depigmentation, all signs suggesting a diagnosis of kwashiorkor. I asked Ventura if I might follow Peter's case. She agreed and we began a relationship which lasted until the time of my departure twelve months later. Despite his malnutrition and lack of development, Ventura's principal concern was with Peter's vomiting. Peter had, according to Ventura, suffered from "mole drop" when he was two months old. He had since been unable to eat anything except cassava starch (a powder obtained from the grated root of the cassava plant). He also received a small amount of Cerelac (a cereal product, largely starch again) in a bottle mixed with water when he could tolerate it. His vomiting had continued daily since his second month. It was his inability to tolerate even cassava starch which brought Ventura to the clinic with Peter.

Ventura reported that when Peter first exhibited the signs of "mole drop" (depressed fontanelle, vomiting), she turned to a cousin who had some knowledge of this illness. He was "nointed" (massaged with oil) and eggs and nutmeg were applied to his head. This, she said, provided some relief though she recognized that he continued to suffer from mole drop. The purpose of the treatment had been to bring the fontanelle to its normal position. Of his current "illness", she explained that the depression of the fontanelle caused him to have pain in his throat, which, in turn, caused coughing. It was the coughing, in Ventura's opinion, which led to his vomiting. Except for the vomiting, Ventura remarked, Peter was well. He was getting injections and "medicine to drink" while at the hospital and was, Ventura said, better at the time of my initial interview in May.

Ventura had many chores to do at home and, in addition, raised cassava on a small plantation in the Carib Block, some distance from Punta Gorda. Still, much of her time was spent with Peter at the hospital. He was released after several days of treatment for "gastroenteritis." No treatment was given or recommended for malnutrition, nor was any record of his general appearance or physical condition noted. If the nurses had shown concern, it was not evidenced in the chart.

I watched Peter for the period of a year following this initial interview and observation. At the age of twenty-two months, he was able to stand with assistance. He could pull himself to a standing position but had to lean against something or someone to remain standing. He could not walk. I could only estimate his weight at that time at approximately twelve to fifteen pounds. He had grown a small amount of soft brown curly hair and had four teeth. He spoke no words and appeared weak and pale at each visit.

The social history surrounding Peter's case bears directly on his medical history and on the treatment of his illness and his lack of development. Peter was the eleventh child born to a Garifuna woman, Nora, who was approximately thirty-four years old at the time of Peter's birth. I visited Nora on several occasions in the small two-room house where she and seven of her children lived. Since all her children had been given her surname it is difficult to say how many *umári* Nora had. Most Garifuna women give each child the surname of the father whether married or not. Nora had broken convention in that regard. She was in several other respects a strong and independent woman.

Two of her children were living with her parents in Punta Gorda, another was with the mother of the child's father. Peter had been "passed over" to Ventura shortly after his birth. When Peter was approximately sixteen months old, Nora gave birth to another child. That infant also appeared considerably underweight and on the last visit in which I saw the baby, his head was covered with a "plaster", a common treatment for "mole drop." Upon my departure, Nora was again pregnant. This was to be her thirteenth child.

Nora reported to me that one child, a daughter, had died in 1976 at the age of eleven months. The child, she said, suffered from vomiting, diarrhea, and fever. The hospital death record apparently indicated that the child was malnourished, though Nora protests this was not so.

When I first began visiting Nora, I noticed that her two year old son, Manuel, had a severe oozing rash over his face and parts of his body. His eyes exuded a thick yellowish fluid. However, he did not otherwise appear unwell and was active. I asked the oldest of the children living with Nora what she thought might be wrong with Manuel. She answered that he had "prickly heat." When, during one visit, I asked Nora if anyone in the family was ill, she stated that Peter had a cold, but otherwise everyone was well. She did not mention Manuel's condition. I asked specifically what had caused Manuel's sores. She stated that she didn't know, but she had obtained penicillin ointment from the hospital for him. The ointment resulted in a temporary subsidence of the symptoms, but shortly after the sores would "come out" again. Manuel, like Peter, was reported to have suffered from "mole drop" when he was younger. His mother said he had been hospitalized several times after he began cutting teeth and had received "drips" (IVs) each time. Nora also stated that Manuel had a "chest problem" from the time he started cutting teeth. She suggested that it might be because he cut his teeth late. Babies delivered in the hospital, she added, often suffer with chest colds because the nurses forget to suction the "cold" out of an infant's chest at birth, as the midwives do. Manuel also had a long history of repeated vomiting, but, according to Nora, had recovered from both disorders when all his baby teeth appeared. She did not connect his sores with any prior condition or event.

Nora reported that most of her children had suffered from mole drop. She explained that she never had sufficient breast milk to nurse them and they were put on a bottle shortly after birth. "They say bottle-fed babies all suffer from mole drop." She suggested that the child may strain too hard on the nipple of the bottle and that this results in the depression of the "mole." Nora told me that she did not use bush medicines and that she "carried" her children to the doctor when they were ill. "But we Carib people, we have our ways." Each of the children who developed mole drop had been treated by a local midwife. Treatment involves sucking on the baby's head to bring the fontanelle up.

Peter lived with Ventura and Emiliano from the time he was approximately two months old until he was approximately fourteen months old. At one point, when he was only a few months old, and before I knew any of the families involved, Nora came to take Peter home. Ventura told me she said to Nora, "If you had told me you were gong to take him back, I wouldn't have worked so hard to feed him. I will miss this baby." Nora started to take the infant, then returned him to Ventura and left the house.

When he was about one year old, Nora sent her oldest daughter to take Peter from Ventura. She had decided that since she must soon quit work because of the imminent birth of her next child, she would be in a position to care for Peter. Further, she felt Ventura had not properly cared for the child. She also remarked to me that she had noticed her older children whom she had "passed over" to her parents rarely came to visit her. It seemed, in fact, to be an incident in which her son who was living with her parents failed to share some fish he had caught with her which precipitated Nora's most recent request for the return of Peter. Ventura, however, refused to give up the child and told Nora's daughter that Nora herself would have to come to get Peter. Ventura was distressed at the thought that Nora might come to demand Peter at any time. A short time later, however, Ventura told me that Nora, now almost due to deliver, was considering giving her this "next" infant as well.

Some two months later, Nora did come for Peter, and Ventura had little choice but to turn him over. She protested that Nora had provided nothing for the child in the year that she had cared for him. Ventura had never had children of her own and Peter received much attention from both Emiliano and Ventura. Ventura reported that Peter's father came to visit Peter occasionally and that, upon request, he would provide what he could for Peter. According to Ventura and Emiliano, Peter's father had made a complaint to the court, at which time he stated he wished the child to remain with the elderly couple. For the most part, Emiliano and Ventura asked for little help from anyone, though neither had any income. Their small two-room house tilted to one side and was in serious need of both repairs and furniture. Peter slept between the couple in a small bed. There was rarely any extra food to be seen in the house. Ventura harvested cassava from her plantation and made it into starch and Emiliano, who was almost eighty, fished when he could to provide for his small family. But when he seriously injured his foot in 1980 he was unable to fish for several weeks.

Apparently a truce was eventually reached between Nora and Ventura as Peter was passed back and forth between them during the last months I was living in Punta Gorda. Ventura was not entirely pleased with this arrangement. It was with excitement that she informed me days in advance of each expected arrival of Peter at their home.

During the year that I followed this case, I recorded the following events:

In June, after his release from the hospital, Ventura reported she had purchased vitamins for Peter and was taking him to the clinic the following day for a "check-up." She said he was no longer vomiting.

A week later Peter seemed far more active and Emiliano seemed pleased. He accounted for his lack of growth by saying he "took after his mother, who is small."

In September, Peter was visited by a *búiai* at Ventura's request. The *búiai* had come from Stann Creek (Dangriga) and was to return to Punta Gorda in two weeks to visit him again. However, by then, Peter had been taken by his mother. The *búiai* reported that Peter's problem was that he had suffered from "mole drop" from birth. Her spirits told her that there was no human or spiritual cause for his illness. Nevertheless, plans were made to hold a small *dugu* (most likely, a *chugu*). The *búiai* pushed up on his palate to raise the fontanelle and "nointed" him. The *búiai* left medicine; additional medicine was obtained from a midwife/healer next door. He now reportedly consumed small amounts of fish, potatoes, and biscuits.

At about this time, Emiliano began to complain of feeling ill. His left eye was oozing matter and he described his vision as "dim." He claimed that he had never been ill before and that he had "never enter no hospital." He added that he didn't "feel so good from inside." He suggested that the sickness in his eye came from a "disorder" with his liver, diagnosed by a physician in Guatemala. He was taking medicine prescribed by this physician for his liver, but felt it wasn't helping. Sometimes, he said, he had to force himself to eat. Emiliano remarked that he had suffered from loss of appetite and a liver disorder for six or seven months, though it was only when he experienced the added problem with his eye that this prior condition was mentioned. Emiliano also reported that his head felt "funny." He believed this was due to the difficulty with his eye. Thus several signs were grouped together and attributed to a single cause ("liver disorder"). The cause of the "liver disorder" was never given. Emiliano's eye eventually improved and no further mention was made of the other problems or symptoms.

A few days later, Ventura told me that Peter had fever, She took him to the hospital for medicine. On her return, Nora was waiting and took Peter from her as she had long said she would.

In November, I visited Peter at his mother's home. He appeared lethargic and thinner than before. His mother insisted that he was improving. She pointed to the fact that he had grown hair and had his first teeth. She had purchased *Glucodin* for him because he had loose stools. She reported that he now was eating rice and tortillas. The doctor gave her "tonic" for him, but he vomited that. She was giving him "vitamins." I gave her eggs and suggested she give him one each day. Nora reported a few days later when I stopped at the office where she worked (she had resumed working) that Peter immediately consumed each egg. She stated that she was now going to get eggs from her father who kept a duck in his yeard. Nora expressed disturbance at Peter's father's apparent lack of interest in Peter. She believed that his father wasn't providing properly for him. The father had recently been admitted to the hospital, suffering from high blood pressure. Nora visited him there and requested additional support, apparently to no avail. He had now taken another "wife."

In December I visited Nora twice. On the first occasion, Nora assured me Peter's condition was essentially the same. Several days later Peter was cutting additional teeth, had a "cold" and appeared extremely lethargic. He wouldn't smile, as he usually did, his stomach appeared swollen and his limbs withered.

Nora said he was unable to swallow large chunks of food and vomited frequently. She believed there was something wrong with his throat. She expressed a desire to take him to Barrios (Puerto Barrios, Guatemala) where they have a "hospital for infants." She said that she believed they didn't care properly for babies at the Punta Gorda hospital.

In January, Peter had an eye infection, a cough, and a runny nose. He was lying face down on the wooden floor on Nora's tiny house when I arrived, but pulled himself up to the doorway and reached for my hand. Nora said he now ate solid food without vomiting. She suggested that the problem with his eyes might have been caused by the bright lights in the house. She stated that she told her daughter to "carry" Peter over to the doctor, but she had failed to do so. Nora said upon this occasion that she now believed that Peter's condition may have been caused by the stress she was under when she was pregnant. She reported that during that period she argued with her father a great deal.

In February of 1980, Manuel became "ill." Nora's father said he believed the child's rash had gone to his throat. Manuel was suffering with a "cold" and was taken to the hospital by his mother. The nurse provided Nora with medicine, but Manuel was not admitted. Nora returned home with Manuel from the hospital. He died at home the following morning. Manuel's death certificate reported the cause of death as measles, with antecedent or contributing causes of kwashiorkor, bronchitis, and dehydration. This was the third such experience for Nora with hospital staff. In 1976 when her daughter, Maria, became ill, Nora's sister, who was caring for Maria at the time, took her to the hospital and reported her illness. The child, however, was not admitted until the following morning; she died that evening. Nora also reported that when Peter was very small and suffering from vomiting and a cough she took him to the hospital. She was given "tonic" and "cough medicine" at the outpatient clinic and sent home. Nora felt Peter would have been well today if he had been admitted on that occasion.

Ventura looked after Peter temporarily during this period. When I visited Peter there she told me that she thought Peter looked bad and planned to cover his body with brandy mixed with egg white. This would give him strength.

In March, Peter was returned to Nora. Emiliano said he believed Peter's problem was due to a "lack of support."

In April, my last visit to Nora, Peter looked much the same as he had, though he seemed to have recovered from his cold. The newest infant (now six months old) appeared malnourished, though Nora seemed to believe he was doing reasonably well. I asked if I might take a picture of all the children. Nora went to some trouble to prepare them all so that they might have their picture taken.

Nora firmly believed that she was doing all she could to care for her children. She was extremely independent and refused to beg for help for her children. She had a responsible position in the town and worked when she was able. She provided for her children to the best of her abilities, as had Ventura. On the last occasion when I visited her, Nora told me that she intended to keep her family together. "I will do the best I can on the money I make, and if that isn't good enough, then we will die."

In Peter's case study, we see general agreement on the diagnosis of "mole drop" and little attempt to alter or "shift" the diagnostic label. "Mole drop" was, of course, not the term employed by biomedical personnel, but no effort was made by the family to negotiate another diagnostic label for Peter's condition with the hospital staff. There was, it should be pointed out, no disagreement between Ventura and the physician or nurses for neither ever communicated a diagnosis to the other. Had the diagnosis of "gastroenteritis" been explained to Ventura, she would likely have rejected it, since gastroenteritis is an acute illness generally of short duration and it was clear to Ventura that Peter had suffered from "mole drop" almost from birth.

There were, on the other hand, a variety of attempts to establish or alter the etiology. Nora utilized several strategies in the process of making sense of Peter's condition. She shifted etiologies or established new etiological chains on several occasions, though the creation of new etiological chains did not necessarily precipitate the rejection of earlier ones. And she incorporated signs into existing etiological chains which had not been mentioned previously. All etiological chains presented by Nora were "naturalistic", and she at no time tried to place Peter's illness in the category of "uncommon illness."

Certain of her explanations emphasized mechanical concepts of illness causation or organ interdependence. For example, she suggested that all bottle-fed babies suffer from "mole drop" because sucking on the nipple of the bottle causes the fontanelle to become depressed. The therapies instituted by a local midwife (sucking on the fontanelle to raise it) and the *búiai* (pushing up on the palate to push the fontanelle into position) are consistent with this explanation. The "plaster" placed on the head of her youngest child represented a similar approach in that the plaster is believed to cause the fontanelle to rise. Her treatment of Manuel's sores was likewise symptomatic therapy. Nora's explanation that Peter could not swallow and vomited large pieces of food referred to a disorder of his throat, again, a basically mechanical concept of causation.

Other etiological chains pointed up the importance of parent-child interactions. In part, she claimed responsibility for Peter's state in her references to her inability to nurse her infants and the necessity of giving them "formula." The inability to nurse was, in turn, blamed on the size of her breasts. Many women who place their infants on "formula" do encounter problems, for few can afford to prepare the "formula" (sold in most stores) according to the directions on the package. That is, far less "formula" is added to a bottle of water than package directions require. Further, there is some question as to the nutritive value of certain products which are sold as "formula." Finally, "formala" is generally mixed with unsterilized water, increasing the risks of gastroenteritis and other gastrointestinal disorders. The government of Belize has, in recent years, made a serious effort to encourage all mothers to nurse their infants and to abandon "formulas."

Nora also spoke of the relationship with her father as one cause of Peter's condition, illustrating the fairly common acceptance of stress as an etiological factor in explanations of illness causation, and again emphasizing the critical nature of parent-child interactions, and, in this case, grandparent-grandchild interactions.

Finally, certain etiological chains stressed the superiority of traditional therapies and practices and the inferiority of biomedicine as practiced in Punta Gorda. Nora, over a period of several years, had a series of unfortunate encounters with biomedicine – specifically the failure of hospital staff to admit first her daughter, then Peter as an infant, and, finally, Manuel to the hospital at times she felt hospitalization was required. The prescription of antibiotic ointment for Manel's "sores" and the treatment of Peter's "gastro-enteritis" without apparent regard for the underlying and precipitating condition suggests that Nora's belief that "they don't care properly for babies here" was not totally unfounded. In additon, "political" medicine and personal prejudices may have played a role as well. That is, the practice of medicine can be highly politicized and a variety of factors enter into its administration. Certainly Nora was never able to effectively manipulate or exploit the biomedical system to the benefit of her family. To do so requires control over a variety of types of information, including the medical paradigms under which biomedicine operates, and, as implied earlier, those least likely to exert such control are the Garifuna and Mayan members of the community.

Emiliano established new etiological chains as well. When Peter had apparently recovered from an acute stage of illness, Emiliano was optimistic and explained that Peter was small because "he took after his mother." When Peter had been removed from their home, he suggested that Peter's problem was due "to a lack of support", an etiological model which assigned responsibility to the parents, and, again, emphasized the importance of parent-child interactions and the obligations of both parents to provide for their children. Peter's illness was thus referred to the failure of one or both parents.

Ventura, unlike Nora and Emiliano, attemped to generate new signs which would both explain the non-responsiveness of Peter's overall condition to a variety of therapies (the actions of the midwife, the treatments prescribed by biomedical staff, traditional herbal and other remedies) and provide an effective therapy. The generation of such signs called for divinatory techniques which, in turn, required the presence of a *búiai*. Despite the fact that the *búiai* reinforced the diagnosis of "mole drop", failed to generate new signs through her *hiúruha*, and let the broad diagnostic category of *lisándi ubaó* stand, the decision was made to hold a *chugu*, most likely as a preventive measure.

As I left Punta Gorda, Peter's condition appeared to have stabilized. It is likely that a combination of factors – Manuel's death, the youngest child's "mole drop", the birth of yet another child, combined with any further deterioration of Peter's condition – will cause a new search for an appropriate and satisfying etiological explanation.[1]

Case Study Two: Mr. John Arzu

Mr. John Arzu is a Garifuna male, living in a small three room house with his wife, seven of their ten children, the common law husbands of two of their daughters and four grandchildren by three of their daughters. Mr. Arzu was sixty-five at the time of my initial contact. About three years earlier, he had developed a numbness in portions of his body. He described the symptoms to his wife and various bush preparations were used to bathe him: a combination of ginger, rubbing alcohol and lime; water obtained from boiling garlic leaf and fever grass; and camphor mixed with rum or alcohol. There was some relief from the symptoms and Mr. Arzu continued his work. After approximately one month, Mr. Arzu mentioned his symptoms to his employer who responded by stating that he didn't believe in bush medicine; he was ordered to see the government physician. Mr. Arzu visited the government doctor. The doctor told him he would be hospitalized for one week for observation. While hospitalized, Mr. Arzu began to experience numbness again and shortly afterwards had a "stroke." He was kept in the hospital for a period of almost four months, during which time he had a second "stroke" and lost his speech entirely. His right side was also paralyzed. The doctor reported to the family that Mr. Arzu had had "the pressure" for many years and that "the sickness had gone to his brain." Eventually, Mr. Arzu returned home. He was on medication and was told to return once a week for a blood pressure check. There had been no noticeable improvement since the second stroke.

Mrs. Arzu heard about a private "doctor" from the States practicing in Stann Creek (Dangriga) who was said to have a treatment for such conditions. The Arzus left for Stann Creek, a trip of several hours by bus, where

Mr. Arzu received treatments for approximately one and one-half months. The treatment involved the use of a machine with a rod which was passed back and forth over his body. At the end of six weeks this practitioner claimed he was being harassed by the government physician in the district and closed his offices. Mrs. Arzu reports there had been some improvement during this period.

The Arzus remained in Stann Creek and next consulted with Sarah, perhaps the most famous living *búiai*. Mr. Arzu, Sarah stated, had an enemy who had disguised himself as a friend. This person had used *obeah* against Mr. Arzu. She prescribed daily baths in a special herbal preparation. Mr. Arzu lived in her temple and spirit center (*dabúiaba*) for three months and received treatment each day. At the end of three months, Mr. Arzu returned home, but the baths were continued for a full year. During this time Mr. Arzu was prohibited from using "doctor" medicine (biomedicine) as the two types of medicine, Sarah explained, cannot be used simultaneously. Sarah asked Mrs. Arzu if she wished the *obeah* turned back on the person who had used it, but Mrs. Arzu replied that she only wished a cure for her husband.

Mr. Arzu showed little improvement when he returned home and eventually the Arzus traveled to Belize City where they had heard of another private physician. Mr. Arzu was given injections and a prescription for medications and told to return in one month and then again one month later. On the third visit a second physician had temporarily replaced the first. He told the Arzus that the illness "wouldn't cure" and it would be best for them to accept the situation, return to Punta Gorda, and continue with the treatment prescribed by the government physician stationed in Punta Gorda. They returned to their home.

Mrs. Arzu tried various remedies in the hope her husband's condition would improve. On the advice of neighbors, nutmeg was placed under his tongue to restore his speech. She utilized a bush known as hammond's leaf to lower his blood pressure. The local Catholic priest visited the family and advised that Mr. Arzu be kept around the children as much as possible, suggesting his speech might return if this were done. A form of "bitters" known as *contrebo* was tried without results, as were several other preparations which Mrs. Arzu no longer remembered.

Mrs. Arzu obtained a leaflet which had been sent to a friend by a self-professed healer in New York City. He claimed that he could help anyone who would "give him their troubles." Mrs. Arzu sent a letter explaining her husband's condition and $1 U S. Several weeks later she received a reply. The man stated if she would send an additional $20 he would send her the materials necessary to treat Mr. Arzu. She sent the $20, a considerable sum in Punta Gorda, and received the following: 1. a handkerchief which Mr.

Arzu alone was to use and which was to be kept apart from all other clothing and washed separately; 2. a cross to be worn around his neck; 3. a medal, specially blessed, which was also to be worn around his neck. The medal, they were told by the healer, "will be God and will help him" 4. powder to be prepared with water in a special way and used to bathe him. A certain amount of this preparation was to be thrown in the four corners of the house. This healer also offered a diagnosis of *obeah*. Mrs. Arzu followed all the instructions but saw no improvement. She wrote the man again. He replied that for an additional $15 U.S. he would send more medicine. Mrs. Arzu consulted with her husband and it was decided not to send any more money. Mr. Arzu still wears the cross and the medal, despite their decision not to continue with this healer.

A lady from La Buga (Livingston, Guatemala) told Mrs. Arzu that she should not think of this as an illness caused by man. Mr. Arzu's condition, she suggested, was due to the fact that in his twenties and thirties he had done much "drinking and playing", sometimes getting wet then drying out without proper concern for himself. She sent medicine from La Buga to be used to massage him. Next, a neighbor told them about a "private" doctor in town. This individual is, in fact, a traditional healer who utilizes a combination of traditional therapies and biomedically justified preparations. The Arzus went to his house. He said he could help if he could get the right medicines, but they were not available in Belize. He gave her some tablets and a "prescription" for medication which she had filled in Guatemala. She said Mr. Arzu showed some improvement after this treatment, but they did not return because the "doctor" had been warned by police to stop giving treatment and prescribing medicine after the death of a man who had come to him for treatment. This practitioner, in fact, continues to practice, but Mr. Arzu walks with a slow, shuffling gait and the family feared his presence at the doctor's house would be noted by the neighbors. I spoke with the doctor about the man who had died after receiving treatment. He said that the man had become ill after he, the practitioner, had prescribed some medicines. He stated that he had warned the man that the medicine would act in this way and he should not be disturbed, that this particular response to the medicine would pass. He explained that the reason the man died was that he became worried and sought out treatment at the local hospital. It was the medicine given to him at the hospital, combined with the medicine given him by the healer, which, the healer stated, had caused his death.

A doctor from Guatemala once came to the Arzu's house and examined Mr. Arzu at Mrs. Arzu's request. He told her he could help. Tablets and injections were obtained from a pharmacy in Guatemala. Mr. Arzu was "nointed" (massaged) with herbal and other preparations as prescribed by this same doctor, but no change was noted.

Mrs. Arzu still hoped for improvement, if not a cure. She had recently heard that a tonic known as Seven Seas could "help in veins." "His veins", she explained, "are stiff and it will help them to move." In the meantime she massaged him with alcohol containing wintergreen and gave him Anacin. She no longer took him to the hospital for blood pressure checks since he was unable to walk that distance and there was no transportation available to them. Mrs. Arzu accepted the physician's diagnosis of stroke, but also believed that Sarah and the healer in New York were correct in claiming that he is a victim of *obeah*. She could see no other reason for his failure to improve.

A local Garifuna bush doctor, familiar with the case, told me privately that it was indeed *obeah* and that he could have helped Mr. Arzu if the family had come to him in time, but the family did not heed his advice nor accept his offer.

The Arzus utilized several alternative diagnostic/therapeutic systems, often employing two or more simultaneously. They consulted with biomedical (state) practitioners in Punta Gorda and Belize City and sought the help of a practitioner (perhaps a *curandero* or Garifuna *surúcia*) from Guatemala. They utilized non-legitimized biomedical personnel, or those claiming, at least in part, a biomedical model, in Stann Creek and P.G. They sought the services of a *búiai* and listened to the advice of friends and neighbors, as well as the local Catholic priest. They sought the assistance of a healer in New York who likely utilized West Indian Creole models of illness causation and therapy.

The case is illustrative of:

1. The potentiality for the simultaneous use of alternative systems and models without concern for inconsistency;
2. the successful integration of two supposedly contradictory models of illness causation through the insertion of one "cause" (*obeah*) as a prior event in the etiological chain containing the events "pressure" and "stroke."
3. strategic techniques for the creation of new etiological chains or for the alteration of existing etiological chains through the generation of signs previously unavailable to them and always inaccessible to biomedical practitioners, and the insertion of previously overlooked signs/events;
4. the fact that neither diagnosis nor etiology necessarily determines a therapy, nor does the failure of a given therapy necessarily lead to rejection of the etiological chain. In biomedicine, diagnosis, etiology, and therapy appear more closely linked. That is, a diagnosis most often implies an etiology and determines a therapy, whereas in Garifuna models of cause-effect relationships, the closer tie is between etiology and therapy. The diagnostic label, in many cases, becomes inconsequential.[2]

Case Study Three: Catalina Noralez

Mrs. Catalina Noralez is a sixty-year-old Garifuna female who lives with her husband, two of the children of their oldest daughter, and a son and his wife in a three building complex.

Mrs. Noralez reported that she had been pregnant nineteen times and had ten living children. Two infants had died within a few weeks of birth, two were stillborn, two were born prematurely and died shortly after birth. She had suffered three miscarraiges relatively late in her pregnancies.

Mr. Noralez was once a school teacher, but when his wife's illness became increasingly debilitating he left the profession to care for her. They were Protestants in a community where the large majority of Garinagu were Catholic and Mr. Noralez was, as well, an assistant minister at a local Protestant church. Though no longer employed in the local school he earned sufficient income from tutoring of children and adults in a variety of subjects to support his wife and two grandchildren. He was a well educated man, fluent in three languages with some ability in a fourth (Kekchi).

In April of 1979, Mrs. Noralez's oldest son approached me. He said he had heard I was studying illness and asked if I would talk with his mother. He was concerned because "she has a strange illness." At times he stated that he believed she was quite normal, but sometimes, he said, she behaved "crazy." The doctor had told him some six years before that she suffered from "premature senility." His explanation was not trusted, however, as this same physician had told the family in 1973 that he expected her to die within a month. "If you have a gray hair in your head", the son added, "they don't care about treating you."

I came to know Mrs. Noralez and her husband well during the next year. Mrs. Noralez had been totally blind for approximately two years. She told me she had seen an "oculist" at one time and that he told her that the optical nerve was destroyed. An American lab technician, who operated the lab at the Punta Gorda hospital, suggested that her blindness was the result of retinal hemorrhaging caused by hypertension. Mrs. Noralez, however, did not accept either diagnosis and stated that it was the pressure the oculist placed on one eye during the examination which caused the blindness. She explained that she had some sight prior to the examination.

Mrs. Noralez also reported that she suffered from high blood pressure, as did her husband, though neither was taking medication at the time of my first visit. She stated that she had gone to the clinic earlier in the week, but the physician had not examined her. The sphygmomanometer was broken and her blood pressure could not be checked on that occasion. The doctor prescribed aspirin, B-complex injections and Lanoxin.

On the first of many visits her husband described to me his wife's most recent symptoms – numbness in her legs, slowness of speech, and difficulty remembering. It was the appearance of these symptoms which had motivated her most recent visit to the doctor, he said. Together they described the initial symptoms and possible causation in this way: Mrs. Noralez had been walking barefoot. Mr. Noralez offered slippers to her and she accepted. That night she felt some numbness. When she first noticed the numbness she reported it to her husband. He started to rub alcohol on her leg and foot, but that didn't provide relief. She believed this numbness was precipitated by walking barefoot in the afternoon. The numbness in her feet and legs worried her, she reported, but not much. She said that she felt like "stretching" and belived this was an indication that something was wrong. It was true that her speech had changed, as Mr. Noralez had reported, but she added this actually happened about one to one and a half years earlier, though this sign had been grouped by her husband with the others. Sometimes when she speaks, she explained, "it runs from me what I was taling about." Now, she added, she "can't remember" and can't walk well. She did not feel much numbness at that time, but stated that she felt as though "there are blunt needles in my foot." She thought she might be improving since obtaining medication from the doctor. The physician had said nothing of continuing with the alcohol massage, so Mr. Noralez had discontinued that therapy. Before receiving tablets from the physician Mrs. Noralez said that she felt a bit frightened because "sometimes when people suffer from high blood pressure, they get paralyzed." "That would be terrible", she added.

She told me she had spoken at length with her husband about her illness. He was said to have stated that whatever God willed for them was right. But, she commented, "not all the time is it God causing the trouble. Sometimes it is the Devil. You can't always tell the difference. When you do somthing very wrong you let the Devil have a piece of you."

Mrs. Noralez also had periodic problems with breathing which she referred to as asthma, though on my initial visit she was experiencing no such problem. During the year which followed, however, she had several episodes of difficulty breathing, usually preceded by a cold.

The family reported use of bush medicines (*sorocee* as a tonic, Billy Web for fever and as a tonic, *contrebo* for fever, China Root to make a tonic-like tea, and sour orange for "cooling in summer."), physician prescribed medications, and a variety of medicinal preparations purchased from the local pharmacy – cough syrups, Aspro, alcohol, Cod Liver Oil Tonic, beef iron and wine, Liquifruta, Vicks, and Bengue.

Mrs. Noralez' illness had an additional unusual feature, one which had first brought her son to me. Mrs. Noralez frequently had visions. She recounted to me that about one year after she became blind she started seeing animals. The animals are sometimes small, she noted, "but when they get together they are huge." They are not animals familiar to her "except when they change form into a child or a large man." As humans they are not people she knows. These human and animal forms often gather around her when she eats "as though they were going to eat with me." She stated that she felt as though she was being haunted. Once she reported that as she awoke she saw a big gobbler, then a big man appeared. She saw dirty salt water being shaken. Something jumped out of the water. At first she thought it was a drake. She said, "Jesus?" Then, suddenly, it was a tall man, but she felt as though she knew the man. She watched, then he disappeared.

At the time of our discussion she reported that she saw snakes moving around her. The snakes were described as hairy with big, long heads and large mouths. The snakes transfigure themselves into other things. The animals, she added, have some human characteristics, but are decidedly not human. The doctor had suggested to her that she simply pay no attention to these animals. The Catholic priest visited and told her there were no animals or spirits, that what she saw were merely psychedelic colors. Her husband read the Bible to her and prayed with her to relieve the visions. Her sister told her the cause was "in her blood." She said she would like to visit the oculist again.

Because of the family's fairly strong orientation toward biomedicine (although they are knowledgeable in bush medicine) and because of Mr. Noralez' position in the church, I had not inquired about the more traditional Garifuna ceremonies which would have seemed an appropriate therapy for such a disorder. A life-long resident of Punta Gorda, however, told me that a *dugu* was held for Catalina at one time; but, my informant added, she was not cured because she did not believe in the ceremony.

Despite her several afflictions, Mrs. Noralez and I often joked about her troubles. In May of 1979, for example, I visited Mrs. Noralez during an "asthma" attack. She said to me: "As I talk about it, it wants to attack me again." I responded: "Maybe we shouldn't talk about it then." She laughed and replied: "It doesn't have ears, you know." In May she suffered again from the same problem and in June I noted, for the first time, her tendency to fall asleep in her chair; in July she was ill again. She said she hadn't felt well on the previous Saturday, but on Sunday her stomach "was stopped up" and she couldn't sneeze. "If one more opening had been closed I probably would have drowned", she added, laughing. In October, she was ill with "high blood pressure." She went to the hospital for medication and reported she was feeling better afterwards. In December I wrote she had been ill with a cold for some time. She sat in the livingroom of their house covered by a blanket to keep off the chill.

Mrs. Noralez' family was extremely solicitous about her health and saw to all her needs. One result of this behavior was that she was quite inactive. I knew of only one occasion on which she left the house, to attend a public meeting at which she was honored for community activities in prior years. She would often fall asleep, almost in the middle of a conversation, and spent much of her time in bed, though I generally found her sitting up when I arrived for my frequent visits. Her sense of humor was excellent and despite the doctor's diagnosis of early senility, she appeared bright, generally cheerful, and her memory excellent.

Mr. Noralez was the therapy manager (Janzen 1981) and assumed all responsibility for Mrs. Noralez' care. He accepted the biomedical diagnosis of "pressure" and attributed her blindness to this. In describing her condition when we first met he combined symptoms which she, in speaking privately with me, separated because not closely associated in time. Mrs. Noralez initiated several attempts at generating etiological signs, but such were rejected by her husband with whom she was generally unsuccessful in negotiating cause-effect models.

Neither Mr. Noralez nor his son who had first introduced me to the family had an explanation for her hallucinations.[3] While her son had stated that his mother sometimes seemed "crazy", no one suggested a diagnosis of *luluti* ("craziness"). Mr. Noralez and I had, in fact, discussed *luluti* which he attributed to extreme emotional stress. He said there were only one or two people in the community who could be described as *luluti*. Mrs. Noralez interjected that there were several such people in a nearby Garifuna village, to which Mr. Noralez quickly replied, "Yes, but there they allow first cousins to marry. Here in Punta Gorda we don't allow .such a thing." While Mrs. Noralez' care took considerable time, her behavior was never disruptive and little energy seems to have been spent in the discovery of either a diagnosis or an etiology for her various disorders, beyond those offered by biomedical personnel. Whenever diagnoses or etiologies were generated, they always assisgned her illness to the category of *lisándi ubaó*.

Others in the community, however, viewed her disorder in different terms, attributing it to the *gubída*. Thus, Mrs. Noralez illness which served in some respect to unify the Noralez family and to produce a therapy manager who extended his management to all aspects of household activities, served within the community to validate Garifuna concepts of cause and effect and the critical nature of the *dugu*.[4]

Case Study Four: Mary Sentino

Mary Sentino is a Garifuna female, age fifty-three. She lives in a small and deteriorating three room house near the "front" with two of her daughters, ages eleven and nineteen, and six grandchildren. Three of the grandchildren are children of an older daughter who lives in Orange Walk, Belize. The other three are the children of her nineteen year-old daughter who lives with her. I was introduced to Mary by her grandson, Ernest, age thirteen. Income for the family was provided by Ernest who shines shoes for the soldiers downtown and by her daughter, Lennie, the mother of the three youngest children in the house. Lennie had been unable to find regular work for some time, but she did take in laundry. When the Irish Guard were stationed in the area she did quite well and clothes were always to be seen drying in front of the house. When the Irish were replaced by the Gurkas, however, she complained that her business declined significantly as the Gurkas always washed their own clothes. The daughter living in Orange Walk occasionally provided some cash, but she has taken a new "husband" and has younger children whom she has to support. She rarely visited the older children in Punta Gorda. On the occasions when she did, Ernest slept under the house, since there was little enough room inside.

Mary had great difficulty walking and rarely left her small home. She was dependent on her children and grandchildren to shop for her and to do much of the housework. However, she rarely complained and was always hospitable and pleasant when I entered her home. She reported that at the age of twelve she suffered a "stroke" and spent approximately one year in bed. She was unable to move for an additional six months. Her left arm and leg were partially paralyzed and her left arm never developed properly. Despite these problems, she had given birth to five children, four of whom were still living. The fifth child died at the age of six months of "thrush."

Mary reported that her daughter in Orange Walk suffered a "stroke" at the age of thirty. This, Mary said, was caused by a "baby cold." After a woman gives birth to a child, Mary explained, she should be careful not to expose herself in any way for three days. Her daughter, however, exposed herself to a breeze and "got coldness" resulting in a stroke. Her daughter, Mary reported, visited the hospital in Orange Walk following her stroke. Her arm, which had been partially paralyzed by the stroke, was "nointed" with oil. She was given a ball to exercise her hand. Then, according to Mary, she came home and used bush medicine. Mary prepared an herb referred to as *siwapat* which she boiled with sour pickles. That, said Mary, helped her a lot. Mary believed that first an illness should be treated with bush; then one could purchase other medicines from the pharmacy. She knew and utilized various bush medicines – *sorocee* as a tonic (prepared as a tea), *Jackass bitters* for fever, *mansinilla* for fever, and a combination of *clavo*, *anise*, *romero*, and other items, all of which could be purchased at the local pharmacy, for "change of life." Mary was knowledgeable about many other bush medicines as well, but, she lamented, much bush had become increasingly difficult to find.

Mary professed not to know the cause of her stroke. She had high blood pressure, but apparently took no medication for it other than APC, though she described to me the appropriate bush to be used to lower "pressure." *Matapalo*, *pia leaf*, and *bokut leaf* are boiled together, and the resulting tea is drunk. She once suffered from "palpitations" but stated she saw a doctor in Barrios (Puerto Barrios, Guatemala), and "got cure."

Mary also stated that she had suffered in the past from "fits." "Fits", she explained, are caused by worries and vexation. "When you worry about life, it causes sickness." When she had "fits", the doctor had said to her "You are the one to get the remedy for yourself. I do not have the remedy." She stated that when she gets "vexed", her tongue "strings up and fall down." "You have to try to forget your problems so the sickness will go away", she added. She referred to a man in town who often had "fits." His problem, she explained, is that both his parents died in a hurricane and then his wife left him and it "rests on his nerves." Though the cause of "fits" is thus seen as an emotional reaction to stressful situations by Mary, herbal treatments can be used. Symptomatic relief involves placing an onion under the nose of the afflicted person or placing salt in his or her mouth. Mint and *rudah* were said to be good for this conditions, as was garlic in rum. Nutmeg was also mentioned as a treatment. She reported she had been cured of her "fits" by drinking rum mixed with burnt mountain cow (tapir) hoof.

Mary, however, did not express concern over her paralysis or her high blood pressure; rather she complained of a severely swollen and often painful leg. Mary said that after the birth of her last child she developed a "black part on my leg where the blood collected." The doctors operated on her leg to cut out the black part, but she had "suffered with it ever since." On my first visit to her house there was a rather large open wound on this leg. Over the fifteen months that I visited her, the wound would periodically grow better and then worsen. She told me she had visited the District Medical Officer on at least four occasions with fever and headache and with pain in her leg. He told her he could help her fever and her headache, but the problem with the leg "will be with you till death." Mary said that her daughter had brought her some ointment from a store in Orange Walk. She washed her leg with "carbonegros" soap and applied the ointment. This had provided some relief. She asked me if I had medicine for her leg. I, in turn, asked the British Army physician stationed at Rideau camp if he would examine her leg. Since Mary had no "transport" and had difficulty walking, the physician came by her house on a trip into Punta Gorda.

Dr. Owens, the physician, reported to me that she had osteomyelitis resulting from a chronic infection. The only possible treatment, he stated, would involve the use of drugs not available in Belize, skin grafts, and a surgical procedure in which a duct would be implanted to drain the fluid from her leg. The ducts of her leg, he explained, were clogged with scar tissue. I told Mary that there was no way that her leg could be treated in Belize and passed on to her the medicine I was given by Dr. Owens.

Approximately two months later the leg, which had at first shown minor improvement, became more swollen than before. Mary told me that she was now using a bush medicine, *messina*, to reduce the swelling. She had sent the children "to the bush" to find this medicine. She said the leg was now "reducing" slowly with the use of bush. After Dr. Owens' visit, she reported she went to the new DMO and asked for help with her leg. The doctor told her there was nothing he could do. At no time during these years had she been provided with a diagnosis of her condition nor a description of the cause. She continued to use the powder provided by Dr. Owens and after two additional months said to me that "by the grace of God and with the medicine" her leg had improved.

Shortly before my departure I again inquired about her health. She said she had suffered from fever recently and had gotten transport to the physician. He gave her aspirin, but didn't give any indication as to what was wrong. Her leg was badly swollen on my last visit and the skin was peeling, as it had been at the time of my first contact with her some seventeen months before. She was not using any medication and remarked simply. "I think it will take me to the grave."

Mary utilized bush (lay), pharmacy (lay), and biomedicine (state) simultaneously. Her concern appears not to have been with the isolation of an etiological chain of signs or a specific diagnosis, but with the identification of a therapy which would have provided relief. There was, during the time I knew Mary, no attempt to view her "illness" as anything other a "worldly" illness, though I did not question her on possible past attempts to identify this as *obeah* or an ancestral or spiritually caused disorder. Had the illness, or any past disorder, been so identified, Mary likely lacked the income to have proceeded with an appropriate treatment. The fact that all treatments she sought were "naturalistic" indicates that, at least in this stage of her illness, she assigned this disorder to the broad category of *lisandi ubaó*. It is likely that this misfortune, like her daughter's stroke, was seen as the result of natural processes – pregnancy and childbirth – with relatively high risks, The production of children is of critical importance to the continuation of the Garifuna social and economic unit; as with any event to which such import is attached, it has inherent risks.

Mary was limited in the diagnostic/therapeutic strategies available to her because of the lack of sufficient income. She was also unable to generate, manipulate, or control information effectively. The use of several alternative systems of therapy either sequentially or simultaneously is one strategy the "therapy managing group" (Janzen 1978) can utilize to generate several diagnoses or etiologies from which the selection of that which is most 'appropriate' in terms of personal and structural needs, consistent or coherent in sociocultural terms, and effective in terms of prognosis can be made. Mary, however, had never been able to obtain even a diagnostic label for her disorder. When, finally, one was offered her, it was of little use for the attached prognosis only referenced her powerlessness.[5]

Case Study Five: Benedicta Reyes

Mrs. Reyes was a seventy-two year old Garifuna female who lived with her husband in a well-kept frame house "to the back." Mr. Reyes had been a cook for the American-owned Esso Company and had spent many years living in the States. The Reyes were relatively well-to-do by local standards because Mr. Reyes had prospered in his work for foreigners. He was no longer working at the time of my initial contact because Esso had left the area, but he talked often of returning to work and perhaps leaving the community again. Mrs. Reyes was admitted to the Punta Gorda hospital in April of 1979 with the following history and diagnosis. "Diabetes and hypertension. History of septic great toe. Right foot swollen and dark." Shortly after her admission to the hospital I conducted an interview with Mrs. Reyes. She stated at that time that she had pain in her toe from January, but the foot had become swollen only the previous week. She had been admitted to the hospital in March with the same problem, had been treated and released. I asked what treatment she had used on the toe prior to her admission on this occasion. She reported she had soaked her foot in hot water with Detol (a commonly used disinfectant). She had also put salt directly on her toe and had rubbed lime on it. This combination of treatments, she stated, had provided relief for several weeks. She remarked that she believed the problem with her toe was directly related to her diabetes. She was, at that time, according to her chart, scheduled for surgery in Belize City and was confident that the treatment to be given her in Belize City would help her condition. She had not been informed of the impending surgery.

Mrs. Reyes, however, was not transferred to Belize City. I have no hospital record of the decision to release her to her home in Punta Gorda, nor of the reasons for the change in plans. She was, however, readmitted to the Punta Gorda hospital in late June with the same problem. A test of her blood sugar level on July 3 gave results of 370 mg (normal range is approximately 60 to 120 mg.). She was sent to Belize City on the following day.

Mrs. Reyes remained in the hospital in Belize City for several months. I followed the case during that period through her husband whom I saw almost daily. In October, he reported that she had undergone not one but several operations. Initially, the decision was made to remove only her toe. The resulting wound, however, became infected or gangrenous. She was returned to surgery two more times, until the surgeons had removed most of her leg up well beyond the mid-thigh. Mrs. Reyes sent word to her husband that she desired a special mass be held for her deceased mother who she believed was unhappy and was responsible for her slow recovery. Mr. Reyes had a special mass said. He also, at her direction, held a *chugu* (similar to a *dugu*, but on a much smaller scale). The total cost to him was approximately $400 B.H. All the food and drink prepared or purchased for the ceremony were buried at the conclusion of the ceremony as is considered obligatory. Shortly after this ceremony, Mr. Reyes left for Belize City to pick up his wife who was now said to be improved.

Mr. Reyes returned from Belize City without his wife. He had been told by hospital personnel when he arrived that she was not yet well enough to travel. Mr. Reyes received several messages during the next two months that his wife was to be released at any time, only to be informed within a few days that she was not yet ready.

In late November, Mr. Reyes gave me additional information on the various ceremonies that had been held to ensure his wife's recovery. He explained that a total of four masses had been said for her at a cost to him of $5 for each one. One was for her deceased mother. He did this on his wife's instructions and those of a male *búiai* hired from Livingston, Guatemala for $45 B.Z. The *búiai* first reported, according to Mr. Reyes, that the father wanted a high mass, then later that the mother desired one as well. The last "mass" cost him between $200 and $400 B.Z., because it was "like a *dugu*." (This apparently was a reference to the *chugu* he had mentioned to me earlier.) Mr. Reyes, who is himself Garifuna, said he didn't believe in *búiai*s and didn't have any idea how they received messages from spirits. He reported that he hired the *búiai* only because his wife requested it. He said the *búiai* came and drank all his liquor. Apparently, the male *búiai* was hired only for a consulation (*arairaguni*) because it was a female *búiai* who reportedly conducted the *chugu*. Still, he said, his wife did not improve. The doctor had assured him that she would get well, but after several operations, she was worse off than before, he complained. Mr. Reyes became discouraged, saying at times that he thought his wife would surely die. The expenses to him were considerable. The blood provided to her during her operations had cost $310 B.H. "I can't give my own blood", Mr. Reyes explained, "because you know how long I work around ranges and heat? My blood is too hot and it would kill her."

In late January, after many delays, Mrs. Reyes was transferred from Belize to the Punta Gorda hospital. I noted that, according to her chart, her blood pressure remained elevated. She complained of cramps in her leg at one point, and had rubbed the leg with Vicks which she kept at her hospital bedside. She assured me that her leg was healing, though her husband seemed less optimistic. "It is still like an open wound", he lamented.

At the end of March, Mrs. Reyes was still hospitalized. Despite nine months of continuous hospitalization, she rarely complained. In mid-March, however, it was noted in her chart that her blood pressure was elevated and that she complained of a headache. The nurses added: "States she is worried over condition. Appears very despondent this morning." In April, Mrs. Reyes was finally released from the hospital and returned to her home. She was learning to walk with crutches at the time I left Punta Gorda and seemed cheerful and optimistic. When I questioned her about the *chugu* she denied that such a ceremony had been conducted.

In early 1983, I received reports that Mrs. Reyes had died. I wrote to her sister's husband who lived next door to ask what the cause of her death had been. The reply read: "The cause of her death was that her leg was removed."

The case illustrates how individuals and their "therapy managing groups" tend to lose control over both the production of signs and the consequent therapeutic strategies when the afflicted individual is hospitalized. From near the outset of this "illness", it appears the Reyes accepted the biomedically generated diagnosis and the biomedically determined link between "sepsis" and diabetes. Mrs. Reyes' utilization of a variety of lay techniques (Detol in hot water, salt and lime juice applied to the wound) between hospitalizations did not indicate a denial of the biomedical model, but more likely the absence of information from biomedical personnel. There was, at no time, a change in diagnostic label, though the family never utilized the term "sepsis." The etiological chain which included "diabetes", "septic toe", surgery, and "further infection" or "failure to heal" was capable of alteration, however, and new signs (the displeasure of ancestors, information generated by one or more *búiais*) were inserted. The therapies required by these signs could be performed without Mrs. Reyes' presence. Such therapies were, of course, the only available to the family in this instance, since hospitalization generally precluded the application of other therapeutic models.

The husband disagreed with his wife's assessment that a *búiai* was required, yet two *búiais* were utilized in the process of seeking a successful therapy. This indicates that the husband was not sole "therapy manager" and shared that responsibility with his wife. This constrasts with the case of Carmelo Ramirez (to follow), the child of a Spanish couple, in which the father assumed all therapy managing responsibilities, and illustrates, to some degree, the difference in relationship between men and women in these two distinct ethnic sections.

The frustration expressed by Mr. Reyes on several occasions was due only in part to his wife's failure to recover and her worsening condition. It was also the result of his almost total inability to produce or control information. Once his wife was removed from the Punta Gorda hospital, this inability became even more manifest. The repeated phone calls telling him his wife was to be released from the Belize City hospital, with subsequent disappointments, only further illustrated the potentiality of "state" medicine to deny the autonomy of individuals and to prevent successful renegotiations of reality by denying access to the model which defines that reality and determines therapeutic strategies.[6]

The case histories which follow are of individuals and families from several non-Garifuna ethnic sections. I have not attempted to review the processes whereby etiologies and diagnoses are assigned or generated as fully as in the preceding case studies, nor have I tried to point out the similarities and differences in the medical models which allow for those processes or the manner in which signs are differentially linked to social, political, and economic structures. In the chapter to follow I have outlined the nature of interethnic transactions in which material goods, services, and information are exchanged and the manner in which limited articulation of codes is achieved.

Case Study Six: Robert Valdez

Mr. Robert Valdez was a sixty-three year old Creole male with a severely ulcerated arm. I became acquainted with Mr. Valdez on my many trips to the Punta Gorda hospital. He spent much time at the home of a friend who lived on the street leading to the hospital. His arm was always bandaged from shoulder to wrist and I would stop to inquire how he was. It was only when I happened to be at the hospital one day as his arm was being cleaned and rebandaged that I realized the extent of the ulceration. Mr. Valdez not only became one of the cases I chose to follow but he also gave me considerable information on bush medicine. He was an occasional practitioner of medicine and it was ironic that he suffered from an illness he himself could not cure.

Mr. Valdez' case is interesting not only because of the several processes or strategies he utilized in his attempts to gain access to or control over various medical resources, but because the case so clearly points up some of the problems with the delivery of biomedicine in Belize.

Mr. Valdez took great pride in his personal history as a *chiclero*, a term which is used to refer to the men who worked the forests of Belize during the days when logging was the principal industry of the country. Logging continues to be of some inportance in the Punta Gorda area, but Mr. Valdez stopped working in the forests several years ago. It appears his reason for quitting was the increasing severity of the ulcerations on his arm. He held a few jobs in Punta Gorda, but had been unable to work in any capacity for approximately one to two years. Upon occasion he drew a small amount of money from the Social Development Department (approximately $2.75 U.S. every two weeks). When he first went to Social Development and told them he was unable to work, he was given $15 B.H. ($7.50 U.S.). This he spent in one of the local grocery-dry goods stores on food. When he returned a week later the Social Development staff wanted to know what he had done with the money they had already given him. They said they could not give him supplemental funds or an additional allowance until some "decisions" had been made in Belize City. Those "decisions" were apparently never made. Mr. Valdez could not support himself or the money alloted to him by the Department. He has been largely dependent on the assistance offered by his friends. He claimed to be related to one of the wealthier Creole families in town, but said that they offered no assistance. He lived in the second story of an old two story house which apparently was provided him by a friend. He had no furniture, appliances, or household goods, and only a mattress for a bed. What food he had was stored under a tin can to keep the rats from it.

Mr. Valdez' medical history is lengthy and occasionally confusing. I recount it here as best I can from the history provided to me by Mr. Valdez and the information I recorded following my initial contacts.

Mr. Valdez reports that he was first troubled with the arm approximately fifteen years ago. He was bitten by an insect. He does not know what sort of insect it might have been. After receiving the bite, which he initially regarded as insignificant, he worked in the water for two weeks. During that time, he noticed that the sore became larger. He had little choice but to keep working; the sore grew in size. Finally, he sought out a doctor in Punta Gorda who, he recounts, never attended to it much. When the sore first began to spread, Mr. Valdez followed the advice the friends and used lime and a variety of herbs or roots on his arm. These were believed to "dry" the sores. He continued working because he had no other income. None of these medicines, however, offered relief.

About five years ago, the arm was treated with some success by a German nun then working at the Punta Gorda Hospital. After treatments lasting approximately one month, she told him the sores were healing and he should wait fifteen days for further treatment. He went back to work and the ulceration spread again. This happened, he believes, because he was wearing a long-sleeved shirt which "chafed" against the sores. He returned to the hospital for additional treatment, unaware of the fact that the sister had left the country temporarily. The doctor who was then stationed in Punta Gorda said he did not know what medicines she was using, and, therefore, could not duplicate the treatment. Mr. Valdez didn't receive any additional treatment until the sister returned for no one else knew the medicines, he explained. The sister, Mr. Valdez states, was giving him injections she made herself. These injections were not made from medicines obtained from the hospital, he believed. They caused him to be sick at his stomach temporarily, but helped his arm. When she returned, the treatments were resumed, but she left the country permanently about one week later. She said she would leave medicines and instructions with the doctor and the nurse, but when Mr. Valdez returned, neither the doctor nor the nurses claimed to know anything of this.

After her departure, he obtained no further treatment for several years. In 1977 or 1978 the British Army physician stationed at Rideau began offering medical services to "locals" and he agreed to examine and treat Mr. Valdez' arm. He told Mr. Valdez before his departure that he would leave medicines at the hospital for treatment of the arm. Mr. Valdez reported that he received four injections, then the remaining medications "disappeared." He insists there were additional doses of the medicine as he had been shown the medicine when it first arrived. He believes the District Medical Officer took the medicine for use in his clinic.

The arm was worse in January of 1979 and was infested with worms when Mr. Valdez decided to seek care again. He explained that he used to work for one of the local merchants as a night watchman and slept on the floor. The arm had been left unbandaged and open to the air. He believes this had something to do with the progressive deterioration of the arm. Friends brought him ointment from Guatemala, but the ointment didn't provide any relief. The District Medical Officer (also the physician at the local hospital) sent Mr. Valdez to Belize City Hospital for treatment. Mr. Valdez remained there for three months. The doctor in Belize City said the arm could be treated and cured. Mr. Valdez asked that the arm be amputated instead. The physician, however, insisted a cure was possible. The physician in Belize City asked him to stay for a skin graft, but there were many patients in the hospital at that time and he said the arm was not yet ready for a graft. Therefore, Mr. Valdez was sent back to Punta Gorda. After a brief period of time the local District Medical Officer sent him back to Belize City for the skin graft. The doctor in Belize City told him, however, that the arm was still not ready. Mr. Valdez spent one month in the Belize City hospital. He was finally told a graft would not be necessary. He was sent back to Punta Gorda. He was, at the time I first met him, shortly after his return to Punta Gorda, receiving no injections as he had been told they had lost their effectiveness. The physician in Belize City said to him there was too much medicine in his blood, and he should go without medication for six months "to get the blood clean." He apparently developed an allergy to tablets which were given to him when he returned to Punta Gorda. In March, when I first became aware of his case, Mr. Valdez was attending the local hospital each day where the arm was cleaned with normal saline and rebandaged. He told me he was also treating it with some "local" medicine which he identified as some form of sulphur. He said the arm would have gotten better if he had not run out of the medicine. He could not afford to buy more.

In July of that year Mr. Valdez told me he was using the leaf of the physic nut tree, boiled with salt, to dry up the arm. I asked how he managed to apply the solution, knowing that the arm was only unbandaged once a day at the hospital. He laughed and said he had gotten the nurse to apply it for him. He had not told her what the solution was.

In late July, Mr. Valdez introduced me to another bush doctor. He explained that this man was attempting to obtain a "series" of medicines from Guatemala which would help him, but the medicines were expensive. He was hoping to save some money to purchase the medicines. He also mentioned that he was thinking of going to Guatemala for treatment. He said the Guatemalans are happy to serve the Belizeans in this way. He said he was still using the physic nut preparation. It caused a great deal of pain, but the arm was improving. In late August, the chief nurse at the hospital discovered Mr. Valdez' 'deception' and put a stop to his use of this preparation. A British Army parasitiologist told me that the leaf of the physic nut tree contained an acid which was very likely promoting some healing. The nurse applied gentian violet.

Mr. Valdez said he experienced some pain at night. The veins and sinews, he explained, are uncovered. Sometimes his fingers became numb and the hand swollen. He put alcohol on the hand to relieve the swelling. When his arm gets better, he told me, he will rub a medicine on it to keep the veins and the sinews supple. This medicine is made from the oil of a *wola* (a small black and white) snake. Only a small amount of the medicine can be used so the oil is applied with a feather every few days until the desired suppleness is reached. To prepare the medicine, he explained, you must first kill the *wola* snake. The fat is fried to extract the oil, then the oil is strained. The oil, he said, penetrates to the affected part.

Mr. Valdez told me that he had never been told what his illness might be. It had been referred to only as an ulcer by the several physicians who had examined him. A Mexican physician who replaced the local District Medical Officer for several weeks in the spring and summer of 1979 examined the arm briefly when Mr. Valdez was in the outpaitent clinic for a dressing change. I was present at the time taking photographs in the hospital, and the American lab technician and I asked him to look at Mr. Valdez' arm. The doctor rendered some medical opinion in Spanish (he spoke very little English) and walked on without any suggestions as to change in treatment. In fact, he never inquired what the treatment at the time might have been.

It was in the late summer or early fall that I first had a chance to talk with a parasitologist stationed at Salamanca camp with the British Army. He was interested in finding local cases of *leishmaniasis* as several soldiers had a mild form of the disease and the physicians were uncertain how it should be treated. The American lab technician, known popularly as "Dr. Lottie", had first suggested to me that Mr. Valdez might be suffering from *leishmaniasis*. The parasitologist was interested in the case and later examined Mr. Valdez arm. He said that it was indeed *leishmaniasis*, though an accurate clinical diagnosis could not be made without specific lab tests. He made some suggestions to the lab technician, but not to the phsyician, as to possible treatments and left.

In September, Mr. Valdez, suffering from an elevated temperature, was admitted to the Punta Gorda hospital "for observation of ulcer left hand." He was given Ampicillin, Vitamin C, and hydrochlothiazide. I visited Mr. Valdez on several occasions. During the third week he reported the nurses had cleaned his arm with medicines that "cut" the flesh and sent pain to his heart. He said the nurses didn't know what they were doing. The chart said "No complaints."

While he was hospitalized, two more British Army physicians, now intrigued by *leishmaniasis* and forced to send their own soldiers home without a cure, visited the hospital and examined his arm. They confirmed the initial diagnosis of *leishmaniasis*. They promised they would send medicine to "Dr. Lottie." Their relations with "Dr. Lottie" were excellent, while relations between the local District Medical Officer and the British physicians remained somewhat cool. I was curious to see how the DMO would react to this 'interference' in his case as at that point the rights and obligations of the British to offer diagnoses and provide treatment to "locals" were unclear. The government had recently announced a "hands off" policy, claiming that it was quite capable of looking after Belizeans. My curiosity was never satisfied for no medicine ever arrived.

Shortly after this, Mr. Valdez was returned to the Belize City Hospital for further treatment. He remained there for three months. On his return he reported to me that the arm was worse than ever. He said he was supposed to come home in November, but there was no "transport" by ambulance available until January. He said he would seek the same treatment at the hospital as before. The physician in Belize City had ordered that injections be given to him in Punta Gorda. However, the local DMO said he didn't have the proper medicine and had no authorization from "Belize" (the Chief Medical Officer) to obtain such medicine. To my knowledge, no attempt was made to obtain any additional medications for Mr. Valdez.

In February he was readmitted to the Punta Gorda hospital with "history of infected wound for eighteen years." He was given Ampicillin, APC, vitamins

B and C. The arm was treated with potassium permanganate soaks and dressed with Eusol. In late February, Mr. Valdez told me he was scheduled to go to the Belize City hospital where his arm was to be amputated. The chart read "scheduled for surgery in Belize at 1 P.M. on February 26." In mid-March, however, I encountered him at his friend's house. He told me it had been decided he would not be sent to Belize as he had developed an allergy to his medication. He had made a decision not to go to Belize City, in any case, as "the food is bad, I get thinner, and the arm gets worse." He was released from the Punta Gorda hospital shortly after the allergy developed and told to return daily for redressing. He believed if he could get thirty to forty quetzales ($30 - $40 U.S.) he would go to Barrios in Guatemala for treatment. He was still hoping for a cure as he very much desired to return to work.

Mr. Valdez' beliefs about the etiology of his illness altered as time passed and as he had opportunity to consider past events and new information. Initially, he mentioned only the insect bite as the source of his difficulty and the fact the arm was not treated properly in the beginning. When the sore first began to develop he attributed it to a beef worm (a common affliction) and later, when it became apparent that there was no beef worm, he came to regard it as a variety of "bay sore." He had, he explained, worked in water for two weeks after receiving the bite and this had worsened what had initially been a minor problem. Avoiding the experience of simultaneous "heat and cold" is critical to the maintenance of health. Once, he reported, he was working in the bush and got sores all over his skin. These became like scales. The cause was that he bathed in the river after working and got in water up to his elbows. A man came along and said: "What are you doing? Your blood is very hot and you are going to bathe in cold water?" About three weeks later, he stated, the sores developed. A Spanish man prepared herbs for him to drink and eventually the scales came off. He was, however, temporarily left with "blue" skin. Gradually the blue skin disappeared but he was now left with large depigmented areas on his arms below his elbows. The physician in Punta Gorda who later treated him told him: "If you hadn't gotten medicine to get the cold out of your blood, you would have gotten a worse disease."

Mr. Valdez told me in the first months that I knew him that he did not believe in *obeah*, though he once pointed out a relative in the streets who he reported had been made crazy by *obeah*. When I asked specifically if the problem with his arm might have been caused by *obeah* he explained that when he was first bitten by the insect there was no one around. "So how could it be *obeah*? Who would do that to me?" Besides, he added, there is no such thing as *obeah*.

> *Obeah*, or what people call *obeah*, is only the work of Satan. The Lord's work is good and bad. Some people sell their souls to Satan or turn to Satan. They can work harm against another through an appeal to Satan. But some might believe it is *obeah*.

He explained further:

If the one who *obeah* [the work of Satan] is directed against, is in the wrong, the *obeah* may work. But if the man is in the right and trusts in the Lord, then *obeah* may turn back on the person who tried to use it. I have a friend who has a bad knee. He has it because he beat his child unnecessarily when the child was telling the truth. His actions turned against him and caused him trouble with his knee. Now it won't go away. Sometimes people believe they have been *obeah*ed and spend a lot of money to have it removed. The sickness usually goes away anyway, but the man attributes it to *obeah*. *Obeah* has led to killing in the past. When a man becomes ill and believes another has done it, he has sometimes killed that man. The Psalms of the Bible may be read against someone and they will be harmed through the power of God. A man turns his soul away from God and towards Satan and that's *obeah*.

Later, in March of 1980, he stated that after some consideration he had changed his mind. He now believed that *obeah* was the only explanation for the failure of the arm to heal. He had, in the fall of 1979, concurred with the British physicians' diagnosis of *leishmaniasis*, adding information which supported his growing understanding of this disease. In accepting an etiology which involved*obeah*, he had not, however, rejected the diagnosis of *leishmaniasis*, but now offered a lengthy description of events which had occurred at the time he first began to suffer with the sore. He had come to believe that a fellow worker, jealous of his skills, had wished him harm and had worked *obeah* on him. He recalled how, at approximately the time the sore began to develop, he had almost been killed by a falling tree and had subsequently been lost in the jungle for several days. His desire, expressed in March after his release from the Punta Gorda hospital, to go to Barrios (Puerto Barrios, Guatemala) was motivated by the belief that in

...Barrios they have people, Spaniards, who know all about *obeah*. They have spirits who help them. They know just what's wrong and who caused the problem as soon as they see you. You don't have to say anything to them. They know when you walk in the room.

In April, shortly before my departure, Mr. Valdez had had the chance to reconsider his case. He said he believed it might be *obeah* but he thought it more likely that the problem lay with his blood, for the state of the blood is critical in determinations of health and illness. His blood has become dirty, he explained, from when he was young; he had worked hard and had bathed in the river while his body was still hot. The river had much lime in it which left white spots on his hands and arms and at the same time made his arm bad. He believed that "cold" had stayed in his blood. He had failled, thereafter, to take anything to purify his blood. It was, therefore, his own ignorance and carelessness which he believed had led him to this state.

Mr. Valdez, for period of time, saw his illness as the result of the actions of someone who was jealous of his skills. He had complained to me that, though he was related to certain Creole members of the town's elite, he had received no assistance from them and they apparently chose not to recognize their relationship to him. His inclusion of *obeah* in the etiological chain emphasized his past as a *chiclero*, one of the few accomplishments to which he could point with pride. His later decision to return his illness to the category of "natural illness" may have been due, in part, to his inability to access a system which would have allowed validation of his incorporation of *obeah*.[7]

Case Study Seven: Viola Gonzalez

Viola Gonzalez was an elderly Spanish woman, originally from Guatemala, who lived with her husband, Domingo, and her "grandson" (son of her husband's son) Juan, age seventeen. Mrs. Gonzalez was ninety-nine years old when I first met her. Her husband was seventy-nine.

Domingo, despite his age and the loss of one eye, worked when he could. He was empolyed by the town on occasion, usually "chopping bush", and for several months worked as a cook and janitor in a local restaurant. The grandson, Juan, had recently graduated from high school (equivalent to 10th grade) and was employed first on a Ranchero run by a group of Catholic nuns, and then at the Army Camp, Rideau. Domingo was often unable to find work and total support during these periods came from Juan. They lived in a small, two-room house built of lumber, with an attached "kitchen." It was modestly furnished with a couple of benches, a table, and two beds. Religious pictures, Juan's diploma, and a few photographs decorated the walls. Viola had a two-burner kerosene stove which failed to operate much of the time. Most cooking was done on a wood-burning "stove."

Viola told me on more than one occasion that she had had seven "husbands." Her last marriage was to a relatively well-to-do dentist in Guatemala. This was corroborated by residents of Punta Gorda who had known the family for some time. Viola also stated that she had given birth to nine children. Each child, she said, had been taken from her shortly after birth, as she became "crazy in the head" for a period of time. She had no idea what happened to any of the children, she said. Viola (who, as of this writing, had celebrated her one hundred and fourth birthday) showed no evidence of senility, nor of psychosis. She gave me no reason to question any information she provided.

I did not seek out Viola because of her age, nor any of her infirmities. Rather, I was introduced to Viola through her husband whom I met shortly after I arrived in Punta Gorda. We became, and remain, close friends. Viola was totally blind. She said that she suffered from high blood pressure and that she had "seizures." She had been blind for several years, but only recently had the blindness progressed to the point where she could not distinguish between light and dark. Despite her various disabilities, Viola was as active as her condition would permit. She could not wander far outside without assistance, and there was rarely anyone to take her anywhere. However, she worked within the house, cleaning, cooking, and washing, and she had on one occasion attempted to mend some used clothing that had been given to her. One evening as I was walking downtown I encountered Domingo and Viola on their way home from a party. Viola said she had consumed seven beers and had danced all evening. Two young men who had been at the party told me later that this was indeed true and they added that she danced well.

Her husband once said to me:

> My wife and I have discussed why people who are young and healthy die and we don't. It is because it isn't our time; God wants us to suffer a little longer. But we are so poor, why doesn't he take us instead of them?

Despite their poverty and their various infirmities, Domingo and Viola struggled on, usually without complaint. Domingo's standard response upon my usual greeting "How are you?", was "Well, I'm fighting it."

Viola and Domingo put great trust in Esquipulas, the Black Jesus of Guatemale. A small picture of Esquipulas had a prominent place within their house. They later insisted that I take the picture with me. Viola explained to me that Esquipulas could help you during illness. If you ask Esquipulas for help when you are sick, he will make you well, she stated. Then, if you recover, you must have a feast on that date each year. She said Domingo couldn't walk for twenty-five years until they prayed to Esquipulas. Then he had fever and pain in his legs for eight days and at the end of this time he recovered and could walk again. She herself, she reported, used to drink a lot when she was young, but she prayed to Esquipulas and he "cured" her. They both continued in their celebration of Esquipulas' Feast Day each January, though they took very little part in the activities the last January that I was in Punta Gorda. One reason seems to have been that at least some of the activities preceding the Feast Day have been moved out of individuals' homes and into the Catholic Church. In previous years, each individual in the town who had claimed a cure by Esquipulas would provide food and drink on one of the eleven days leading up to Esquipulas Day. Others would attend; there was, in this sense, a circulation of the responsibilities for completing the obligation to Esquipulas. The great cost involved in providing food and drink for a large group of people on even one evening may also have been a factor in their decision not to continue the celebration, although it had not stopped them in prior years. Apparently attenuated festivities continued in at least one individual's home with attendance by some of the more prominent Creole and Spanish families in town.

Initially Viola and Domingo stated that they did not believe in *obeah,* although it later became apparent that they accepted some beliefs about the potential effectiveness of *obeah*. Viola eventually confided that she had once used *obeah* to bring Juan back when he was lost, but her reference is most likely to benign "magic" for the term *obeah* refers to one's attempts to harm another. After I had known them for several months, they disclosed that the Indians (Maya) knew about *obeah* and there were as well people in Punta Gorda in the past who knew how to use *obeah*. One *obeah* man died, they said, because there was a woman in Punta Gorda who had stronger *obeah*.

Domingo had been told at one time that the trouble with his legs might be due to *obeah*, but he rejected this diagnosis. He had tried all sorts of medication without success and finally went to Esquipulas. He begged Esquipulas to help him and Esquipulas cured him. I asked how he could be certain it wasn't *obeah* which had caused the initial problem. He replied: "Because it got better." "But couldn't Esquipulas fight *obeah*?" "Well, yes, he has the power and if he wants he can cure you of *obeah.*" Viola interjected at that point, before we had completed our discussion, that someone had once tried to kill her with *obeah*, but all she got was ant bites.

As time progressed, I was used as 'negotiator' in several situations. Viola called upon me to stand with her in chastizing Domingo. When there were other family crises, Viola would often confide in me, apparently in the hope that I might be able to intervene. I was used to "negotiate' in another sense too, as I will later recount. I was also called upon occasionally to intercede if there was some medical problem which they seemed not to have the knowledge or the networks to deal with.

At one time, in the early months of my stay in Punta Gorda, an elderly Creole-Spanish woman and prominent citizen of the community, was hospitalized and said to be dying. She had for many years been a friend to Viola and Viola was deeply disturbed at the thought of her friend's death. I was invited for lunch one day at Viola's house and arrived to find everyone upset, for their pet parrot was ill and wouldn't eat. Viola explained to me that the parrot was suffering because "Miss Dina" was ill. The spirit of Miss Dina was said to be troubling the parrot. "When Miss Dina dies, the parrot will also die", she explained. She said that she herself felt "Miss Dina's illness in my heart." They still hoped that Miss Dina might recover. I did not tell them that I had just come from the hospital and Miss Dina had died the previous hour.

Viola and Domingo used a variety of medicines – bush, popular or "patent" remedies, and medicines obtained from the local hospital. They used *skagineal* for headaches, *cancer bush* for sores, *piñon* for blisters in the mouth, alcohol, Vicks, aspirin, and Red Lavinda and Florida Water (obtained from Guatemala) for Viola's "blood pressure" and heart. When Juan had a boil on his arm, Viola made a salve out of blue soap, *malba leaves* and sweet oil and applied it to the boil. Domingo was at one time given a bottle of medicine (possibly a local concoction known as *gangwao*) which Viola told me secretively was "for men who couldn't perform with their wives."

When I first visited them, Viola said she had not been to the doctor in seven years. In the year which followed, however, she, Domingo, and Juan went to the clinic on several occasions. Viola told me when I first began to visit that she suffered from high blood pressure. She explained that once she had held a cold chicken in her hands and had received a "shock." She had suffered with the pressure ever since. She believed nutrition was also a contributing cause. The less food you eat the better off you are, she reported. "The pressure don't want you to eat too much. The nourishment is too high for the pressure. The blood gets to much nourished. And that's what causes it." A doctor had told her at one point, she stated, not to eat rice, beans, or fat. Knowing that these are principal components in the diet of most Punta Gordans, I asked what she did eat. "I don't eat", she replied. In fact, there were many days in which her diet consisted of nothing more than tea and tortillas. She enjoyed the occasional cold beer I brought her and said the beer helped keep the pressure from "catching her." Once when Domingo was ill with a "cough, cold and fever", she prepared bananas in coconut milk for him because rice is "cold" and would make him cough more. In malaria, she once said, the blood becomes too weak and begins to turn to water. "You must eat properly to bring the strength back to the blood. Greens are good for this. Onions and garlic are good for the heart and lungs. Some people say pepper is bad for you, but small amounts have a cooling effect."

Viola enjoyed cake, but said she had to be careful because if the cake contained a large number of eggs, it would make the blood hot. In general, the only treatments she sought for her "pressure" were either dietary, baths to "cool the body", or Red Lavinda or Florida Water which helped one to "cool" off. One teaspoon of epsom salts in water was also said to cool the blood. She also attempted to avoid getting vexed if she could, though Domingo and Juan seemed to provide her with numerous opportunities for "vexation."

Eventually, Viola attended the clinic and returned with medication. The slip which she brought back recorded her blood pressure as 140/80. I suggested to her that her blood pressure was excellent for someone her age and that her symptoms might be more easily seen as the result of a heart condition. She had previously mentioned to me that a physician had once told her that her heart was weak. This physician advised her not to "get mad or too hot and to rest a lot." Viola seemed to accept this information after I explained to her how the heart beating irregularly could account for her "seizures." Later, however, she returned to discussing her illness in terms of her "pressure."

The "seizures" which Viola mentioned were episodes which would begin sometimes, but apparently not always, with physical or emotional stress. They occurred more frequently during the dry season when it was both extremely hot and humid. Viola would suddenly "drop" to the floor and become "fixed." She said that during these periods "I don't know myself."

The pressure, she added, "had her tight" and caused shaking or convulsing. After the attack of pressure "took her", she stated she began to "feel myself" again.

Having never seen Viola during one of her "seizures", I remained somewhat skeptical of her description of their nature and severity. One Saturday afternoon I went to visit Viola. Her husband, Domingo, came to the door as I arrived and said, "Come in quickly, the old lady is dying." I entered and found Viola lying in bed. Her eyes were rolled back, she could not speak and did not seem to understand anything said to her. Her fists were clenched and her arms drawn up. She was groaning and rigid. I asked a friend who had a vehicle to drive me to the doctor's residence. I hoped to bring him back to Viola's house. He was not in but was said to be at the hospital. We then drove to the hospital. At the hospital I was told by the nurse in charge for that day that she didn't know where he was. I described Viola's signs and asked what I should do. The nurse informed me that Viola should have come to the outpatient clinic that morning. I explained that she hadn't become ill until afternoon and she could not have walked to the clinic in any case. The nurse's reply was: "Well, then she should have relatives." I felt what I can only assume was an emotion similar to those felt by so many of the residents of Punta Gorda who have confronted the state biomedical system and have lost.

Fortunately, Viola recovered. I visited Viola again twice that evening. Later in the evening, she was able to talk but was very weak. She said she had taken Florida Water and that had helped. Later she said the pressure had "caught" her because she was vexed with Juan. The following morning I returned, expecting to find her in bed. Instead she was up and doing her usual chores. Knowing I had a cold the previous week, she immediately questioned me as to my health and told me she had been worried about me.

Viola rarely asked for my help. She had learned to deal with the "pressure" and with the seizures and had accepted them. But on one occasion she asked me to intercede. Viola had a small ulceration on the instep of her foot. It had begun as a minor cut but had worsened. She said she needed a shot of penicillin, but, because of the difficulty of getting to the hospital, she had taken some penicillin pills prescribed for Domingo. She thought the foot was now better. Since Domingo had never received a prescription for penicillin tablets, I could only assume that the pills she took were aspirin, which had been prescribed recently for Domingo. Several days later, when I visited again, I noted that the ulcer was fairly serious, but that the area of infection seemed smaller. She was soaking the foot as I had suggested. She would then put Vicks on the ulcer and a small piece of cloth over that. She said she had also applied candle wax. A few days later, Viola finally asked for my assistance. She stated that the foot was hurting her and she asked if I could get some medicine from the doctor at Rideau (the army camp). She also complained of a headache. I left her some aspirin and promised to check with the physician at Rideau if I could get a ride out to the camp. A few days later I had still been unable to obtain the requested medication and Viola had Domingo buy her some tablets which she refered to as "sulphur" tablets. She said they could be applied directly after being dissolved in water or they could be swallowed. She swallowed them because she felt direct application to the foot was too drying. Some time after that, Viola made the decision to apply the tablets directly. Eventually the foot did heal.

Viola's use of biomedicine did not always conform to Western expectations. On one occasion, during the period when her foot was bothering her, she stated she was feeling ill with the heat and had a bad headache. I asked what she had done. She said she didn't want to go to the hospital so she had taken some capsules which she had been given by the doctor some months or possibly years earlier. She didn't remember what the capsules had been prescribed for, but she said she was feeling better. She explained that when she and Domingo attended the clinic they always got pills but put them away. I asked if it was different with injections, if they returned to the hospital as instructed. She replied that they did not. Later, when Juan had a boil on his arm, he went to the hospital and was given an injection. He was told to return for three more days for injections. He returned the first day, but not the second or third.

On another occasion, Viola had been given a prescription for 10 mg. of Librium daily. What prompted the physician to give her Librium is unclear to me. In any case, she was also given several other packages of medicine, with varying instructions – take one three times daily, take two two times daily, and so on. For most people, such instructions may present a minor logistical problem. But Viola was blind. She could not read the package instructions. She knew only that she was to take two of one kind, one of another, and so on, but she had no way of telling from which package she was drawing. When I appeared one morning and she complained she had been sleeping all day for two days, I checked the packages and discovered that she had been taking 20 mg. of Librium every morning.

Since Viola had so much difficulty on this occasion, I suggested to her that in the future, she have someone in the house sort out the pills in the morning for her before they left for work, and that each set of pills be separated from the others. On a later occasion when she was again ill and had acquired prescriptions from the physician, she 'solved' her problem by having Domingo count out the appropriate number of pills for the day (this time she was taking antibiotics) she then took all the pills at once.

Domingo had a variety of complaints as well. He had lost one eye in an accident some years earlier. The artificial eye given him had also been lost.

The eye socket would occasionally become red, swollen, and painful. Vision in the other eye was not good. In the years since I left P.G., Domingo has lost all sight and, in Viola's words, "sees with his foot."

Domingo had a severe cold on one occasion. Viola said the cause was that he had gone out in the breeze without a jacket after having been in a hot kitchen. Another time, Domingo exhibited the symptoms of a mild stroke – slowness of speech, numbness of his tongue, and difficulty in walking. Despite these signs, he went to work. Viola and Domingo told me they were both planning to go to the hospital the next day. Viola also said that she had meant to go the previous week, but had cooking to do.

In December of 1979, Domingo had a severely infected foot. The infection began with bites received while working for the city chopping grass in the cemetery. His niece, a Catholic nun who lived at the novitiate outside of Punta Gorda, gave him some medicine, but he reported that the foot hadn't improved. Finally, he went to the hospital and was given a prescription for three injections. He was given the first that day, returned for the second the following day, but didn't go for the third, as he claimed the foot was better. Domingo also complained of a sore neck. He attributed it to the way he slept. Viola, however, believed it was due to high blood pressure because it "catches me the same." Domingo's pressure was recorded on one visit to the clinic as 190/90.

Domingo occasionally took a half packet of epsom salts in water to purge himself. He reported you can also purge with castor oil but it is dangerous if you have abdominal pain for the purge may be too strong. His daughter died of a burst appendix after taking castor oil, he explained. The epsom salts and castor oil are used to clean the liver; salts should be taken every fifteen days if you drink much alcohol. Viola added that brandy, vermouth, and whisky are good for you, but rum has something in it which is harmful. She said she knew of treatments for illness in which the prescribed medicine was a certain amount of vermouth every day. She said she drank a bottle of beer every two weeks if she could afford it to keep the pressure from "catching her."

Domingo and Viola made several trips to the hospital during the period of time I lived in Punta Gorda. That behavior may have been partially influenced by my presence and the belief that I "worked" at the hospital. In the early days of our relationship, Viola and Domingo expressed to me the belief that the hospital was a dangerous place to go. They stated that the "only way you go out is dead", that the nurses "don't know what they're doing" and that the nurses may give you an injection "which will kill you." Even those who were consistent users of the clinic and hospital often expressed beliefs not far removed from these.

In March, not long after my introduction to the family, Domingo complained that he had been ill for several days. He said he had pain in his neck, heartburn, weakness in his knees, an inability to sleep, and "giddiness." He had been working and had become weak while at work. He approached his employer and was told to go to the doctor. After waiting for several hours at the clinic he received a prescription for Benadryl elixer, procaine penicillin, aspirin, and 10 mg. tablets of Valium. He was told the "green pills" (Valium) would help him sleep at nights. The physician asked if he had fevers in the night. He replied that he did. The physician offered a name for his illness, but Domingo couldn't remember what it was. It was, he said, "like malaria." Viola interrupted at this point to say that he had *goma*, the common word for a hangover. She complained that he didn't want to admit to the drinking as a part of the problem. Domingo had not mentioned any drinking when describing his symtoms to me. Domingo, after a brief period of harrassment in my presence, accepted the drinking as part of the sequence of events leading to his illness. There was no further discussion of some "malaria" like disease and the benadryl was admitted by Domingo to be a tonic which "puts things back in the blood which have been drained out by drinking." In this manner, they negotiated the etiology in my presence, using me to test each new theory about cause-effect relationships. Lacking clear information from the physician as to the cause of Domingo's problem, they had been free to seek an etiology in a sequence of events. Negotiation allowed them to decide which events to include in the sequence and at what point in time the sequence was to begin.

My personal relationship with Viola was a close one and she told me on one occasion that she believed I was the spirit of an ancestor come back through her mother. She sometimes referred to me as "mama." In this manner, I was drawn into the position of "protector" and negotiator and Viola expected me to support her assignment and interpretation of signs.

Domingo and Viola Gonzalez viewed their situation as the result of God's will. Domingo believed that "God wished them to suffer a bit longer." This did not prevent them from seeking therapy wherever they might, and Viola's occasional seizures likely referred not to God's desires, but Domingo's incalcitrant behavior. Domingo and Viola had few material resources. Domingo's drinking left those resources depleted; that, combined with his sometimes unpredictable behavior, often precipitated Viola's spells which she assessed as signifying Domingo's failure to perform appropriately his accepted social role. That Domingo never accepted personal responsibility for Viola's illness was a result of the fact that he defined such a role differently than did Viola. In addition, Domingo's illness episodes were often attributed by Viola to his drinking and carelessness. He suffered from a cold because, she explained, he had worked in a hot kitchen and then had gone out in the breeze without a jacket. The later appearance of a number of signs simultaneously ("giddiness", "heartburn", and so on) was attributed by Viola to his consumption of rum on the previous day. When Viola's personal support system was seriously jeopardized by the illness of her best friend, the threat was manifested not in the illness of any of the human members of the household, but in Domingo's parrot. Thus, Domingo was not to be left untouched by Viola's loss.[8]

Case Study Eight: Thomas Cowo

Mr. Thomas Cowo, a forty-five year old Mopan Maya male from the village of San Antonio, was admitted to the hospital in Punta Gorda in February of 1979. He was referred by the American Peace Corps nurse stationed in San Antonio who stated, in a brief note to hospital personnel, that he had been running a high fever for some time, but had not complained of chills. The District Medical Officer said that the Maya did not use or know the term "chills", however, and admitted the patient with a diagnosis of "possible malaria." The patient was to be examined for typhoid fever as well, though the treatment prescribed was that usually prescribed in cases of malaria. Mr. Cowo's wife and several of their twelve children accompained him to the hospital and were frequently at his bedside in the days that followed. It was clear that Mr. Cowo, whatever the nature of his sickness, was quite ill.

Two days after his admission the nurse noted in his chart that the patient "was trying to run away." On the same day, the remark was made by one of the nurses that the patient appeared "confused." Early the next morning, the following information was recorded:

> Patient come on floor and roll all over ward. Patient reacted as psycho [?] .... Medication given with force. Patient taken over asleep lying on floor. With aid and great force patient placed to lie in bed. I.V. injection ordered. Patient pulled out I.V.

Two days later it was noted that the patient "still appears disoriented." On the following day, I wrote in my notes:

> Mr. Cowo is still disoriented. Today is market day and there are fifteen people in his room. He is now asleep or semicomatose and does not respond. Everyone stands quietly by the bed without speaking. His wife is seated but everyone else stands. The nurse reports to me the family is very concerned, but no one from the group has asked about his condition today. There are several small children and babies in the room. I spoke with the wife briefly. She began crying when another patient (Maya) reported her husband's behavior during her absence.

It was at this time that I asked for and received permission from Mrs. Cowo to follow her husband's case when he was released from the hospital. I noted on the following day that Mr. Cowo seemed improved but that his temperature was still elevated (102°F). The nurse disclosed that a relative of the family had said the family might remove the patient from the hospital and take him to a bush doctor.

On February 28, nine days after his admission, Mr. Cowo's family took him from the hospital "against medical advice." There was no doctor present at the hospital to counsel the family against the action as the District Medical Officer had been transferred to another town in Belize and the new physician had not yet arrived. Hospital personnel who had known the patient reported that Mr. Cowo was taken by his family to a bush doctor in the largely Kekchi Mayan village of San Miguel. Many Mopan believe that the Kekchi are more knowledgeable about healing, though there are Mopan healers as well. It should be noted that the Kekchi are said to be best at the employment of medicines for evil intents as well and are sometimes feared for this reason. In this case, as I later learned, the family desired to take Mr. Cowo to a Mopan healer well known to them, but the healer of choice was unable to perform the tasks necessary to Mr. Cowo's treatment at that time.

I left for San Antonio on the first available truck out of Punta Gorda three days after Mr. Cowo's departure from the hospital, and arrived in San Antonio some two hours later. There was no hotel in the town. I was told to see the American Peace Corps nurse by those who knew the village, but she was in Punta Gorda for the day buying vegetables. I rented a small "house" used to store corn and proceeded to try to locate the Cowo family. I found their house and spoke with the children. Mr. and Mrs. Cowo were, according to one of their children, with the bush doctor some ten miles away. I returned to my "house" and, with the assistance of the owner's children, strung up a hammock loaned to me by the village's Catholic priest. A short time later, the priest came to tell me that Mr. Cowo's sister was now home. I returned to the Cowo compound. Mr. Cowo's sister, who had just come from work, talked with me of his treatment and prognosis. The bush doctor cautioned the family from the beginning that Mr. Cowo should have been brought to him earlier in the week as these were "bad days in which to collect herbs." The bush doctor advised he would treat Mr. Cowo for three days, but stated if he had not improved in that time, the family should take him to the hospital in Belize City. Mr. Cowo's sister, Darla, said that the bush doctor was not optimistic about a cure, but that he, Mr. Cowo, had appeared stronger on her previous day's visit. The local Catholic priest (an American) had offered to take the children from San Antonio to San Miguel to visit their father, but the bush doctor said that was not wise as it might disturb the cure.

The decision to remove him from the Punta Gorda hospital and take him to the bush doctor, she explained, was made by the wife and oldest sons, and he was moved directly from the hospital to San Miguel. The sister stated the family's decision was based on the doctor's failure to provide a diagnosis. She added that when her son was sick the doctor "said right away what was wrong and he got better." This sequence of events, – appearance of signs, diagnosis, and recovery, – had occurred as well when her brother's sister was ill. It was the ambiguity of the situation which was most troubling to the family.

The sister explained that the family had never used this bush doctor before. The bush doctor to whom they would normally have turned had injured his foot and was not able to collect herbs. The fee of the bush doctor in San Miguel was $100 B.H., but the family was to pay only after Mr. Cowo had recovered. According to Darla, Mr. Cowo was bathed in herbal teas on the first day of treatment. On that day his sister said he "appeared to be dead" and she was certain she would never see her brother again. On the second day his son reported that he was better, could take some food, and was talking. The bush doctor's wife explained to the family that "sometimes the patient gets worse before getting better because the body attempts to fight the bush medicine." She assured the family that he would improve. On the second and third day of treatment, a *Ramada* (a Catholic ceremony apparently of Spanish origin) was held in the house of the bush doctor. The family sent food for the ceremony; the family and friends spent the night praying.

Mr. Cowo's sister told me that some people had said to her that this illness was due to *obeah*. Darla had lived for several years in Belize City and had a responsible position within the town of San Antonio. She was skeptical of the proffered diagnosis of *obeah* and equally skeptical of the skills of bush doctors. She explained to me that "the bush doctor works on you and if God is willing you get better." As Darla and I sat speaking in the family's home, the second eldest son appeared on his bicyle, having just returned from San Miguel. "Ah" she said, hurrying to the door, "now we shall find out what is happening." The boy approached the house crying. The bush doctor had sent word that Mr. Cowo was dying and that the family should come for the body. The sister immediately went for the priest. Within a short time, the priest, the older sons of Mr. Cowo and several male villagers left in the priest's truck.

Preparations for the wake and funeral began immediately. Darla and I went to a small store to buy white candles. The villagers had already begun to gather. Darla suggested that I spend the night with the family as "it is dark outside and the children may stone you if you go out." The Maya were always friendly and I was little concerned about the children, but I had no desire to return to my "storage" house. I was given a hammock in another small house in the family compound, but remained with the family much of the night.

Approximately two hours after their departure, the priest and the others returned with Mr. Cowo's body. The body was wrapped in a burlap bag and was dragged from the truck up a small hill and into the house where Mr. Cowo had lived. The body was laid on a large sheet of cardboard. I left briefly and by the time I returned, the men had redressed Mr. Cowo in a pair of pants and a white shirt. The body was surrounded by burning white candles placed on the edges of the cardboard. Certain items, such as his shoes and his machete, had been placed beside him. There was no coffin, but other villagers would begin to task of building a simple wooden coffin early in the morning.

The priest returned within an hour and remained much of the night. Villagers came to the house and were offered food and rum. Most stayed throughout the night. A room at the back of house was set aside for the babies. Most of the conversation that night and through the next day was in Mopan. When possible, however, I spoke with the sister. Mrs. Cowo repeated many times that her husband had asked to be released from his suffering. He had become coherent prior to his death and spoke at length with his wife. He said that it was his time to die and he was willing to go. He asked only that his suffering end.

He was buried the following morning in the cemetery approximately one-half mile from his home, and, as is traditional, the grave marked with a large plant with a single red flower. This is the only manner in which graves are marked and a cemetery can be identified by the presence of these unusual plants. The men, many of whom had been drinking throughout the night, attended the ceremony, and then returned to their drinking for the day. Little work was done in the village that day.

Darla told me that Mr. Cowo had been ill for weeks prior to his hospitalization. He sweated profusely and complained of severe headaches. He told Darla that the fever would come when his teeth began hurting. He said he would like to go to the doctor to have his teeth pulled as he believed that was the cause of his problem. Darla said to me that she regretted that she never asked which tooth was troubling him. She concluded that it was the pain of the toothache and the headache and fever which killed him. She pointed to her own teeth and said, "Maybe the infection of the tooth traveled up into his head and made him crazy." Darla stated that for a while, prior to his hospitalization, he behaved strangely. Mr. Cowo's wife once came to her and asked: "What is happening to your brother? He is crazy!" Darla went to check on him, but reported that she was afraid to go near him. She feared that, in his state, he might beat her. They got the Peace Corps nurse at the clinic, which is no more than a few hundred yards away, to give him some medicine. The following day he was said to be much improved. Then, according to Darla, the fever and pain and sweating returned, though there were periods of temporary improvement. He was apparently ill for at least two weeks before the decision was made to take him to the hospital. The nurse had been recontacted during this interval as he arrived at the hospital with a note from her requesting his admission. Darla states that at no time during his hospitalization had anyone mentioned to the physician his original complaint concerning his teeth.

Nor, according to Darla, had the physician ever spoken with the family about his case. Treatment was provided (antibiotics, IVs, and anti-malarial medication), but little was ever communicated to the family about his progress or the possible causes of his illness. His wife was informed that the blood sample sent to Belize City to test for malaria was "too thick" and another had to be sent. A second sample was reported to be negative. Little other information was provided.

I spoke with the new physician, just arrived, about Mr. Cowo on my return to Punta Gorda. He was unfamiliar with the case and I told him what I could. He said that no one dies of malaria until three or four years after developing the disease, and malaria, he argued, had only entered Belize one and one-half years ago. Therefore, Mr. Cowo could not have died of malaria. He referred to the milder form of malaria which has become common in Belize in recent years; the more severe form is said not be present. He believed Mr. Cowo might have died of dehydration connected with fever and sweating, or typhoid fever or of an infectious endocarditis. There was no additional information in his chart which might have allowed a diagnosis.

In March I had occasion to speak with one of the Catholic sisters who served the village of San Antonio. She reported to me that both Mr. Cowo's wife and Darla now believed that he was *obeah*ed. The bush doctor had warned them that he was not certain he could help Mr. Cowo because he thought the cause to be *obeah* from the beginning. The nun explained that Mr. Cowo was amassing land and others were jealous of his wealth.

In late March I visited Mrs. Cowo again. She was, at that time, several months pregnant with her fourteenth child and had not been well. She explained that when her husband first became ill, it was her intent to take him to a Mopan bush doctor in the village of San Antonio. However, the bush doctor, as stated previously, was troubled with a swollen foot and could not go to the bush to collect the medicines necessary to Mr. Cowo's treatment. After the family had him admitted to the Punta Gorda hospital, she said many people came to her and told her to "take him out right away." But she said the physician refused to release him and she did not know what to do. It was only the physician's departure from Punta Gorda that allowed her to take some action.

She stated that the blood tests were returned from Belize City prior to his removal from the hospital and that she was told there was no evidence of malaria. The negative results of the test for malaria simply reinforced the information she had received that this was indeed *obeah*. She believed he was *obeah*ed because "the village is bad and people don't like it if you live well." The bush doctor, however, later told her the *obeah* was done by someone outside the village and Mr. Cowo should have been brought to him right away. I asked Mrs. Cowo if many people suffered illness from *obeah*. She responded, "Oh, yes, plenty."

I continued my contacts with Mrs. Cowo over a period of another thirteen or fourteen months. Despite her disturbance over her husband's treatment when hospitalized, she returned to the hospital several months later, at the urging of the Peace Corps nurse, to give birth to her daughter. Very few Mayan women enter the hospital voluntarily to deliver children. On the other hand, most Mayan women expect assistance from their husbands with the birth.

When Mrs. Cowo suffered what the physician labeled *thrombophlebitis* in April of 1980 she returned again. At that time she told me that this illness was called *disapella* in her village. *Disapella*, she explained, occurs "when you walk on a hot day and find *disapella* in the water." "You can also pick it up from the ground. It is like an insect but you can't see it." Self treatment prior to admission to the hospital included Phrensic for pain (aspirin and caffein), Paludrin for fever (an anti-malarial medication) and cold water applied to the affected part of her leg. She believed the pain worsened while hospitalized because the nurses no longer applied cold water to her leg. She remembered a bush medicine used in the village to treat children when they suffered from *disapella* but she did not know the name of the medicine.

When she and her children were ill, as they frequently seemed to be, she often saw the Peace Corps nurse who operated a small clinic in the village. On one occasion, she sought treatment from a PAHO medical team doing research in the village. She had, in the past, taken one of the children to the "coolie doctor" in Punta Gorda (also referred to as the "private doctor") for treatment when the government doctor wasn't in and when medicine given her by the Peace Corps nurse failed to "cure." She was quite pleased with the "private doctor's" treatment and she related that she planned to take another of her children to him. Sometimes, however, she chose to seek no treatment at all, though the severity of the symptoms seems not to have been a factor in this decision. Once she reported that one of the children had "almost died." The symptoms she described were those of gastroenteritis which kills a sizable percentage of young Mayan children. However, no therapy had been attempted. At that time, I also noted that one of her younger daughters was perspiring heavily though the day was not especially warm and the child was inactive. I asked Mrs. Cowo why she perspired so. "Well, maybe she has prickly heat. Maybe she has heat in her body. Maybe she want to go to river to bathe."

As the time for my departure grew near I visited Mrs. Cowo one last time. She told me that she had heard of a widower in another village with many children and wondered aloud whether she might marry him, though they had never met. Despite the absence of a husband, she and her children seemed to be doing well. One son worked at the army camp, Salamanca; others worked their father's "plantation." The oldest son was married and he and his wife lived in a house only a few feet from the main house. Mr. Cowo's sister and aunt maintained their residence in the compound. The older children showed me a large sheet of wood on which their late father's declaration of loyalty to the government, expressed when he joined the People's United Party, had been recorded by his sons. This had assumed a place of prominence within the house.

Mrs. Cowo eventually accepted the interpretation of *obeah* and claimed it came from someone who resented the family. *Obeah*, in this case, sufficed as both diagnostic label and etiological explanation. Had the physician at the P.G. hospital offered an alternative diagnosis, such diagnosis might initially have been accepted but ultimately rejected if Mr. Cowo had failed to recover following treatment determined by that diagnosis. In any case, a biomedical diagnosis offered by a physician neither supercedes nor displaces a diagnosis of *obeah* though, in this instance, the failure to provide any diagnosis simply supported the assessment of *obeah*.

The Creole Catholic sister who spoke with me later about Mr. Cowo's death appeared to concur in a diagnosis of *obeah* and suggested that the people of San Antonio had resented the large amount of land which Mr. Cowo had amassed. His death was attributed by the family and the social group to his success by one measure and his failure by another. He had, by community standards, not fulfilled his responsibilities to the larger social group. His illness and death functioned to remind the villagers of their obligation to one another and to restate an obvious fact of their social reality – that success may be ephemeral. The bush doctor's assessment that the *obeah* was done by someone outside the community relieved Mrs. Cowo and her sons of the responsibility for taking action against a fellow villager.

Case Study Nine: Carmelo Ramirez

My introduction to the Carmelo Ramirez case occurred when Carmelo, then eleven months of age, was admitted to the Punta Gorda hospital with fever and convulsions. The diagnosis offered by the physician was "meningeal reaction." The chart offered very little additional information. Carmelo had suffered a convulsion prior to admission to the hospital. His temperature fluctuated. He was given antibiotics. After a brief period of treatment, Carmelo was released from the hospital asymptomatic. Three months later, Carmelo was readmitted with the same symptoms. He again recovered quickly and was hospitalized for only a brief period of time. His primary treatment was, as previously, a course of antibiotics. Neither the first DMO nor the second who had replaced him by the time of Carmelo's second admission was able to explain to the family the source of Carmelo's problem. Carmelo's family was Spanish and had come from Guatemala, but had long been resident in Punta Gorda. They had twelve children, of whom Carmelo was the youngest. Mr. Ramirez' brother and his family also lived in Punta Gorda. Though not especially well-to-do judging from external appearances, Mr. Ramirez' primary associations were with members of the town's elite and with other family members. Mr. Ramirez' subsequent actions in managing Carmelo's case suggest that he had greater financal resources than did any other individual or family, with the possible exception of the Cowo's.

The mother spoke very little English; most of my discussions about the child were, therefore, with the father. But it was also the father who was largely responsible for case 'management' and for all decisions about Carmelo's care. Roberto, Carmelo's father, explained to me that Carmelo frequently developed fevers and then would suffer from convulsions. He said Carmelo had been ill since birth. "Maybe it is something in his head", he suggested, explaining that Carmelo's mother had been hit in the stomach by a ball when she was pregnant with Carmelo and was hospitalized briefly in Guatemala. He believed this injury to Carmelo's mother might be the cause of Carmelo's "sickness." "No one here", he stated in frustration, "knows what's wrong." He as disturbed that no satisfactory diagnosis had ever been offered, for "meningeal reaction" did not explain the origin of Carmelo's disorder. After the second hospitalization, the father decided to visit a physician in Belize City. Within the month Carmelo had been taken to Belize City. The physician they saw had been recommended by the local District Medical Officer. The doctor ran many tests, but, after one week, reported he could find nothing wrong. Roberto informed the doctor that he intended to stay in Belize City for more tests, as he wanted to find out why the child kept having fevers. Roberto suggested to the physician that Carmelo's head should be x-rayed, for he still identified the injury as the likely source of Carmelo's illness. Roberto was told to take the child's temperature four times daily for three days. Additional X-rays and other tests were done. The results were the same. The physician reported that Carmelo's urine was somewhat darker than should be expected but did not believe this indicated anything of importance. Roberto took the child to a "Hindu" physician. This physician treated him for "small seizures", apparently without success. Roberto sought out another doctor, described as a "private" physician. This physician checked the child carefully and announced that Carmelo's tonsils were swollen and this was the cause of the fevers. He prescribed thirty days of treatment at home and told Roberto to bring Carmelo back in three months. Apparently Roberto did not return to this physician, nor, apparently, was he willing to accept this diagnosis. When I last spoke with him in April of 1980, more than one year after the first hospitalization, Roberto reported that he had instead taken Carmelo to a pediatrician in Barrios (Guatemala).

He stated that all tests conducted by that physician had been negative. Carmelo was taking vitamins and "suspension" for fevers, but suffered only "poquito" fevers. The child appeared healthy and the father at last seemed convinced that Carmelo would recover fully, though he had never received a diagnosis with which he was totally satisfied.[9]

Roberto was one of the few "therapy managers" (Janzen 1978) I encountered who actively and persistently sought a diagnostic label for an illness. His continued search for an acceptable diagnosis within biomedicine was facilitated by the variation in available biomedical models and his control over the financial resources necessary to such a search. His extensive and expensive effort was ended not with the successful generation of pathognomic signs, but with the pragmatic realization that Carmelo was improving. His utilization of an exclusively biomedical model (or at least of biomedical resources) also illustrates the tendency of P.G.'s "elite" to reject etiologies which include *obeah* or other evil spirits as an explanantory model in childhood illnesses. Most do appear, however, to believe that *obeah* may be employed to cause illness in adults. Nevertheless, there are exceptions. An infant in one prominent family of Creole and East Indian background was said to have been "possessed." The local Catholic priest was called in to perform an "exorcism" of the spirit. (See fn 9 for Roberto's final solution and the emphasis on family ties expressed by this explanation).

Case Study Ten: Elias Pratt

Elias Pratt was a six-year-old East Indian boy admitted to the hospital in Punta Gorda in August of 1979. His home address was given as Mafredi Village, a small East Indian settlement approximately fifteen miles outside of Punta Gorda; his religion was listed as Methodist. His admitting history read: "History of elevated temperature." His hemoglobin on admission was 5, his hematocrit was 14, and his white blood count was 17,700. His skin and eyes were yellowed. His liver function tests were abnormal. He was given procaine penicillin in large doses upon admission and Tylenol syrup. Elias was a very quiet child; most of the interviewing was done with his mother, Ortelia, and with his grandfather. These two, the mother and grandfather, functioned as the therapy managing group.

According to his mother, Elias had been hospitalized twice before in Belize City with the same illness. The mother, however had never been told what his illness was. She had been informed only that his spleen was enlarged. She knew that he ran fevers occasionally, and that periodically he became very weak and could not walk. When he was younger, she reported, he fell down the steps of his house several times. She believed that these falls might have been the cause of the swelling in his side. Ortelia recounted that the current District Medical Officer sent Elias to Belize City once in the past where he was "cured." Elias' father's brother, she added, suffers from the same illness. The doctor, Ortelia reported, conjectured that the illness might be "in the blood." I asked Ortelia what treatment had been provided for Elias in Belize City. She stated that they drew off blood every couple of days. Since Elias' illness was now somehow identified with the state of his blood, she thought that perhaps this procedure had been used to remove the sickness.

Elias lived with his grandparents, mother, and his grandparents' youngest daughter in Mafredi. The grandparents operated a small farm where they raised approximately eighty head of cattle. Elias had lived here for many years. When his mother and father separated shortly after Elias' birth, Elias' mother moved to the village of San Pedro Columbia several miles away, but Elias was left with his mother's parents. Divorce is uncommon among East Indian families and most children are raised by their parents. Ortelia explained of her separation that she didn't like her husband any longer. She returned to live with her family when Elias began to show signs of illness. She related that while Elias was often "sick" as a small child, this current illness had only appeared recently.

Further discussions with Ortelia disclosed the following etiological sequence. His first symptoms, she stated, appeared early in the year when he fell and hit his side. He was sent to Belize. The mother was told by the doctor in Punta Gorda at that time he might need a blood transfusion, but, she reported, he received only "liquid medicines" in Belize. He was "sickly" as a baby, the mother remembered, but "not like now." Now, she reported, he had difficulty recovering from colds. Sometimes he cried in the night because of the pain. She believed it was his spleen that was swollen. The nurse on duty told me that the child was scheduled to receive blood tranfusions at the Punta Gorda hospital when his liver size was reduced.

On this particular occasion, Elias had shown signs of "illness" on the previous Monday. However, it was not possible to "get transport" out of Mafredi until Wednesday. Since Elias was too weak to walk, his mother carried the six-year-old approximately three-quarters of a mile from the location where the trucks had stopped to the outpatient clinic of the hospital. He was admitted from the outpatient clinic.

The lab technician who had run most of the tests on Elias suggested to me that the boy might be suffering from leukemia. She noted that the red blood cells had an abnormal appearance, but she was unable to determine what this signified. No diagnosis was entered into his chart on this or any other occasion. No test that had been run indicated a diagnosis. An ambulance driver for the hospital who was East Indian and knew the family came to tell me that Elias' parents were first cousins. He suggested that this might be the cause of Elias' illness.

I asked Ortelia if anyone had suggested treatment with bush for him. She said that in Belize City an East Indian woman had told her to cut a piece of bark from a particular tree. The size of the piece was to correspond to the size of his left foot. It was to be hung over a hearth to dry. "As the bark shrinks, the spleen will shrink to the same size." "Plenty of people tell me that", she added. She expressed concern over her son's condition and added that sometimes at night she thought about his illness a lot. "I don't know if he will live or die." Nevertheless, she hesitated to speak to the doctor about a diagnosis, his future treatment, or a prognosis, and asked if I could talk with him in her behalf. Elias was released from the hospital after an extensive period of hospitalization. He appeared considerably improved though still suffering from anemia.

In December, I visited the family at Mafredi. Ortelia and Elias had just returned from three weeks in Belize City where Elias had been hospitalized for four days because of "poor blood." The DMO had advised his admission to Belize City hospital for further tests and treatment. He had been given transfusions and medications and appeared well. The family had been told to return in January so that Elias might receive further treatment. The family asked me to intercede to obtain records held in the Belize City hospital to determine what sort of treatment he was to receive. They wished to know if the same treatment could be given to him in the hospital in Punta Gorda, as the expense of the trip to Belize and a hotel were great, even though the family was relatively well off by local standards.

I asked Ortelia again if she knew what was wrong with Elias. She said the doctor had told her it was some sort of anemia, but she couldn't remember the precise name. I asked her if the term might be *thalessemia*. The mother brightened and said, "Yes, that was it." The family appeared relieved that someone seemed to have some understanding of his illness. I tried to explain what little I knew about the illness to the family. The concept of an illness which "runs in the family" is understood, but the idea of a genetic disorder is not. They asked me if his sickness could be cured. I responded that it was treatable, but not curable. The grandfather replied that they would like very much to find a cure.

In April, I spoke with the grandfather again. He remarked that Elias was not doing well. He had been in Belize City once again for injections. He was told to return but the family had turned to bush medicines to treat the swollen spleen. The grandfather explained that the medicines, supplied by an East Indian woman in the Mafredi area, had reduced the enlarged spleen for a while, but that his condition had since worsened. The family now considered bring Elias back to the doctor at Punta Gorda. They hoped for a cure this time, the grandfather confided.

The Pratt family had failed to mention to me that the father and mother of the afflicted child were first cousins. They may have felt this to be unrelated to the sequence of events leading to the appearance of Elias' "sickness." Nevertheless, a member of the East Indian community, with no knowledge of the genetic basis of thalessemia, felt it important to inform me of this relationship. This suggests that the community or larger social group had seen in the signs of this child's illness one further indication of the correctness of their prohibition against first cousin marriages. While no ethnomedical model utilized by the inhabitants of the southern Toledo provided for the notion of illnesses caused by recessive or dominant genes, all groups did appear to recognize illnesses or traits which were inherited from other family members. In general, such illnesses are thought to be incurable. The Pratt family's persistent search for a cure further suggests that the family had chosen not to explore my statements about the role of inheritance in Elias' illness.[10]

Case Study Eleven: Mr. Juan Sho

Mr. Juan Sho age thirty-four, and two of his brothers moved to the town of Punta Gorda from their native Mopan Mayan village. Each was accompanied by his family and each proceeded to set up a small grocery and dry goods store. The brother who first arrived was able to help the other two with the establishment of their stores. Each of the families experienced numerous illness episodes and business problems. At least two of the brothers, including Mr. Sho, consulted an American, Mr. Evans, who had lived in Punta Gorda for several years and who had developed a reputation for accurately reading cards and analyzing dreams (see Therapeutic Specialists, Ch. IV).

Mr. Sho visited Mr. Evans several times over a three year period seeking advice about illness in the family and business troubles. In mid-1979 Mr. Sho sought out Mr. Evans again. At that consultation Mr. Evans said the cards indicated that Mr. Sho would soon have trouble with business and the cause would be carelessness. Mr. Evans visited Mr. Sho's shop and gave him advice on the management of the small business. He also noted at the same time that the family wasn't eating properly. They ate, he reported to me, the same foods at each meal – broth with peppers, onions, and tomatoes, and corn tortillas. He said he had never seen them eat meat. Mr. Sho, however, replied that he used sardines and fish powder "made by the Indians." Mr. Evans reported he took the family to the pharmacy for multiple vitamins with mineral supplements and advice from the pharmacist.

Mr. Sho returned to Mr. Evans five days later and said he had had terrible dreams. He had dreamt he was lost in the bush or trying to get over an unfordable river. He wanted to know if more vitamins would stop his dreams.

Evans told him to see the doctor or the pharmacist. He saw the pharmacist and was given Librium. This, Mr. Evans assumed, must have helped because Mr. Sho did not come back for some time. He did return one month later, however, and requested that Mr. Evans read the cards for his wife. Mr. Evans did so and said he could seen only confusion and disorganization within the family unit. The wife admitted that there had been much trouble. Mr. Evans said each person was trying to "point at the other." Mr. Evans said at that time he also saw fraud in the cards.

Some two weeks later, a "government inspector" appeared at Mr. Sho's shop and said the prices for the goods Mr. Sho offered were "wrong." There is price control in the country and prices of most items are regulated. He stated that for $300 B.Z. he would not report this to the authorities. Mr. Sho gave the man $200 B.Z. Mr. Sho then consulted Mr. Evans. Mr. Evans told him he had done the wrong thing. Mr. Sho wanted to know if they could burn candles to bring the man back. Evans replied that he couldn't do that. "Maybe some can, but I can't", he told me later.

About two weeks later Mr. Sho appeared again for another card reading. He said the police had found the man and Mr. Sho wanted to know if the cards indicated the police had the right man. If so, Evans reported Mr. Sho planned to kill him. Mr. Evans told him that he couldn't be absolutely certain with the cards that the police had the proper man. He suggested to Mr. Sho that if he killed the man he surely wouldn't get his $200 back. "Vengeance is mine, saith the Lord", cautioned Mr. Evans to Mr. Sho.

Some time later, Mr. Sho reappeared. He complained of nightmares, continuing thirst, hunger and frequent urination. He asked Mr. Evans to read the cards to determine if his illness was one "of God" or "of man." Mr. Evans advised him to see the government doctor immediately and to pay the fee for a private consultation with the doctor. Mr. Sho, however, did not go to the doctor's residence. Mr. Evans later heard that he was using bush medicine for the treatment of his symptoms.

Mr. Evans left Belize for a period of several months and during that time Mr. Sho became progressively worse. Eventually he visited the government doctor in Belize City and was told that he had diabetes. He was given a prescription for tablets which he had filled in Belize City. However, he apparently did not understand or was not told that the prescription was to be refilled and that he was to continue on the tablets. Once the tablets were gone the symptoms reappeared. He finally returned to the doctor and was told to have the prescription refilled. He was again taking the pills and reported he was feeling better when I first visited him in his small store. I provided him with the material to test his urine for sugar content and then returned a few days later. He told me had had eaten turkey the day before, had become ill, and had much sugar in his urine. I asked what else he had eaten and he replied he had eaten tortillas with the turkey. I wrote out for him a list of foods which he should avoid, suggesting that the tortillas, not the turkey, had made his condition worse.

In the meantime he had solicited the advice of a Mennonite farmer who had stopped in the store. The Mennonites are known to have their own medical supplies. The man told Mr. Sho that he required insulin, but that the Mennonites had none. Mr. Sho and his wife considered a trip to Guatemala to obtain insulin (none was then available in Belize), but they could not leave the store nor did they speak Spanish. A short time later I visited again. Mr. Sho had continued to use the test material for urine sugar but his prescription for tablets had run out and he expressed no interest in refilling the prescription. He stated he was feeling quite ill and had suffered considerable loss of weight. He was, at that time, using *sorocee*, a local bush medicine. He was concerned now only with finding a "cure" for his illness rather than further treatment of the symptoms. I stated that there were several ways to treat the illness, but there was, to my knowledge, no cure.

As I left the shop, his wife asked me to look at the children. She sat in the yard pulling lice from the hair of one of her sons. She asked if I knew of a treatment for lice. I suggested that she contact the American lab technician who occasionally provided both medicines and advice for simple problems.

On my next visit, I found Mr. Sho in considerably better health. He was taking no pills, had resumed all his normal activities, had not returned to the doctor, and had not radically altered his diet. He reported he had obtained some medicine from a bush doctor in the Maya village of San Miguel. He did not know the name of the medicine and was only able to refer to it as "bitters", a term used locally to refer to several varieties of herbs and roots. He indicated that he continued to use the test material and that his urine showed only a trace of sugar.

On a later visit, he reported he had obtained another form of "bitters" known as Billy Web bark from a local woman whom he identified as Carib or Creole, and he had sent a request to his native village for an additonal supply. He stated he was feeling quite well, but had found that both tortillas and soda biscuits made him ill. He was hoping shortly for a cure and said that he believed a cure was possible as, according to the government physician, the illness had reached his kidneys and his urine, but had not yet reached his blood.

It appears that Mr. Sho accepted the diagnostic label of "diabetes", but not the prognostic assessment that the illness was incurable. This is an attitude commonly held by members of all ethnic groups in Punta Gorda toward most illnesses and not, as we have seen in other cases, unique to the Maya. An affliction may persist for several years before the individual or the therapy managing group revises the prognosis. In fact, the Maya suffer from few illnesses which are not "curable." The incidence of chronic or progressive diseases, such as cardiac disorders, diabetes, hypertension, arthritis, asthma, cancer, and so on, is extremely low, whereas the incidence of acute illnesses, generally easily treatable, but often resulting in death if untreated, is relatively high, reinforcing the belief that most illnesses are of short duration. Mr. Sho was the only Mayan individual I encountered in a period of seventeen months who had been diagnosed as having diabetes. This was an illness, therefore, with which the Maya had had little experience.

It is likely that Mr. Sho's diet was altered to some extent when he and his family moved to P.G., though there was little evidence of this. The fact that all three brothers left the same village to move to Punta Gorda suggests they may have experienced problems in the village. Some Mayan people who came from the Mayan villages to shop in town or to sell products avoided Mr. Sho's shop, expressing the belief that he "cheated" them just as they felt the other merchants did. This apparent rejection, as well as other problems described to and by Mr. Evans, may have affected Mr. Sho's physical condition; there may well have been a strong psychosocial dimension to Mr. Sho's illness.[11]

Case Study Twelve: Mr. Jose Choc

Mr. Jose Choc was a thirty-five year old Kekchi Maya male admitted to the Punta Gorda hospital in April of 1979. This was his first visit to a doctor and his first stay in a hospital. He gave his address as Moho River near Santa Elena and his religion as Pentecostal. I became interested in the case largely because of the unusual nature of his illness. His chest was covered with large, oozing sores. His admitting record read: "Patient admitted with a history of lesion in chest on and off for five years now. Also complains of pain in both knees since two weeks ago." He was slightly anemic and his white count was elevated. His treatment during the period of hospitalization consisted of cleaning and dressing the lesions, APC, B-Complex, and propen with strep daily. He was discharged after a stay of five days. The discharge diagnosis stated that he suffered from a tubercular chest and neck. However, the physician informed me the diagnosis was never confirmed. The nurses recorded that he had no complaints during his stay.

I interviewed Mr. Choc shortly after his arrival at the hospital. In addition, I encountered him on some twelve to fifteen occasions after that and had several opportunities to speak with him. When initially interviewed he explained to me that he had a "sickness" on his chest. He said that these "boils" had first appeared about five years earlier. He had used bush medicine obtained from a bush doctor to "keep it under control." He did not know what sort of medicine was used. He could only describe its preparation and use. The medicine was mashed until soft and applied directly, he explained. He said he believed bush medicine could help until one could reach a doctor. When asked if he was improving under the physician's care he replied, "Well, I don't know. Only the doctor can say. But it looks worse to me."

He told me that the continual pain had often made it difficult for him to work and that he had decided to seek out help for his condition when a small team of British soldiers on patrol in the jungle arrived at the settlement where he lived (such settlements usually consist of one to four or five houses; in his case, his house may have been isolated from any others as he told me there was no one to care for his wife and children in his absence). He approached the soldiers and asked if they could help him. They replied that the only help they could offer was to take him back with them and leave him at the hospital in Punta Gorda. He consulted his wife and, with the family's approval, left with the soldiers. He believed he would receive treatment at the hospital and would be able to return home on the same or the following day. He had not realized, having had no prior experience with physicians or hospitals, that he might be detained. His wife had once seen the doctor in the past, he reported, but he did not remember why she had sought out help.

When I spoke with Jose in the hospital he told me his major concern was his family. Since he had not expected to be hospitalized, he had left his family with neither food nor money. Nor did they know at that point where he might be. He said he had no relatives in the immediate vicinity who might look after them. He was uncertain how he might return to his home once he was discharged as the soldiers who had provided him with transport to town were not available to transport him back. He also expressed concern about his ability to work. He had farmed a small plantation, but in recent years had had difficulty working because of his illness. He stated he did not know how he would be able to provide for his family. His wife was then expecting their eleventh child and she, too, had been ill.

He and his wife had eight living children. Jose delivered all the babies without assistance. He explained that what was required of him was that he keep his wife warm, give her black pepper and the soup of a fowl. Black pepper is believed to ease the delivery; a physician suggested to me it may make the contractions stronger. Two of their children had died. One died shortly after birth; the other, a male, died at the age of approximately seven years. Jose told me that this child died of "loose stools and vomiting." He says that the child climbed onto a roof and fell off. "His body got soft all over. Then he got fever and loose stools which didn't stop." Jose attributes the child's death to the fall which he believes provoked the loose stools, vomiting, and fever.

A few weeks after his discharge, I spoke with the soldiers who had first brought him to the hospital. They said they had recently seem him again when they were on patrol. He approached them once more and asked for their help. The soldiers said the lesions had now spread to his legs. They explained that they could only take him back to hospital. He refused. One of the soldiers asked him if he had a "social disease." He replied that he did. He would, of course, have had no idea what this diagnostic or etiologic label signified; the term is not in use among Belizeans and venereal disease is, in any case, extremely uncommon among the Maya. The same soldier stated that Mr. Choc appeared to be suffering from advanced stages of syphilis.

Within a few months Mr. Choc and his family had resettled outside Punta Gorda. He said he had been given the use of a small house by a local businessman. The house was in very poor repair but he reported that it was temporarily adequate. He was looking for some sort of work in town. He often stopped by my house to ask for jobs or to ask if I had extra food. Though he wore a shirt, the lesions were obvious and there was considerable drainage. However, he did not mention his "illness" to me, nor did he indicate that he was utilizing any treatment at that time. Now living in Punta Gorda, he never again sought treatment at the local hospital for himself.

In September his wife was admitted to the hospital. The following comments were entered into her chart: "Patient refused to stay in hospital. History of swollen feet and pain in lower abdomen and in legs. Fundus 30 weeks." She apparently did agree to remain in the hospital and later returned for the birth of her child. One of the nurses at that time, a Creole woman, recalled Mr. Choc's illness and remarked: "They say it's *obeah*. I don't know if it's true."

In late September I asked Mr. Choc if he believed his illness was due to *obeah*. He had previously told me he didn't know how the sickness started. "It just came out from my skin", he said. It was not "inside", he added. This time, however, he responded that some people said his illness was *obeah*. We continued our conversation:

S. How can it be treated if it is *obeah*?
C. Well, there are bush doctors who know how to cure it
S. What is the treatment?
C. The doctor mixes medicines and applies them.
S. What kinds of medicines?
C. I don't know
S. Do they (the bush doctors) ever tell you who did the *obeah*?
C. Sometimes, and sometimes they won't
S. What happens to the person who did the *obeah*?
C. Nothing
S. Do the bush doctors use prayers?
C. Sometimes
S. Catholic or Kekchi prayers?
C. Well, I don't know

In October, Mr. Choc came by my house to see if I had work. He reported that he had just taken his son to the doctor for "pain on belly." I asked if he'd gotten medicine for his son. He replied that he had. I asked what sort of medicine it was. He answered "Well, it is for pain on belly." During the period of time since his release from the hospital he had sought no further treatment for his own illness.

In February, Mr. Choc expressed a desire to return his family to the Moho as he been unable to find work in Punta Gorda. He was looking for some way to finance the trip back. Within a few weeks he had left Punta Gorda. I saw him shortly before my departure on a road some distance from Punta Gorda. From all appearances his condition remained unchanged.

Mr. Choc admitted to a possible diagnosis of *obeah*. I had not explored with him the possible interpretations he attached to that etiological assignment. Certainly his illness, in a very different sense, was a constant reminder of his total inability to effectively access any social or therapeutic network. His move to Punta Gorda reinforced his status as a marginal individual unable to develop even kin ties that could be exploited with any success. He agreed to the interpretative decisions of the British soldiers (a "social disease") only in order to gain access to a potential network for the exploitation of a therapeutic resource. He thus contributed to an evolving sterotype of the Maya held by British soldiers in which certain illnesses were said to be the result of "immoral" behavior and ignorance.

Summary

> Healing everywhere concerns the human intervention in disorder; culturally specific attempts to mend the physical, conceptual, and social breaches entailed in illness. Illness, in turn , is a particular expression of a universal feature of human experience, that of threat to the normal state of being, or to survival. This implies an eclipse of man's *social* being by his *natural* state, and hence frequently poses a challenge to existing order. As such, it touches upon universal paradoxes of human existence, and their symbolic expression in particular cultural schemes. These paradoxes center upon the unity and, at the same time, the duality of body and mind, the ambiguity of self as subject and object, and the opposition of natural and social being (Comaroff 1981:368).

The interpretive process is both guided and constrained. Signs of physical disorder may refer to some dysfunction at the organismic level but they may also indicate far more, for such signs are polysemous. They generate many interpretations, each linked to some cultural, social, political, or natural domain in a way often barely understood by healers and physicians and, at best, tenuously incorporated into or subsumed under some explanatory paradigm. As I stated in the first chapter, not all possible signs of disorder are utilized within any single interpretive system. Both the presentation and experience of disorder are affected by the cultural values and practices which one accepts as a member of a specific ethnic or cultural groups. The domains from which signs are drawn or generated are defined by other than natural parameters.

The signs of illness and illness as a sign, as a communicative device, are overdetermined. That is, they have many potential interpretants. Any exposition of a system of causality which imputes one meaning or interpretation to a sign or series of signs (syndrome) likely does an injustice to the data; certainly this is the case in pluralistic medical systems for alternative explanations are always available. To state that the link between the illness sign and its signification(s) may be arbitrary, as I have suggested, is to assign such signs to the category of symbols, and symbols become highly manipulatable objects which can be turned to a variety of uses. Illness and medicine (therapy) are not 'state' and 'system', respectively; rather both are on-going interpretive processes.

In each of these cases, the significance attached to the illness by the patient, the therapy managers, and the larger social group can be clearly distinguished from that of the biomedical practitioner. And, in each of these cases, the meaning or significance attached to the illness can be referred to the domain of personal and social relationships, to ethical or moral concerns, or to concerns about the self and its relationship to other selves.

Illness episodes, as I stated at the outset of this chapter, are stories, myths composed at least in part of past experiences of the social collectivity now re-expressed both concretely and symbolically through the suffering of an individual. New meanings are added to prior meanings, and earlier significations may be lost. The total set of all possible meanings (or interpretants) is never accessible to either participants or observers. An interpretant functions as a sign which, in turn, must be interpreted. We analyze these various interpretations as a sequence of events and explore the diachronic and synchronic relationships among signs, but may, in the process, lose much of the mythical quality of the experience, perhaps even its 'true' significance. We can, at best, only initiate an archaeology of the sign. The fact that we perhaps cannot penetrate to the core of even a single sign should not deter us from the effort, for we thus begin to examine ourselves, to explain the paradigms which govern our explorations.

NOTES

1. On my last visit to Punta Gorda, Peter was said to be attending school. Peter's mother stated that she sometimes had to carry him, but that he was otherwise well. She had given birth to two additional children during my four year absence, and with her own funds had built a second small house.
2. Mr. Arzu is now deceased. I did not ask the cause of his death.
3. Visual hallucinations sometimes accompany or are part of that syndrome known as narcolepsy in which the afflicted individual suffers from "sleep attacks." The biomedical model unites signs (the sudden onset of sleep and visual hallucinations) which would not be perceived as associated within the Garifuna model.
4. Mrs. Noralez died in July of 1984, though her condition had not changed substantially in March of that year when I visited with her again.
5. The wound on Mrs. Sentino's leg had healed though the leg was still severely swollen. Mrs. Sentino's daughter, Lennie, now has three children and has established her own separate household. Mary's grandon, Ernest, still lives with her and works when employment is available. An older son had returned immediately prior to my visit in 1984 and stated that he planned to stay to look after his mother.
6. Mr. Reyes has moved and I obtained no additional information on Mrs. Reyes or the cause of her death.
7. I encountered Mr. Valdez on several occasions during my visit to Punta Gorda in 1984. His arm was almost entirely healed. He explained that he had gotten funds to go to Guatemala where he was kept in the hospital for a seven month period and 'cured.' He now owns a small chicken farm "to the back."
8. I visited Viola and Domingo many times in 1984. Viola's condition remained largely unchanged. Domingo, as reported in the case studies, is now totally blind. Still, the two of them manage to cook, clean, and do the washing without assistance. An American Peace Corps worker sometimes helps them with their shopping. On one occasion, I saw a young boy guiding Domingo to the market to make his purchases. Neighbors and relatives sometimes drop by to bring small amounts of food or to run errands for the couple.
9. I spoke with Carmelo's father on my return to Punta Gorda. He reported that his son was now very healthy and there had been no recurrence of the "fits." He stated that on his last visted to Guatemala to seek treatment for Carmelo, the cause of Carmelo's illness was explained to him. Roberto had a daughter who had been seriously injured in an automobile accident in Guatemala and later died. Roberto's wife, who was then pregnant with Carmelo, stayed with the daughter while she was in the hospital. Roberto explained that the daughter was "fretting" all the time, "turning this way and that." Carmelo had picked this up from the dying girl and hence had been born with "fits." This, Roberto said, had been explained to him by the physician, thus allowing to establish a non-biomedical explanation which he stated was generated by a biomedical physician.
10. I was unable to obtain additional information on Elias' condition.
11. I returned to Mr. Sho's shop in 1984 to see how he was doing. He had lost a considerable amount of weight, complained that he never had strength, that he felt as though his feet and legs were being "stuck with needles" and that his eyesight was bad. He said he had tired of taking bitters and had never returned to the local physician. I told him that he would lose his eyesight altogether, his family would have to take care of him, and he would no longer be able to provide for his children if he did not seek care. I asked a friend of mine, a nurse at the local hospital and son of prominent Garifuna bush doctor, to visit Mr. Sho and explained to him what he must do. I was recently told that Mr. Sho is now receiving treatment after visiting with a specialist.

CHAPTER 8

Health Seeking Transactions in a Pluralistic Society

Like ethnomedicine's interpretive models, the paradigms governing biomedicine have a long and complex history; there is no reason to assume that evolution has forced upon biomedicine a consistently logical form. "Modern" medicine is, in fact, constituted of several interpretive models which are only superficially integrated through reference to the scientific approach. Horton (1967) distinguishes Western science from traditional systems of thought by referring to the one as "open" and the other as "closed." Yet, the ethnographic data suggests that ethnomedical systems are not impervious to change and that there are many innovators among indigenous therapists, while the history of "scientific" medicine clearly shows that there have been periods in which biomedicine was strongly wedded to certain paradigms or metaphors which were dogmatically defended. The suggestion of certitude seems to evolve as an act of faith on the part of users; the aura of certainty surrounding biomedicine has not been entirely perpetuated by biomedical personnel who often recognize the limitations of the biomedical model or models.

Whatever the source, the notion of a coherent and well-integrated body of thought is brought into question by examination of modern medical theories and the history of the development of scientific medicine. Coulter (1975) defines two major and distinct models that govern not only the interpretive process but therapeutic intervention, and he traces the early expression of both to the Hippocratic corpus. The one, Empiricism, has it modern expression in homeopathy, in Coulter's view; the second, Rationalism, in today's allopathic tradition. Copeland (1977) describes two very different explanatory models (*xenochthonous*, *autochthonous*) used to account for the origin of disease and its manifestation in the individual. The former describes disease as the interaction between a healthy host and an extraneous cause and attempts to classify disease, in part, according to the extraneous cause. This approach, Copeland claims, first emerged in the seventeenth century with Sydenham's "ontologic theory of disease." The latter model treats disease as the net effect of cause and response by the host.

> If we conclude that there is nothing innately pernicious in any of the environmental agents we identify as the cause of disease, then the origin of disease is in the limitations of our own adaptive capabilities.... Disease thus becomes a description of some limitation in the inventory of adaptive resources, or genotype, of the organism (Copeland 1977: 532).

While this latter theory is, by implication, relatively recent, elements of it are evident in fourth century B.C. Greek medical thought.

Norton (1969) identifies several explanatory frameworks which are currently part of biomedicine. These include germ theory, allergy theory and focal sepsis theory, all of which have, in Norton's words "been cut down to size." He describes as "closed systems, rooted in unshakable faith", the following: osteopathy, acupuncture, radiesthesia, naturopathy, Christian Science, and homeopathy. And he lists three "hypotheses" emerging in recent decades: the psychosomatic hypothesis, the stress hypothesis and the hypothesis of autoimmune disease, each hypothesis used to explain the orgins of a certain category of disease and/or the manifestation of illness in a particular individual.

There is, finally, the mind-body distinction which still divides modern medicine into two broad categories encompassing both theory and therapy. Psychosomatic medicine's attempts to eliminate the dichotomy have been only marginally successful.

Finding common elements which unite all components of the predominating medical model is difficult. To isolate common understandings which unite all theories claiming to be part of biomedicine is even more difficult. Nevertheless, certain concepts would seem to undergird the predominating paradigm, if we exclude the purely psychological or psychotherapeutic models. 1. organs and structures are interdependent; 2. the understanding of disease processes necessarily involves a knowledge of events at the cellular level; 3. there are chemical and structural changes in blood, tissue, and bone which result from the disease process and these changes are ultimately detectable, that is, blood, tissue, and bone, as well as body products or components, become the source of signs, the structures whereby the invisible can be made 'visible'; 4. all disease originates in natural causes; and 5. all diseases are ultimately "knowable"; biomedicine has as its philosophical basis that set of tenets known as logical positivism.

These basic precepts govern biomedicine as its is delivered in Belize. Yet, biomedicine is susceptible to alterations or changes in focus and 'modern' health care has not remained untouched by the various systems with which it must compete or the social and political environment in which it functions. In general, medicine becomes an offensive action taken to control invading organisms. The emphasis is on organism-organism interactions, not on the failure of the body to regulate environment-organism interactions. Certain more "sophisticated" aspects of the biomedical model – such as the "stress model" of illness causation – have little place in the practice of medicine in

Punta Gorda. Further, with the exception of the various physicians who serve the Toledo District (most are present for a few months or years and then move on to another assignment), biomedical care is delivered by individuals who are themselves members of Punta Gorda's many ethnic collectivities and who serve in a social context in which their identity as members of specific ethnic sections affects their personal acceptance of the predominating biomedical paradigms, the manner in which such models are made consistent with medical models which may be socially and morally more compelling for them, and the actual techniques whereby care is provided.

Despite marked differences in the theories which distinguish biomedicine from traditional therapeutic models, there are similarities between and among systems. For example, the signs (objective) and symptoms (subjective) presented by the individual are subjected to evaluation in both, though the biomedical practitioner seems to place less emphasis on the patient's production of symptoms than does the healer and proportionately more on the objective signs produced through physical examination or clinical analysis. The signs, in both ethnomedical systems and biomedicine, do not refer directly to a disease state, but require interpretation (Barthes 1972, Kahn 1978, Foucault 1973, Hecht 1889, Eco 1976). The physician, with a variety of diagnostic techniques at his disposal, may choose any of a number of ways to generate new signs inaccessible to the traditional therapist. The ethnomedical therapist, on the other hand, generates or evaluates signs not considered by the physician. But the generation of signs for both is based on certain *a priori* models and neither diagnostician generates all possible signs. While the consideration of a variety of personal and contextual factors in establishing a diagnosis and prognosis has been urged for several centuries, biomedical personnel far too frequently have neither the time nor the inclination to take these into consideration. The healer, on the other hand, may find in these his chief source of signs.

Further, each medical model must generate interpretations which are consistent with the social and moral philosophies from which the models have evolved. Thus, individuals, and the social collectivities in which they live, must be held responsible for their illnesses in ways which support and confirm existing models of appropriate conduct and supernatural intervention.

Each medical model, whether biomedical or ethnomedical, provides, in theory, the means and material for the successful completion of four processes. 1. the generation and interpretation of signs which establish an etiology, 2. the generation and interpretation of diagnostic signs, 3. the generation and interpretation of prognostic signs, and 4. the intervention in bodily and social processes in order to produce the signs indicative of health. However, political, economic, and technological constraints imposed on state biomedicine prohibit it from effectively completing any of these processes in a sizeable percentage of cases.

The biomedical diagnostician, as the ethnomedical therapist, must collect or elicit signs and symptoms, must group those which are not diagnostic into syndromes according to some pre-existing model which anticipates the simultaneous or consecutive occurrence of certain signs and the occurrence of certain diseases, and must determine the syntagmatic and paradigmatic relationship of signs to one another, including those signs which have not yet appeared. The biomedical practitioner proceeds by applying a diagnostic label where possible to the appearance and expected appearance of signs, though symptomatic therapy can be undertaken without the application of a disease name. Often, in fact, the therapy itself becomes the principal diagnostic tool. An individual complaining of lower abdominal pain, fever, and diarrhea may be given antibiotics. If the patient improves, the therapy implies a diagnosis, that is, it suggests, in broad terms, that the patient was the victim of the invasion of the lower intestinal tract by bacteria. Thus, state biomedicine as delivered in Punta Gorda, Belize, is constrained in terms of the range of diagnoses which can be generated not only by the absence of diagnostic equipment and supplies but by the limited range of therapies available as well.

In ethnomedical models, the etiological chain of events (signs) which precedes the illness episode may be critical. If it is not evident in the existing signs, it must be elicited in questioning. Diagnosis is of less importance than ascertaining etiology, and ethnomedical therapies are often directed at an alteration in etiological events, rather than at a change in an organic process. If an illness is due to *obeah*, for example, the physician may provide symptomatic and temporary relief, but the sequence of events leading up to the expression of illness must be carefully examined and treated. In the case of common and easily resolved episodes, however, neither diagnosis nor etiology may be of great concern.

In every medical model, etiology and diagnosis are closely linked though either may be altered as new signs are produced. The cause-effect relationships of biomedicine are not always susceptible to alteration because the techniques for generating new signs are affected by the lack of diagnostic equipment and supplies, the shortage of experienced technicians, and the large number of patients who must be seen daily.

The biomedical practitioner examines a certain number of limited domains in his search for diagnostic signs. The boundaries of the body may, in fact, define the territory. The healer commonly looks beyond the physical body to the social body in his search for signs. This is perhaps a basic distinction between the healer and biomedical diagnostician; it is a distinction which almost totally disappears, however, when we examine the activities of the psychiatrist and compare them to those of the traditional therapist.

While biomedicine focuses on the interdependence of organ systems, the

Garifuna medical model tends to focus on the interdependence of the afflicted individual and other beings, including those who no longer live and the various spirits who are believed to inhabit the universe. Biomedicine emphasizes metonyms, that is, parts which stand for wholes. It utilizes blood and tissue and urine and iconic representations which we call X-rays to analyze the patient's condition. The patient becomes a collection of components, the analysis of each alteration in tissue or product thus standing for the patient and the disease. Ethnomedicine, on the other hand, tends not to make interpretations based on metonyms alone. Rather, ethnomedicine is metaphoric as opposed to metonymic in that the afflicted person comes to stand for something else. That is, the union of illness and individual symbolically reinforces important understandings about the natural and spiritual world as that reality has come to be known.

Biomedicine as practiced in Belize is subject to additional constraints. There are, first of all, the ecological or epidemiological constraints which partially determine the physician's expectations as to the likelihood of the appearance of any given disease. These constraints lead the physician to interpret the signs first on the basis of what he has come to believe should exist. Additionally, ecological factors determine not only the range of diseases which may manifest themselves in the individual (tuberculosis, gastroenteritis, dysentery, leishmaniasis, malaria, parasites, and so on), but, in part, determine or influence the type of therapy which may be prescribed. High temperatures, high humidity, contaminated wells, periodic shortages of water, lack of refrigeration, impassable roads, and so on, are givens the physician cannot avoid. The physician must recognize that the dietary staples of the people he serves are rice, beans, tortillas, cassava, and fish, and individuals are unlikely to radically alter their diets. He must accept that individuals will continue to use well water, especially in the dry season, and that Mayan women are not likely to begin wearing shoes in the near future. And he must be cognizant of the fact that ethnically derived interpretive systems will affect the patient's perception of the physician's explanations and his understanding of both proscriptive and prescriptive therapies.

There are, as well, the social constraints on interpretation and therapy which are imposed on every healer. The biomedical physician is not exempt from them. The physician in Punta Gorda is subjected to very little community pressure or pressure from particular social networks to provide an interpretation consistent with or supportive of local beliefs or sentiments. His position as an employee of the State prevents that, as does the usually short term physicians serve in Punta Gorda. However, to maintain his legitimacy as a diagnostician and therapist within his own profession, he must generate interpretations and utilize therapeutic techniques more or less consistent with biomedical models.

There are linguistic constraints on the interpretive and therapeutic processes in Punta Gorda. Few persons in the south of Toledo are fluent in all the languages in which the illness experience may be expressed. Sharing a language is often essential to the success of the therapeutic endeavor and language plays a substantial role in the choice of therapist and diagnostician. It does, however, seem rarely to stop an exchange across ethnic boundaries where other considerations necessitate such a move. Each ethnic section possesses members knowledgeable in the use of medicines. They speak the language of that ethnic section as a first language and their basic assumptions and values are those of the majority of the members of that section. Most bush doctors are, additionally, fluent in at least one other language. The East Indian bush doctor referred to earlier is fluent in Spanish, English, and Kekchi. A Creole bush doctor I interviewed is fluent in both Spanish and English. All Garifuna bush doctors are speakers of English and most are also fluent in Spanish. One Garifuna healer was fluent in Garifuna, English, Spanish, Mopan, and Kekchi and served patients from each of these sections. Language is rarely a barrier to seeking care from healers. Language was, however, a frequent and serious barrier to effective transactions between biomedical personnel and patients or potential patients.

The District Medical Officer in charge when I first arrived was fluent in Spanish but spoke poor English. The second understood only English among the several languages his patients spoke. The replacement for the second who served the District for several months spoke almost no English at all. This led to frequent communicative failures. A two-year old Garifuna girl was brought to the hospital by her grandmother. The grandmother was distraught by the time she reached the hospital for the child had died in her arms as she walked. The physician looked briefly at the child, still held by the grandmother, and said something in Spanish. An American who worked at the hospital supplied her own translation: "Oh, you're saying her problem was that she had no mother" (an assumption based on a rather negative attitude held by many Americans of the Garinagu), a statement, of course, heard by the grandmother. "Si", replied the doctor, who clearly had not understood her translation. His comment, however, had been to the effect that when he had seen the child in the outpatient clinic she had been only a "little sick." One can only marvel that a cure might be effected in a context in which the patient may speak only Kekchi, the nurse only English, and the physician only Spanish!

Individual healers within ethnic sections are largely autonomous and incorporate skills, materiel, insights, and understandings into their therapeutic practices not necessarily possessed by others, even within their own sections. Flexibility and adaptability are essential traits of the healer in southern Belize and each responds in his or her own manner to changing conditions.

Healers within Punta Gorda are always identified with a particular ethnic section and they are believed to have acquired the skills and understandings of cause-effect relationships specific to that section. For that reason, their clients are most often members of that section as well. But individuals within one ethnic section believe that the healers of other sections may have access to materiel and models unknown to or unused by the healers of their own group. These healers possess methods for generating and interpreting signs not available within every section or to every practitioner.

Though each ethnomedical therapeutic system exhibits the characteristic of adaptability and healers are autonomous and independent entrepreneurs capable of altering the shape and style of health care delivery, social, cultural, and technological constraints impose a basic and more inflexible contour upon system and practice. Each healer serves as a "moral agent" (Kramer and Thomas 1982:189), a reservoir of moral precepts, the perpetuator of social and cultural convictions held by the group as a whole or dominant subgroups within an ethnic section. Whatever his or her diagnostic techniques and therapeutic methods, the range of interpretations generated is constrained by this specific characteristic of the healer's role.

There are, as well, important political constraints which affect both the availability of interpretive models and access to therapeutic resources. By the term political I mean here the macrostructure evident at the national level which permits for the collection, transformation, and distribution of resources and which exists separate from the sociopolitical structures of ethnic sections and communities. Examples of the impact of this political macrostructure on the health-seeking decisions of citizens of Punta Gorda and the therapy-rendering behaviors of healers are not difficult to find. Role legitimacy is denied by the state to unlicensed midwives and to bush doctors; no mechanism for distribution of resources to non-biomedical healers exists. Licensed midwives are prohibited from delivering babies outside the hospital setting if they are also employed by the hospital, thus forcing most women to give birth in the hospital. Medicines and supplies sent from a missionary group in the States to the American lab technician who, in turn, distributed these supplies to nurses in the villages of San Antonio and Crique Sarco were, as she had predicted, confiscated and turned over to the local District Medical Officer. The British Army physician ended his attendance at the clinic in San Antonio as the Belizean government altered its policy on delivery of health care by non-government personnel. The American Peace Corps nurse found herself in disagreement on several occasions with one or more of the District Medical Officers to whom she was subordinate.

Technological constraints are also imposed on the interpretive and therapeutic process. No single medical model allows for the production and evaluation of all the signs which would indicate illness and permit a diagnosis or determination of an etiology. In general, however, ethnomedical models incorporate the methods and the means for the generation and observation of signs which lead to diagnoses/etiologies consistent with that model's ideological system. This is an important point, too often overlooked in examining competition and conflict between biomedicine and other medical resources in third world countries. Ethnomedical models not only provide culturally appropriate explanations for all illness signs, but they provide the methods whereby additional signs necessary to a successful interpretation can be generated. Biomedicine often fails in that regard. It must admit diagnostic failures, occasions on which the existing technology and the interpretive paradigms are inadequate for the generation and transformation of all signs. Mr. Cowo's family complained because the tests failed to show the cause of his illness. He was removed from the hospital setting and taken to a bush doctor who provided a contextually appropriate and meaningful diagnosis and had both the materiel and the means to generate such an explanation. That Mr. Cowo died is inconsequential to the success of the basic diagnostic paradigm which was employed. Mr. Valdez believed his problem might have been caused by *obeah*. Biomedicine possesses no technology for the determination of such an object. Hence, Mr. Valdez planned to seek affirmation of his assumptions from another health care provider. It is clear, on the other hand, that state medicine succeeds in the generation of signs which cannot be produced or evaluated by ethnomedical systems.

If, as one elderly man put it, the hospital is regarded as a place "where you go to die" and interethnic health care transactions are facilitated by a variety of factors, why do individuals continue to utilize the hospital clinic, agree to admission to the hospital, and pay a substantial fee to see the doctor privately? The most obvious response is that biomedicine often "works." It effects the desired results, especially in cases of acute infectious diseases. Further, state biomedical personnel exert control over information, diagnostic technologies and techniques, and therapies not accessible to other groups. An afflicted individual, seeking relief from the signs and symptoms of a distressed state, views state medicine as one additional therapeutic system in a range of alternatives. He adjusts, to the extent he has the skills to do so, his strategies for exploitation of any given resource. The physician, overworked and undersupplied, a stranger in this community, has far less need to 'succeed' in this diaglogue. The knowledgeable patient will develop techniques to overcome this asymmetry. However, few patients in Punta Gorda have the information necessary to this resolution. In transactions with state biomedical staff, the following set of behaviors and expectations inhibit the discourse:

1. Patients do not automatically report all signs and symptoms.
2. It is expected that the physician will have his own techniques for

generating signs. If the physician fails to ask the appropriate questions, patients may never report specific signs. In addition, they will frequently leave out important events in the etiological chain, and they will most likely, in describing their illness, remove the illness experience from the social context in which it occurred. Many persons expressed distress at the fact that the physician had neither questioned them sufficiently, examined them thoroughly, nor provided them with a diagnosis or a prognosis. Yet in a situation in which patient and physician are clearly distinguished in terms of class, status, and role, and most commonly, ethnic group membership as well, the zero sign (Barthes 1972) comes to dominate and no additional communication occurs.

3. Patients very rarely gather information which will substantially affect their understanding of their disorder from a biomedicial perspective.

4. When information is presented or acquired, it is frequently reinterpreted to conform to more 'accessible' models and a preferred prognosis.

The trend toward increasing intersectional or interethnic transactions aimed at the maintenance of or return to health both facilitates the articulation or merging of codes and is a direct result of such processes. But, for a variety of reasons, the codes required by the patient drawn into the biomedical system in Belize are generally not made available to him. He is most often unable to gain access to the communicative code or interpretive models utilized by the physician. Under such circumstances, there emerge several possibilities for the patient; that is, there exist several communicative and exploitative strategies. One of these strategies is the presentation of a partial list of signs which are known to be acceptable to the physician. As each group gains experience in dealing with state biomedical practitioners, they become more efficient at presenting the signs which they believe to be of importance to the physician; the others, signs and events not recognized or accorded significance by the physician, are reserved for the members of the therapy managing group, close friends, family members, and healers.

Where common understandings exist or where certain elements of a medical model are shared, these may be exploited by both sides. Expressing concepts in a more familiar idiom (*code switching*) is also a common practice, both for physician and patient. Biomedical practitioners frequently find it convenient to speak "in terms understandable to the patient", that is, to utilize the patient's code or portions of it in explaining illness or suggesting therapeutic interventions. For example, Mr. Arzu's wife was told that her husband had a "sickness" which had "gone to his brain"; Elias Pratt's mother was told that young Elias' illness might be "in the blood." As we have seen, such attempts may yield little useful information, or, as in the Pratt case, lead to additional misunderstandings. Blood samples, Elias' mother believed, were taken to "draw off the illness." A Mayan man explains that his small daughter has "fever", a term which is acceptable to the physician though the set of signs which are indicated by the term "fever" is different for the two major participants in this transaction.

In Belize, efficient exploiters of the biomedical system had learned to use the terms and concepts acceptable to the physician even while lacking an understanding of the models from which they were derived. This also meant that the physician was presented with an incomplete list of all signs which could have been offered. Efficient exploiters of the biomedical system also tended to use intermediaries or "brokers" who were assumed to be sympathetic to the patient's case while able to communicate effectively with biomedical personnel. For example, Viola asked me to obtain antibiotics from the Army camp for her. The Pratt family requested that I get the records on Elias' case from the Belize City hospital. Within the hospital setting, Garifuna patients most commonly turn to Garifuna aides or nurses to gather information or to make a request even though these individuals may themselves have to pass on the request to others.

But biomedicine's codes are often intractable, barely open to exploitation or co-optation. Another communicative strategy exists and it predominates in transactions between the physician and patient in Punta Gorda. I can only refer to this approach as the *strategy of silence* for it involves both verbal and kinesic silence. Perhaps Barths would have used here the term *zero sign.* The absence of the sign is itself full of significance. In this mode of communication, two or more distinct codes or models are left to stand – those of the physician and those of the patient and his or her larger social group. Neither set of interpretations is challenged. Therefore, neither therapist nor patient finds his code in conflict with that of the other. The patient selects and presents his symptoms. The physician may, but very often does not, ask questions. Questions, in any case, generally shed little light on the patient's condition from the patient's perspective, for he has no understanding of the model on which they were predicated. Quite frequently no part of the patient's body is touched. His temperature and blood pressure have been recorded by nurses or their aides and this may constitute the only physical contact between personnel and patient. The patient may utter no sound when examined. A treatment may be prescribed, but the patient is rarely advised as to the full nature of the treatment and almost never as to the reasons for the treatment. Nor, in turn, does the patient ask these questions. Only infrequently is his condition given a name. He is simply handed a prescription to be filled, told to return for a certain number of days for injections, or ordered to present himself to the nurses for admission to the hospital. This strategy allows the physician to make an interpretation which is not communicated to the patient, the family, or to the social group. It also allows for interpretive 'failures', that is, the inability of the physician to produce a diagnosis, to occur without comment. Both patient and physician are allowed the freedom to construct an interpretation according to a given model or models without challenge to the judgment, rationality, and competence of the other. Each preserves some degree of freedom that might have been yielded in a true dialogue. For example, the failure of the physician to explain to Mr. Sho the nature of diabetes allowed Mr. Sho to pursue a cure since his understanding was that the illness "was only in my urine." The strategy of silence does not inhibit further negotiation between patient and social group nor between the afflicted individual and other therapists.

Bases for Transactions Across Ethnic Boundaries

Beyond a need shared by patients and healers in all ethnic sections to generate effective therapies, what bases exist for transactions across ethnic and lay/professional boundaries and what strategies are employed to control the communicative process?

In fact, the techniques for establishing both etiology and diagnosis are similar if not identical across all groups, though the physical and social boundaries of the areas which may be explored vary considerably. The "diagnostic approach" presented below is taken from a standard biomedical text on diagnosis and treatment. It outlines the method for determining the appropriate assignment of a single subjective sign – dizziness. It describes, in broad outline, the same process which healers, diviners, and physicians use everywhere to properly label illness signs, though the diagnostic/etiologic categories generated differ.

Though the model here involves the production and interpretation of subjective signs alone, practitioners in all groups utilize both subjective and objective signs. The biomedical approach, however, tends to restrict the generation of signs to those which are produced by and about the body.

In some cases, an attenuated diagnostic approach is thought to indicate the skill of the diagnostician. Mr. Valdez, for example, stated that healers in Guatemala could instantly diagnose *obeah*. This does not imply that the diagnostic process has been ignored, but rather that the signs utilized to produce an etiology and diagnosis are "visible" to these highly skilled practitioners while they remain "invisible" to others. The *hiúruha* of the Garifuna *búiai* often possess knowledge about etiology unknown to either the 'victim' or to healers and physicians, and the diagnostic process may be abbreviated in the sense that the usual question and response pattern may be unnecessary.

It is likely this belief that all healers, including biomedically trained physicians, share in this special ability to generate and interpret signs, to make "visible" that which is "invisible" (Foucault 1972) that leads many

DIAGNOSTIC MODEL

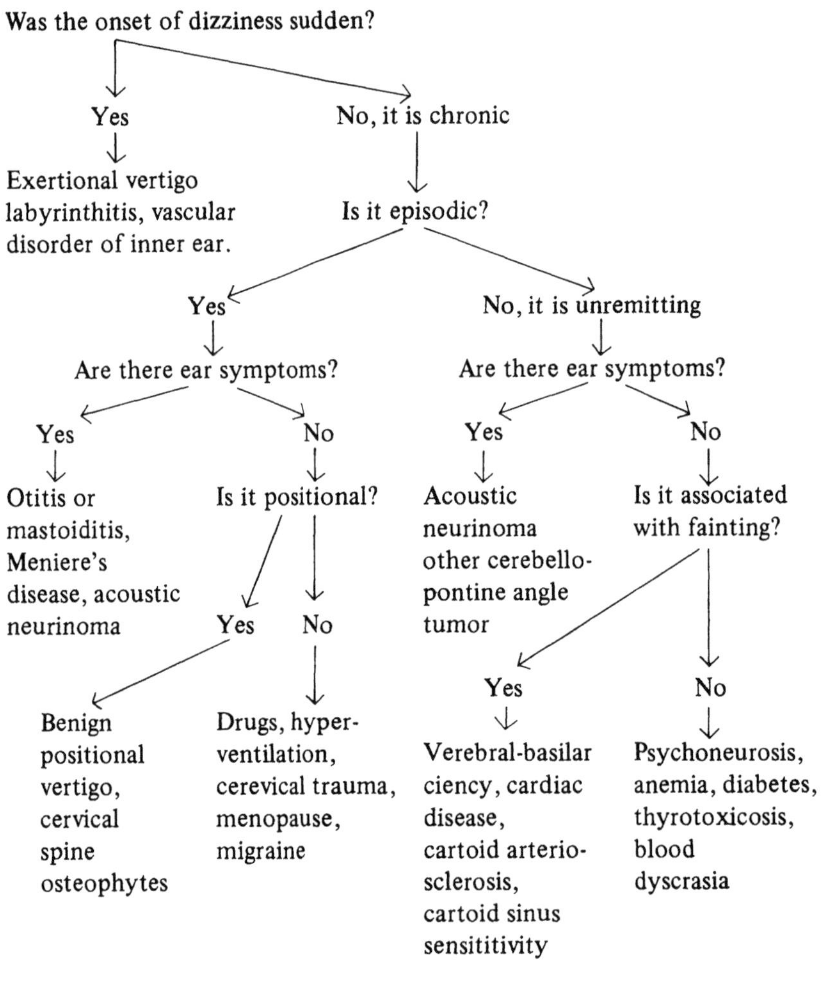

From: Current Medical Diagnosis and Treatment 1981 Marcus Krupp and Milton Chatton, eds). Los Altos, Calif.: Lange Medical Publications, p. 567.

patients or therapy managers to fail to describe all the signs the biomedical practitioner regards as essential to the diagnostic process.

The biomedical diagnostician may produce an explanation which identifies a *biological* object, as, for example, the District Medical Officer did in Mr. Arzu's case (a "stroke"), but because of the infinite regressive character of the sign, an earlier 'cause' may be sought by the healer, the patient, or the therapy managing group as well. This prior object may be determined to be physiological or anatomical (for example, high blood pressure), or the object may be judged to be *social* in nature (e.g., poor relations with one's fellow man). Biomedical personnel generally fail to understand that these seemingly contradictory diagnostic/etiologic labels represent the fulfillment of the sign process – to the extent any sign is ever complete – as Evans-Pritchard pointed out nearly half a century ago.

The Toledo's ethnic groups have had contact with one another long enough to have developed networks for the exchange of information. As intersectional transactions increase there is increasing motivation for the *articulation of codes* governing concepts of causation and therapy. Articulation of codes is a process whereby similarties in codes (a *co-incidence of codes*) are emphasized. The understanding of blood as a source of illness as well as a source of signs and as a substance which permits therapeutic intervention (see below) is an example of such an articulation. So, too, is the "semantic shift" (Kay 1979) made in applying the term *obeah* to all ethnically derived beliefs in man-caused illness or misfortune. In addition, the transfer of information which now occurs with increasing frequency has led, in some instances, to an identity or uniformity of codes. That is, as time passes, there is a growing tendency to merge or adapt codes so that they become indistinguishable from one another. The system of lay medicine to which I have referred appears to have its basis in both processes. But the development of uniform or partially articulated codes or models does not necessarily lead to the creation of a single 'system' of ethnomedicine which will be espoused by all ethnic groups, for the maintenance of a variety of diagnostic and therapeutic options will continue as an important strategy.

There is a clear tendency to seek traditional therapies without crossing ethnic boundaries. One major reason for the persistence of such behaviors is the accessibility of the interpretive model; that is, patient and healer share certain assumptions concerning the nature of illness and the range of appropriate therapies. However, if a patient and/or his/her therapy managing group wish to avoid the labeling of certain signs with significations which reflect negatively on the moral or social behavior and motivations of patient or group, then the likelihood that other interpretive models will be used is significantly increased.

There are broad areas of agreement among the five major ethnic groups in the southern Toledo (Garifuna, Creole, Spanish, Maya, and East Indian) which provide the basis for mutual understanding and communication. No two groups hold all beliefs in common, though each shares some beliefs with each of the others. The discussion which follows focuses on the similarities among models rather than the differences which still distinguish one group from another.

1. Illness may be either natural or unnatural in origin, although almost every illness is, at least initially, assumed to be natural. Unnatural illnesses are the result of the work of man (*obeah*, *idáhadu*), or of evil spirits, ancestral spirits, or ghosts. A belief in the efficacy of *obeah* is ubiquitous and binds, in one sense, all ethnic groups. Unnatural illnesses cannot be effectively treated by a physician, though "doctor" medicine may temporarily relieve some of the symptoms. *Obeah* can be diagnosed and treated by some but not all bush doctors. *Obeah* can be turned back on the perpetrator. The more powerful of the bush doctors are sometimes thought to be knowledgeable in both bad and good medicines and, therefore, may be both feared and respected.

2. Physicians can sometimes treat illnesses more effectively than can bush doctors, but bush doctors are believed to excell in the treatment of many disorders. Healers also 'specialize' and there are recognized distinctions among healers in terms of their skills and therapies. Many illnesses which cannot be cured by the physician (e.g., asthma, diabetes, and cancer) are reported to have been successfully treated by traditional therapists.

3. Individual symptoms, rather than a cluster of symptoms organized into a syndrome, are very often the focus of attention and each symptom may be regarded as indicative of a separate disease process. For example, an individual reporting symptoms to the diagnostician may state that he has fever, cough, and fresh cold (sneezing, runny nose) rather than to imply that these three necessarily constitute elements of a single disease by labeling them with a single designatum.

4. The terms germ, virus, and bacteria have not entered the lay language of illness and they are not incorporated into any theory of disease. Nor is any concept of contagion consistent with the biomedical model. There is no understanding of the genetic basis of any illness, though there is the recognition among all groups that certain disorders "run in the family." Chronic illnesses are not well understood. No clear explanations of illnesses such as hypertension, cancer, and diabetes have yet emerged. In general, most illnesses are regarded as curable, though the appropriate cure may remain unknown or inaccessible.

5. Many, if not most, illnesses are thought to be the result of some sort of imbalance. Imbalance in the body may result from improper diet, from physical stress, or from exposure to environmental stimuli antagonistic to

the body in its state at that point in time. An 'imbalance' in relations with one's ancestors, with other spirits, and with one's fellow man may also result in illness.

6. Some illnesses have mechanistic causes – pressures may be exerted externally or internally upon organs, an infant's fontanelle may fall from excessive sucking, the heart may be under strain because the blood is too thin, and so on.

7. Every group recognizes the following as causes of illness or disorder: the contrast of heat and cold in the body, strain or overwork, worry, seasonal changes in environmental conditions, contagion (without a biomedical basis), female sexuality, ghosts or ancestral spirits, and *obeah*. All groups believe that emotional stress (worry, vexation) causes or influences illness states. Most believe that the mind and body interact to produce alterations in physical and emotional states. While the belief exists among the Maya that worries can lead to sickness, there seems to be less emphasis than evidenced among the other ethnic sections. Physical stress, most commonly attributed to overwork, is regarded as the cause of a variety of physical disorders.

8. Each group believes the newborn to be susceptible to illness. Infants may be born with disorders but there is no understanding of the genetic basis of any illness. Many lump "inborn", "familial", or inherited illnesses with disorders which are said to result from actions or events in the life of the mother prior to the birth of the infant.

9. Discussions of illness almost never reference the aging process. There are few illnesses which are believed to be the illnesses of advancing age.

10. The body may accumulate various 'toxic' substances. This may occur as the result of drinking, improper diet, or prior illness. These substances generally accumulate in the blood or liver. Health may be maintained or restored by "cleaning" out the body. This is most commonly done with purges or herbal teas made from "bitters."

11. Blood is the source of much sickness and careful attention must be paid to it. It can overnourished, too thick, too thin, or depleted of important elements.

12. "Cold" may enter different parts of the body, including the blood, abdomen, womb, brain, and so forth. "Cold" may refer either to the accumulation of "mucus" or analogous body fluids or to a change in temperature. Garifuna men and women may refer to the signs of veneral disease as a "cold in the private parts", the discharge seen as analogus to the mucosal secretions of a cold.

13. Diet and climatic or other environmental conditions are important determinants of health and illness and must be closely watched. Few individuals hold notions of nutrition similar to those evolving out of biomedicine's understanding of biochemistry or to "modern" notions of nutrition currently

popular in the States. Proper diet is critical to the maintenance of health for at least four of the five major ethnic groups. Maya, while apparently de-emphasizing the importance of diet, are careful to avoid taking cold liquids when their bodies are in a certain state. It is important to avoid exposure to cold when one's body (or blood) is hot and vice versa, or to bathe in cool or cold water while still perspiring.

14. Every group utilizes preventive therapies or behaviors. The use of purges and tonics, the avoidance of physical stress to the degree possible, a reasonable level of sobriety, and the maintenance of appropriate and respectful relations with deceased ancestors, other spiritual beings, and one's neighbors and community members assist individuals in maintaining health and preventing illness.

15. Herbs, roots, and other such materials are the natural source of medicine. All ethnic groups utilize these extensively, though most Maya appear not to be knowledgeable about "bush." Responsibility for knowledge of bush lies with the Mayan healer or midwife. These "natural" medicines are generally regarded as superior to "doctor" medicine, with some exceptions. Many believe doctor medicines are simply the synthetic, processed, or concentrated forms of bush medicines.

16. "Pharmacy" medicines are used by almost everyone and are generally thought to be effective in the treatment of minor illnesses or in the provision of symptomatic relief. Medicines available at the local pharmacy include some of the items used in the preparation of lay or bush remedies (mansinilla, achote, cloves, romero, etc.) as well as drugs which would, in the States, require a prescription, such as tranquilizers and antibiotics. The pharmacy and most of the local grocery/dry goods stores also sell a range of proprietory preparations, such as cough syrup, cold capsules, tonics and vitamins, rubbing alcohol, worm medicine, salves, metholatum products, and products containing aspirin; these have generally been extremely popular.

17. While bush doctors most frequently prepare medicines in a form which is to be drunk, massage (known among some groups as "nointing"), bathing and manipulation of body parts are also practiced by all groups.

18. Models of body functions and the interrelation of body parts are simple. Internal functionings and distinctions among organs are not well understood. Certain organs were rarely if ever mentioned in discussions of illness (for example, pancreas, gall bladder, lungs, and intestines). There is a tendency to use a single term to refer to major portions of the anatomy. The term "stomach", for example, may be used by the Garinagu in reference to any portion of the anatomy from mid-chest to lower abdomen. "Foot" may refer to any portion of the anatomy below the knee or mid-calf.

19. The language utilized to describe illness episodes often includes references to the social context in which illness occurs. Illness represents

for every ethnic group an attack upon both the physical self and the social self – the social self is defined here as that self which emerges out of the acceptance of specific social roles and the interaction with other social beings.

20. To refer to an individuals as "crazy" is generally to make reference to specific behavioral abnormalities which would normally be considered as indicators of psychosis in the States as well. Individuals who roam the streets talking only to themselves or who cannot carry on a contextually appropriate conversation ("they talk crazy", "she always answers the opposite") are most likely to be judged insane. In other words, serious deficiencies in communication skills are the principal criteria. Occasional outbursts of violent behavior may not be considered indicative of any mental disturbance though repeated attacks on others would likely lead the community to describe the individual as "crazy." Heavy use of alcohol was not regarded as an illness. Extreme alcohol abuse which resulted in alcoholic psychosis led to the label of "crazy" in some cases, but it was not clear that the individual's behavior was necessarily associated with his drinking patterns. Marijuana use, which was becoming increasingly common among younger adults and some adolescents was considered potentially more dangerous. As one healer stated: "These days many young fellows act like they are crazy because they smoke marijuana and their brains aren't strong enough for it." Interestingly, a tea made from marijuana (called *gangi* by the East Indians) was used by some in the treatment of asthma.

An obvious case of mogoloidism was not mentioned when I interviewed family members about prior illness. Moderate to severe mental retardation was never discussed when the topic was physiological or psychological disorders. A diagnosis of "neurosis" was occasionally entered into the chart of a patient by the District Medical Officer. It would appear that the DMO used this term to refer to cases in which there seemed to be no organic basis for the patient's complaints. The DMO in residence at the time of my departure from Punta Gorda stated that neurosis was more common among the Maya because of their greater fear of *obeah*. "Neurosis" would not be recognized by the people of Punta Gorda as a disorder; the 'signs' which indicated neurosis to the physician would generally not be incorporated into any ethnomedical model of illness, excepting as such signs were interpreted as indicative of *obeah*.

An Example of the Articulation of Codes: Blood as Metaphor and Metonym

Codes governing indigenous concepts of the body are culturally derived, but in ethnically heterogeneous societies, codes must be changed or articulated for any one group or individual to obtain desired resources under the control of another group. This is as true for medical resources – technologies, skills, knowledge, materiel, drugs, facilities, roles – as for other sorts of resources. This means that individuals in heterogeneous societies may need to learn several body schemata in order to efficiently participate in and exploit the medical resources of others.

In many cases, body-parts, rather than body-systems or vague subjective signs become the convenient focus of attention (Ellen 1977). They are perceived as the source and generator of signs, or in Peirce's terminology, as the dynamic object motivating the representamen, and they may be probed, examined, or ritually evaluated in order to obtain further information (signs). Body-parts, a term used here to include both products of the body usually separable from the body, such as feces, sputum, sweat, semen, menstrual blood, etc., and various organs generally considered inseparable from the body, such as the heart, brain, blood (under most conditions), etc. become body-metaphors, or, for the diagnostician/therapist, body-metonyms. They are utilized by both diagnostician and layman to talk about a variety of physiological and nonphysiological concerns.

In the ethnically heterogeneous situation which existed in the town of Punta Gorda, blood became a convenient body symbol, a metonymic and metaphoric device, whereby various ethnic/professional codes could be articulated. There were, however, important distinctions between the biomedical view and the lay conception of blood. Blood was perceived by almost everyone in the community not as the *source* of signs of health/illness states exclusively (the general biomedical concept) but rather as the source of the state or illness itself, a view seemingly held by all ethnic groups and intentionally or unintentionally perpetuated by biomedical personnel. Thus therapies performed directly on the blood were regarded as most effective (see Pratt case study).

The belief that blood could become "bad" or unclean" was ubiquitious. Concepts concerning the release of bad blood as a therapy existed among at least three major ethnic groups – the Garinagu, Creoles, and Maya – I did not determine whether this represented an attempt at articulation of codes and the adjustment of various ethnically/culturally derived body schemata to the necessity of interethnic transactions or the previous existence of parallel beliefs.

Weak blood was perceived by many as a possible consequence of certain disease states, but it was more commonly regarded as the cause of illness. Weak blood left one susceptible to a variety of problems, including heart trouble, trembling, fits, weakness, shortness of breath, and attack by ghosts. The Garifuna phrase *heratina nitau* expresses the idea that one's blood (*híitau*) is strong. *Meratina nitau* (literally, my blood is sick), is generally believed to result from improper nourishment. *Matatina nitau* (literally, I have no blood) indicates a belief in the lack of sufficient quantities of blood. *Duna nitau* (literally, my blood is water) was said by one informant to occur in cases of malaria. Tonics and certain roots and herbs, generically known as "bitters" (Jackass Bitters, Contrebo, Sorocee, Billy Web bark, etc.) could be used to "build" the blood, but it was often believed to be necessary to "cleanse" the blood prior to this with herbal purges. *Achote* could be used to remove biliousness from the blood. Dirty blood manifested itself as sores or boils; "heat" in the blood might cause the same signs, the lesions allowing the release of heat from the body. Measles were also said to appear because of "heat" in the blood. In one case of possible *leishmaniasis* which had not responded to biomedical treatment, a Garifuna bush doctor suggested to me that the man's blood was bad and had to be "replaced", a process which he said required the use of two bush medicines simultaneously.

To "build" the blood was equivalent to increasing its volume in many cases. Therefore, to overdose with bitters could cause an excess of blood which could, in turn, result in high blood pressure or nosebleeds. Some suggested that high blood pressure was caused by blood that was too thick. Viola stated that "the pressure" which "catches" her periodically resulted from over-nourishment of the blood. Consequently her diet much of the time consisted of nothing more than tea and tortillas since most other foods were considered too strong for the blood. Locals often expressed the idea that high blood pressure (*inuiti hítau* in Garifuna, literally, high blood) came with "civilization" and was unknown in the past. A Creole bush doctor told me that too much cold in the blood could lead to thick blood which, in turn, swells the veins. Swollen veins, he stated, could burst, causing a stroke.

Several individuals indicated a belief that improper circulation of the blood could cause a variety of problems. Improper circulation might result from thick blood or thin blood, or it might be due to a failure of the heart to pump the blood properly. Because water and blood are of approximately the same consistency, medicines made by boiling "bush" and drinking the water were said by one East Indian bush doctor to be most effective since the water could "penetrate" the blood as tablets could not. Cancer was thought by some to be as a poison affecting the blood. It could be treated with a plant known as the "cancer bush" which was said to purify the blood. Another East Indian and Miskito Indian bush doctor, widely renowned for his treatment of snakebite, had reached a similar conclusion. Believing cancer to be an analog of the poison released by the snake, he had experimented with the same medicines used in the treatment of snakebite on persons who had been told they had cancer. The cause of death in snakebite, this healer reported, was the growth of a large blood clot around the heart. Unless this clot could be "broken up" and vomited out, the victim stood no chance of recovering. A Creole bush doctor suggested that the release of blood from a bruise could prevent the later occurrence of cancer.

The East Indian healer referred to on several occasions previously, used a variant of penicillin in some of his treatments, insisting that "regular" penicillin was too strong for the blood of his anemic patients (diagnosed through a complaint of weakness) and a "weaker" form of penicillin was more appropriate. The same man treated diabetes with roots which "drove the extra sugar from the blood" through sweat and urine. Patients with diabetes were told to avoid salt (but not sugar) because salt thickened the blood, rendering the medication less effective. Failure to respond to therapy indicated to the therapist the patient must have eaten outside his own home and had consumed salt.

"Blood" also functioned as a convenient metaphoric device in explaining interpersonal relationships. Viola claimed I was drawn to her in her moments of crisis because we "shared blood." She eventually came to refer to me as "mama." A Garifuna bush doctor suggested to a disheartened friend that the reason for his wife's infidelity was to be found in the fact that their bloods "no longer matched."

This use of a single body component to discuss a variety of illness states thus minimized communicational barriers, facilitated 'understanding' and provided a single lexical item around which could be grouped many concerns not restricted to alterations in the physiological self.

Class, Ethnicity, and Health-Seeking Behaviors

Within the town of Punta Gorda there is a partial coincidence of class membership and ethnic section affiliation; yet ethnicity alone does not serve to structure most relationships. It is, nevertheless, a factor in the success of exploitative strategies and in the accessibility of or control over medical resources. No single ethnic section has exclusive rights to state medicine and the models and networks and political linkages upon which it is predicated, though, overall, members of some are more effective in accessing or manipulating the paradigms and structural relationships utilized or evolved by the state.

When alternative medical models are available for exploitation, class, and status are partial determinants of the choice of paradigm or resource. This is not to deny the complex interweaving of class and ethnicity in Punta Gorda, but to state again that a variety of factors, only one of which is ethnic group membership, affect health and illness care decisions. Roberto Ramirez' choice of resources and his final etiologic conclusions which he supported with the statement of a biomedical practitioner, were likely affected by his identification as one of Punta Gorda's elite. The exclusive utilization of biomedicine may function as a marker of status, or is assumed by some to function in this manner. As a member, even if marginally, of the town's elite, Roberto was constrained in his actions by certain community expectations. The elite were frequent users and strong advocates of biomedicine, though not always state medicine. They often traveled to Belize City or Guatemala, as Roberto did, in the search for better care which was also deemed to be socially appropriate. Few among the elite made much use of bush medicine, though there were a number of popular remedies in use and pharmacy medicines were often employed. Roberto sought help locally from state biomedical staff, but was disappointed; however, he was able to mobilize the fiscal resources necessary to his continued exploitation of biomedicine's diverse resources and his proffered image as a competent father.

It might be assumed that class distinctions prohibited Roberto from seeking care from a member of a lower ranking section. While this may have been a factor in determining Roberto's health-seeking behaviors, it does not always inhibit other members of Punta Gorda's elite from utilizing resources often identified with other ethnic sections, most of which are regarded as subordinate. The elite, as a group, seem to have evolved a set of medical practices and beliefs which is highly syncretistic, but there seems little question that the movement of women and other goods has also meant the sharing of components of medical models. Several women from this group were participants in and major supporters of the cult of Esquipulas. As least some, especially among the younger generation, believed in the efficacy of *obeah*. In fact, their economic and social position is assumed to make them especially susceptible to *obeah*. One young man was said to have sought protection against *obeah* from a Garifuna bush doctor because he felt he had many potential enemies. Another blamed his occasionally erratic behavior on *obeah* used against him by a former girl friend.

Summary

For most of the fifty or so years which constitute the history of medical ethnography, researchers have described indigenous medical systems which were, or appeared to be, largely unaffected by contact with other socio-medical systems. Even in those instances in which previous contact and integration or assimilation were acknowledged, the medical beliefs and practices of the society under examination were treated as coherent, well-integrated, and effectively isolated. While ethnographers recognized that the individual sign might have multiple referents, even within a single indigenous system, therapeutic intervention was generally believed to follow from the assignment of a diagnostic label. That is, there were seen to be a limited set of options in terms of health-seeking behaviors and this set was defined by the parameters of the total cultural system. The cognitive categories which accounted for relationships among etiology, diagnosis, prognosis, and therapy were said to be logically related and the medical "system" was considered interdependent with the economic, political, religious, and social systems. Intra-cultural variations, to the extent such existed or were acknowledged to exist, were considered inconsequential or ignored altogether.

More recently, however, ethnographers have turned to an examination of the complexities introduced into medical systems by contact with other peoples or societies, whether that contact be exclusively with the cognitive assumptions and therapeutic interventions of biomedicine or with those of other "traditional" sociomedical systems. They have begun to look carefully at a variety of phenomena, including the processes of conflict, competition, subordination, incorporation, integration, interaction, and accommodation. As the recognition grows that no medical system exists in isolation, the subjects of alternative coping strategies, changing medical paradigms, patterns or hierachies of resort, legitimation of "traditional" therapists, and so on have emerged as significant issues, with the focus on the effects of multiple or alternative therapeutic systems on the health seeking behaviors of a given population or populations (Beals 1977; Boswell 1969; Buxton 1973; Chrisman 1977; Cobb 1976, 1977; Dominick 1981MS; Fabrega 1974, 1977; Feierman 1981; Foster and Anderson 1978; Frakenberg and Leeson 1976; Greenwood 1981; Hessler et al 1975; Jansen 1973; Janzen 1974, 1978a, 1978b; Kimani 1981; Kleinman 1980; Kleinman, Eisenberg and Good 1978; Leslie 1977a, 1977b; Lieberman and Dressler 1977; Lin et al 1978; Locker 1981; Mahaniah 1981; Nichter 1978; Paul 1955; Press 1978, 1980; Reid 1982; Romanucci-Ross (Schwartz) 1977; Staiano 1981; Sussman 1981; Tuwumasi 1979; Woods 1977).

There are considerable advantages to the continuation of several systems of causality and therapy in the village of Punta Gorda. From the patient's point of view, the potential for negotiation, for re-evaluation of signs and their meanings, and for a realignment of signs into different syndromes (etiologic or diagnostic shifting) increases the likelihood of exploiting a resource which will be perceived as effective in the treatment of illness. This means, in turn, that the patient and his therapy managing group gain increasing control over the course of therapy. Some patients avoid being drawn into the biomedical system because they feel loss of control over their options, especially if hospitalization occurs. At the same time, the possibility that a healer may determine that an ancestor is seeking placation through an expensive ceremony may cause some to seek help first at the local clinic in order to avoid or delay a morally and financially burdensome obligation.

The existence of several therapeutic/interpretive systems allows for the maintenance of esoteric specialities, even while code-switching, the articulation of codes, and the development of some degree of conformity in codes allows for increasing communication among ethnic groups already forced into transactions of a political, social, and economic nature. The continuation of ethnic specific therapeutic roles, and, therefore, of ethnic specific therapies, such as that provided by the *búiai*, allows for the rentention of psychologically important boundary markers. Participation in the *dugu* and *chugu* are distinctive signs of ethnic identity not likely to disappear in the near future.

Health-seeking behaviors, as illustrated by the case studies, have been changed by the addition of financially and geographically accessible alternatives to traditional therapeutic resources. While a few individuals claim that they have never utilized the local clinic, the vast majority of the citizens of Punta Gorda have sought help from the providers of state controlled biomedicine. There is, at the same time, a growing "lay" therapeutic system which incorporates elements from many models, including, to a limited extent, that of biomedicine. This 'system' is largely independent of and immune to the intervention of professionals and allows for and results from increased interethnic transactions. But increasing intersectional transactions among members of various ethnic groups have also resulted in the utilization of traditional models of illness which are outside the confines of the ethnic specific model of the patient.

Interethnic transactions and the confrontation with biomedicine have impacted each ethnic section differently. Garifuna medical beliefs and practices, which have been the major focus of this study, have been altered, but the broad parameters of the model as reflected in the four domains of cause-effect relationships have not been significantly affected. The key to the survival of the interpretive paradigm lies in its flexibility and adaptability.

In comparing the data generated in this study and that of Coehlo and Taylor from the 1940s and 1950s, it appears that an increasing number of illnesses are being moved from the domains which incoporate "uncommon" (*wamálisian*) illnesses to those which incorporate "common" illnesses. There are at least three possible explanations for these changes:

1. The success of certain biomedical therapies has often meant the quick and positive resolution of acute illnesses which were, prior to the introduction of antibiotics and methods of rehydration, frequently fatal. The rapid course of these illnesses and their indiscriminate assault on individuals from all age groups most likely required explanations which referenced spirits or the immoral intentions of other members of the social collectivity.

2. With the increasing exposure of Garifuna people to American and British beliefs and practices which have their primary basis in biomedical explanations of illness causation, there has been a move away from the

'traditional' explanatory models towards the acceptance of biomedical and "westernized" explanations.

3. Finally, uncommon illnesses are often attributed to human intervention in the affairs of others. With the development of state and local institutions for control and regulation of a limited range of behaviors, the need for recourse to the supernatural has diminished.

While acute illnesses have been lessened by preventive medicine – for example, immunizations – and their impact made less severe through the introduction of antibiotics, chronic illnesses can be expected to increase as the life expectancy of the average citizen increases. State biomedicine cannot deal with these failures of the human organism as effectively as it can with the invasion of bacteria, particularly in a nation in which diagnostic equipment and treatment facilities are limited. This may be expected to result in an increased utilization of those medical models which best explain such conditions, regardless of the effectiveness of the therapies which are produced by these models.

There are, as I stated in the introductory chapter, psychosomatic components to all illnesses and this seems particularly true of the long-term and non-resolvable sequences of illness signs which are typical of chronic illnesses. Traditional models of illness causation have historically generated satisfying explanations, and ethnic specific therapies successfully treat the psychosomatic elements of such illnesses, while therapies are often expanded to include the social collectivity as well. The "self" which is affected during the course of an illness is a social self which requires therapeutic interventions solidly based in culturally generated models.

The signs of illness and illness as a sign, as a communicative device, are polysemic, overdetermined. That is, they have several interpretants. Any exposition of a system of causality which imputes one meaning or interpretation to a sign or series of signs ignores the contextual variables and the multidimensional nature of the sign. This is especially evident in the case of pluralistic medical systems in which alternative interpretations are available.

Attempts to establish a taxonomy of Garifuna (or other) disease terms based on ethnosemantic eliciting techniques would have been frustrated by several conditions characteristic of pluralistic systems:

1. the recognition and employment of alternative interpretive models either simultaneously or sequentially
2. the fact that newly recognized or experienced illnesses (e.g., cancer) may be incorporated into a taxonomy in ways not fully consistent with the original principles of cataegorization;
3. the exploitation of the greater range of 'disease' or illness types to suit the needs of the patient, the social group, or the therapist.

Categories or domains of cause-effect relationships constitute a set of possibilities, exploitable according to context. The signs or symptoms that the patient (and the social group) exhibit may be referred to one syndrome or category of illness rather than another depending on the total social, cultural, historical, and political context in which the signs are manifested and the understandings of cause-effect relationships held by the healer consulted. The *object* which provoked the occurrence of the *representamen* may have little or no relation in physiological or absolute terms to the *interpretant* to which it is linked, nor to the therapeutic action which follows.

In all social systems, the conceptualization of the disease process or of bodily functions is linked to a variety of natural and supernatural phenomena. There is assumed to be a cultural code which links etiology and therapy to social, moral, religious, and political systems, This interrelationship of systems is an *a priori* of the anthropological discipline and it is the tendency or drive toward consistency that leads us to speak of medical "systems." Intracultural diversity has considerably complicated the decisions that anthropologists must make in the reporting and analysis of data; to present coherent and internally consistent models means to ignore some of that diversity. However, diversity within systems is as much a characteristic of certain systems as are the patterns or regularities which we attempt to identify. As I argued earlier, "systems" are often granted greater coherency than is justified by the data. The "codes" or paradigms then of which I have spoken should not be regarded as sets of rules which determine and make predictable specific responses, but a set of constraints limiting the range of interpretive and therapeutic options.

No one medical model generates the technology to produce and evaluate all signs. Where alternative models exist, each can and will be exploited in the search for a culturally, socially, and personally satisfying explanation. The tendency toward an articulation of codes and the similarity in structural position of healers in all ethnic sections makes movement across ethnic boundaries to exploit the interpretations and technologies of another group or a specific healer a relatively simple process. The case studies present what initially seems to be an almost random selection of therapeutic behaviors in the often desperate search for a resolution. Closer examination, however, reveals that the choice of therapy usually depends on the degree of accessibility of the "system" or resource. Accessibility must be defined not in terms of physical and financial access alone, but in terms of the communicative models and cultural assumptions employed by the healer and the afflicted person. The more important distinctions, in this sense, are not between biomedicine and bush or ethnomedicine or some other healing resource, but distinctions between resources defined by accessibility to both the interpretive models and the therapeutic means of healing.

The healer, now, as in the past, produces knowledge, but he does so in accordance with the broad constraints placed upon him by his personal acceptance of the ethnically derived symbols which define his role and justify structural relationships within and among ethnic collectivities or sections. The healer's ownership of specific therapeutic resources results from the evolution of ethnic strategies developed to produce signs, i.e., information, about the body which were in conformity with overall moral and social values, as well as derived from and supportive of economic and political processes. That is to say that the production of knowledge and the production of goods are essentially governed by the same processes. With increasing competition from biomedicine and other medical models, including those controlled by sacred specialists, Garifuna healers have developed strategies to exploit new or more specific econoiches, but they continue to provide therapies which are more appropriate to the personal and social context in which illnesses occur. Just as Garifuna people have never allowed any group to dominante them, so too do they modify the potential power of healers through the maintenance of several therapeutic options. Though state delivered biomedicine generally functions or attempts to function by subordinating individuals to the grander medical scheme, the exploitation of biomedical therapies becomes one method whereby an additional degree of independence may be maintained.

Bibliography

Ashcraft, Norman (1973). Colonialism and Underdevelopment: Processes of Political Economic Change in British Honduras. N.Y.: Teachers College Press, Columbia University.

Bär (Baer), Eugen (1975). Semiotic Approaches to Psychotherapy. Bloomington, Ind.: Indiana Univ. Publ., Studies in Semiotics, Vol. I.

Baer, Eugen (1982MS). Medical Semiotics

Baer, Eugen (1982). The medical symptom. Amer. Jour. of Semiotics. 1(3):17-34.

Barnes, J.A. (1972). Social networks. Addison-Wesley Module in Anthropology, 26, pp. 1-29.

Barth, Fredrik (1969). Introduction. In: Ethnic Groups and Boundaries (Fredrik Barth, ed.) Boston: Little, Brown and Co., pp.9-38.

Barthes, Roland (1972). Sémiologie et médecine. Les Sciences de Folie (Roger Bastide, ed.) Paris: Mouton, pp.37-46.

Bateson, Gregory (1968). Psychiatric thinking: an epistemological approach. In: Communication: The Social Matrix of Psychiatry (J' Ruesch and G. Bateson) N.Y.: W.W. Norton, pp. 228-256.

Beals, A.R. (1977). Strategies of resort to curers in south India. In: Asian Medical Systems (C. Leslie, ed.), Berkeley: Univ. of Calif. Press, pp. 184-200.

Bennett, John (ed.) (1975). The New Ethnicity. St. Paul: West Publ. Co.

Bolland Nigel (1977). The Formation of a Colonial Society. Belize, From Conquest to Crown Colony. Baltimore, Maryland: Johns Hopkins Univ.

Bolland, Nigel (1979). Slavery in Belize. BISRA Occasional Publication 7, pp.3-37.

Boswell, D.M. (1969). Personal crises and the mobilization of the social network. In: Social Networks in Urban Situations (J.C. Mitchell, ed.) Manchester: Univ. Press, pp. 245-296.

Bouissac, Paul (1976). Circus and Culture: A Semiotic Approach. Bloomington, Indiana: Indiana Univ. Press.

Buhler, Richard O., S.J. (1976). A History of the Catholic Church in Belize. BISRA.

Bullard, Mary Kenyon (1973). The Recognition of Psychiatric Disorder in British Honduras. Unpubl. Ph. D. Diss., Univ. of Oregon

Buxton, Jean (1973). Religion and Healing in Mandari. Oxford: Clarendon Press.

Celan, Eugen and Solomon Marcus (1973). Le diagnostic comme langage, I. Cahiers de Linguistique 10: 163-173.

Chrisman, Noel (1977). The health seeking process: an approach to the natural history of illness. Culture, Medicine and Psychiatry 1: 351-377.

Cobb, Ann K. (1976). A Theory of Medical Pluralism in the United States. Unpubl. Doctoral Dissertation, Univ. of Kansas.

Cobb, Ann K. (1977). Pluralistic legitimation of an alternative therapy system: the case of chiropractic. Medical Anthropology, 1 (4):1-23.

Coehlo, Ruy Galvao Andrade (1955). The Black Carib of Honduras: A Study in Acculturation. Unpubl. Ph.D. Dissertation, Northwestern University.

Cohen, Abner (1974). Introduction: the lesson of ethnicity. In: Urban Ethnicity (Abner Cohen, ed.) N.Y.: Tavistock Publications

Comaroff, Jean (1981). Healing and cultural transformation: the Tswana of southern Africa, Social Sci., and Medicine 15B(3): 367-378.
Conzemius, Eduard (1928). Ethnographical notes on the Black Carib (Garif). American Anthropologist, n.s., 30(2): 183-205.
Copeland, Dana D. (1977). Concepts of disease and diagnosis. Perspectives in Biology and Medicine, 20:528-538.
Cosminsky, Sheila (1976MS). Medicinal plants of the Black Caribs (Garifuna). Paper presented at the International Congress of Americanists, Paris, Sept. 2-6, 1976.
Cosminsky, Sheila (1976). Birth rituals and symbolism: A Quiche Maya-Black Carib comparison. In: Ritual and Symbol in Native Central America (Philip Young and James Howe, eds.) Univ. of Oregon Anthro. Papers, No. 9.
Cosminsky, Sheila (1977). Inter-ethnic relations in a southern Belizean community. Ethnicity 4:226-245.
Coulter, Harris (1973-77). Divided Legacy: A History of the Schism in Medical Thought. 3 vols. Washington, D.C.: Wehawken Book Co.
Crookshank, F.C. (1923). The importance of a theory of signs and a critique of language in the study of medicine. The Meaning of Meaning (Ogden and Richards, eds. 1938). N.Y.: Harcourt, Brace and World, pp. 337-355.
De La Borde. (1888; orig. 1674). History of the origin, customs, religion, wars, and travels of the Caribs, savages in the Antilles in America. Translated and reprinted in Timehri, Jour. of the Royal Agricultural and Commercial Society of British Guinea. Vol. 5:224-254.
Deeley, John (1976). The doctrine of signs: taking form at last. Semiotica 18(2): 171-193.
Deeley, John (1982) Introducing Semiotic. Its History and Doctrine. Bloomington: Indiana Univ. Press.
Dobson, Narda (1973). A History of Belize. London: Longman Caribbean.
Dominick, Paul (1980). On discovering the semiotic organization of the lexicon: state of health as a multifaced domain. Proceedings of the Fifth Annual Meeting of the Semiotic Society of America. M. Herzfeld (ed.) Plenum Publ., Inc.
Dominick, Paul (1981MS). The domain of health: several views. Paper presented at the Conference on Culture and Communication, Temple Univ., Philadelphia, Penn., April, 1981.
Douglas, Mary (1971). Do dogs laugh? A cross-cultural approach to body symbolism. Jour. Psychosomatic Research 15: 387-390.
Eco, Umberto (1976) A Theory of Semiotics. Bloomington: Indiana Univ. Press.
Eisenberg, Leon (1977). Disease and illness. Culture, Medicine and Psychiatry 1(1) 9-23.
Fabrega, Horacio (1972). Medical anthropology. Biennial Review of Anthropology. Stanford: Stanford Univ. Press, pp.167-229.
Fabrega, Horacio (1974). Disease and Social Behavior. Boston: MIT Press.
Fabrega, Horacio (1977). The scope of ethnomedical science. Culture, Medicine and Psychiatry. 1: 201-228.
Fabrega, Horacio (1979). Elementary systems of medicine. Culture, Medicine and Psychiatry 3: 167-198.
Feierman, Elizabeth Karlin (1981). Alternative medical services in rural Tanzania: a physician's view. Social Science and Medicine, 15B(3): 399-404.
Foster, George and Barbara Anderson (1978). Medical Anthropology. N.Y.: John Wiley & Sons.
Foucault, M. 1965 (1961). Madness and Civilization. N.Y.: Random House
Foucault, M. 1973 (1963). The Birth of the Clinic. London: Tavistock.
Frankenberg, Ronald and Joyce Leeson (1976). Disease, illness and sickness: Social aspects of the choice of healer in a Lusaka suburb. In: Social Anthropology and Medicine (J.B. London, ed.) N.Y.: Academic Press: 223-250.
Freud, Sigmund (1926) Inhibitions, symptoms, and anxiety. In: Standard Edition.

Gonzalez (Solien) Nancie (1959). West Indian characteristics of the Black Carib. Southwestern Journal of Anthropology 15: 300-307.
Gonzalez, Nancie (1963). Patterns of diet, health and sickness in a Black Carib community. Tropical and Geographical Medicine, 15: 422-430.
Gonzalez, Nancie (1969). Black Carib Household Structure: A Study of Migration and Modernization. Seattle: Univ. of Wash. Press.
Gonzalez, Nancie (1970). *Obeah* and other witchcraft among the Black Caribs. In: Systems of North American Witchcraft and Sorcery. D. Walker (ed.) Moscow, Idaho: Univ. of Idaho Press, pp. 93-109.
Good, Byron J. (1977). The heart of what's the matter: The semantics of illness in Iran. Culture, Medicine and Psychiatry 1(1): 25-58.
Grant, C.H. (1976). The Making of Modern Belize. N.Y.: Cambridge Univ. Press.
Greenwood, Bernard (1981). Cold or spirits? Choice and ambiguity in Morocco's pluralistic medical system. Social Science and Medicine 15B, (3): 219-236.
Gregory, James R. (1972). Pioneers on a Cultural Frontier: The Mopan Maya of British Honduras. Unpubl. Ph.D. Dissertation, Univ. of Pittsburgh.
Gregory, James (1976). The modification of an interethnic boundary in Belize. Amer. Ethnologist 3(4):683-708.
Greimas, A.J. and J. Courtés (1982). Semiotics and Language: An Analytical Dictionary. Bloomington: Indiana Univ. Press.
Guiraud, Pierre (1975). Semiology. Boston: Routledge and Kegan Paul.
Gullick, C.J.M.R. (1976a). Exiled from St. Vincent: The Development of Black Carib Culture in Central America up to 1945. Malta: Progress Press.
Gullick, C.J.M.R. (1976b). Piaye and Pia Manadi. Belizean Studies 4(6):7-12.
Gullick, C.J.M.R. (1979). Ethnic interaction and Carib language. Journal of Belizean Affairs, 9: 3-20.
Hadel, Richard E. (1972). Carib Folk Songs and Carib Culture. Unpubl. Ph. D. Dissertation, Univ. of Texas
Hammond, Norman (1975). Lubaantun. Peabody Museum Monograph 2, Harvard University.
Hammond, Norman (1977). The earliest Maya. Scientific American, March, pp. 116-133.
Hannerz, Ulf. (1974). Ethnicity and opportunity in urban America. In: Urban Ethnicity (Abner Cohen, ed.). N.Y.: Tavistock Publ., 37-76.
Hawkes, Terence (1977). Structuralism and Semiotics. Berkeley, Calif.: Univ. of Calif. Press.
Hecht, L. (1880). Séméiotique. In: Deschambre's Dictionnaire Encyclopédique Des Sciences Médicales, pp. 560-573.
Helms, Mary (1975MS). Household organization in eastern Central America. A comparative study. Paper presented at the AAA meenting. San Francisco, 1975.
Hessler, Richard M., Michael Nolan, Benjamin Ogbru, and Peter Kong-Ming New. 1975. Intraethnic diversity: Health care of the Chinese-Americans. Human Organization, 34(3): 253-262.
Horton, Robin (1967). African traditional thought and Western science. Africa 37:50-72; 155-187.
Illich, Ivan (1976). Medical Nemesis. New York: Random House.
Jandar, Rudolf (1981). General semiotics and biosemiotics. In: Semiotic Themes (Richard DeGeorge, ed.). Lawrence: Univ. of Kansas Press, pp. 225-250.
Jansen, G. (1973). The Doctor-Patient Relationship in an Africal Tribal Society. Assen, The Netherlands: Van Gorcum and Co.
Janzen, John (1973MS). Signs, symptoms and symbols: A semiotic interpretation of Kongo illness and therapy. Paper presented at Amer. Anth. Assoc. meetings, New Orleans.
Janzen, John M. (1974). Pluralistic legitimation of therapy systems in contemporary Zaire. Rural Africana. 26: 105-122.
Janzen, John M. (1978a). The Quest for Therapy. Medical Pluralism in Lower Zaire. Berkeley: Univ. of Calif. Press.

Janzen, John (1978b). The comparative study of medical systems as changing social systems. Social Science and Medicine, 12: 121-129.
Jenkins, Carol (1980MS). Maluntrition and spirits: *Umeo* among the Garifuna (Black Carib) of Belize. Paper presented at Amer. Anthrop. Assoc. meetings, December, 1980. Washington, D.C.
Kahn, Joan (1978). A diagnostic semiotic. Semiotica 22/1-2:75-106.
Kay, Margarita (1979). Lexemic change and semantic shift in disease names. Culture, Medicine and Psychiatry 3: 73-94.
Kerns, Virginia (1977). Daughters Bring In: Ceremonial and Social Organization of the Black Carib of Belize. Unpubl. Ph.D. Diss., University of Illinois, Urbana.
Kerns, Virginia (1984). Past and present evidence of interethnic mating. In; Current Developments in Anthropological Genetics: The Black Caribs, Vol. III (Michael Crawford, ed.). New York: Plenum Press.
Kimani, Violet Nyambura (1981). The unsystematic alternative: towards plural health care among the Kikuyu of central Africa. Social Science and Medicine 15B(3): 333-340.
Kleinman, Arthur (1973). Medicine's symbolic reality: On a central problem in the philosophy of medicine. Inquiry 16:206-213.
Kleinman, Arthur (1980). Patients and Healers in the Context of Culture. Berkeley: Univ. of Calif. Press.
Kleinman, Arthur, Leon Eisenberg and Byron Good. (1978). Culture, illness, and care: Clinical lessons from anthropological and cross-cultural research. Annals of Internal Medicine, 88: 251-258.
Krupp, Marcus and Milton Chatton (1981). Current Medical Diagnosis and Treatment. Los Altos, Calif.: Lange Medical Publishers.
Leslie, Charles (1977a). Pluralism and integration in the Indian and Chinese medical systems. In: Culture, Disease and Healing (David Landy, ed.). New York: MacMillan Publ. Co., 511-517.
Leslie, Charles (ed.) (1977b). Asian Medical Systems. Berkeley: Univ. of Calif. Press.
Lieberman, Dena and William W. Dressler (1977). Bilingualism and cognition of St. Lucian disease terms. Medical Anthropology, 1 (1):81-110.
Lin, Tsung-Yi, Kenneth Tardiff, George Donetz and Walter Goresky (1978). Ethnicity and patterns of health-seeking. Culture, Medicine and Psychiatry 2: 3-13.
Locker, David (1981). Symptoms and Illness: The Cognitive Organization of Disorder. New York and London: Tavistock.
Lotman, Ju M. (1976). Culture and information. Dispositio, 3(1): 213-215.
McCaffrey, Colin (1967). Potentialities for community development in a Kekchi Indian village in British Honduras. Unpubl. Ph.D. Diss., Univ. of Calif. at Berkeley.
MacCannell, Dean (1979). Ethnosemiotics. In: The Semiotics of Culture. (I.P. Winner and J. Umiker-Sebeok, eds.) The Hague: Mouton, pp. 149-172.
MacCannell, Dean and Juliet Flower MacCannell (1982). The Time of the Sign. A Semiotic Interpretation of Modern Culture. Bloomington: Indiana Univ. Press.
Mackenzie, W.J.M. (1976). Foreword. In: The Making of Modern Belize (C.H. Grant), pp. ix-xi.
Macklin, Catherine L. (1976). The Garifuna 'Thanksgiving'. Belizean Studies, 4(6): 1-6.
MacRae, Donald G. (1975). The body and social metaphor. In: The Body as a Medium of Expression. (Benthall and Polhemus, eds.) London: Allen Lane, pp. 59-73.
Mahaniah, J. Kimpianga M. (1981). La sturcture multi-dimesionnelle de guérison a Kinshasa, capitale du Zaire. Social Science and Medicine, 15B(3): 341-349.
Maranda, Pierre (1972). Introduction. In: Mythology (Pierre Maranda, ed.). Baltimore: Penguin Books, pp. 7-20.
Meillasoux, Claude (1981). Maidens, Meal and Money. Capitalism and the Domestic Community. New York, Cambridge Univ. Press.
Morris, Charles (1964). Signification and Significance. Cambridge, Mass.: MIT Press.
Morris, Charles (1971). Writings on the General Theory of Signs. The Hague: Mouton.
Nichter, Mark (1978). Patterns of resort in the use of therapy systems and their signifi-

cance for health planning in South Asia. Medical Anthropology, 2(2): 29-56.
Norton, Alan (1969). The New Dimensions of Medicine. London: Hodder and Stoughton.
Palacio, Joseph (1973). Carib ancestral rites: A brief analysis. National Studies, 1(3).
Palacio, Joseph (1982). Food and Social Relations in a Garifuna Village. Unpubl. Ph.D. Diss., Berkeley: Univ. of Calif.
Paul, Benjamin (ed.) (1955). Health, Culture and Community: Case Studies of Public Reactions to Health Programs. N.Y.: Russell Sage Foundation.
Polhemus, Ted (1975). Social bodies. In: The Body as a Medium of Expression (Jonathan Benthall and Ted Polhumus, eds.) London: Allen Lane, pp. 13-35.
Peirce, C.S. (1931-1958).Collected Papers of Charles Sanders Peirce, 8 vols. Cambridge Mass: Harvard Univ. Press.
Press, Irwin (1978). Bureaucracy versus folk medicine: Implications from Seville, Spain. In: Health and the Human Condition: Perspectives on Medical Anthropology (Michael Logan and Edward Hunt, eds.) North Scituate, Mass: Duxbury Press, pp. 376-387.
Press, Irwin (1980). Problems in the definition and classification of medical systems. Social Science and Medicine, 14B: 45-57.
Reid, Marlene (1982). Patient/healer interactions in Sukama medicine. In: African Health and Healing Systems: Proceedings of a Symposium. (P. Stanley Yoder, ed). Los Angeles: Crossroads Press, pp. 121-158.
Roberts, Christopher Davis (1981). *Kutambuwa Ugonjuwa*: Concepts of illness and transformation among the Tabwa of Zaire. Social Science and Medicine, 15B(3): 309-316.
Romanucci-Ross (Schwartz), Lola (1977). The hierarchy of resort in curative practices: The Admiralty Islands, Melanesia. In: Culture, Disease and Healing (David Landy, ed.). N.Y.: Macmillan Publ. Co., pp. 481-487.
Rubenstein, Edward (1980). Diseases caused by impaired communication among cells. Scientific American 242(3): 106-113.
Sanford, Margaret (1976MS). Disease and folk-curing among the Garifuna of Belize. Paper presented at Intnl. Congress of Americanists, Paris.
Sebeok, Thomas (1976). Contributions to the Doctrine of Signs. Bloomington: Indiana Univ. Publications: Studies in Semiotics, Vol. 5.
Sebeok, Thomas (ed.) (1978). Sight, Sound and Sense. Bloomington: Indiana Univ. Press.
Sebeok, Thomas A. (1984). Symptom. In: New Directions in Linguistics and Semiotics (James Copeland, ed.) Houston: Rice University, pp. 211-230.
Sedgwick, Peter (1973). Illness – mental and otherwise. Hastings Center Studies 1(3): 19-40.
Shands, Harley C. (1970). Semiotic Approaches to Psychiatry. The Hague: Mouton.
Shands, Harley C. (1978). Verbal patterns and medical disease: Prophylactic implications of learning. In: Sight, Sound, and Sense (T.A. Sebeok, ed.). Bloomington: Indiana Univ. Press, pp. 175-200.
Shands, Harley and James Meltzer (1973). Language and Psychiatry. The Hague: Mouton (Janua Linguarum V. 165).
Shands, Harley and James Meltzer (1977). Unexpected semiotic implications of medical inquiry. In: A Perfusion of Signs (T.A. Sebeok, ed.). Bloomington: Indiana Univ. Press, pp. 77-89.
Shedlin, Michele G. (1977). Body image and contraceptive acceptability in a Mexican community. Paper presented at the Symposium: Body Concepts and Implications for Health, AAA Annual Meetings, Houston.
Skidmore, Arthur (1981). Peirce and semiotics: An introduction to Peirce's theory of signs. In: Semiotic Themes. (Richard DeGeorge, ed.). Lawrence; Univ. of Kansas Press, pp. 33-50.
Sidel, Victor and Ruth Sidel (1972). The human services in China. Social Policy, March/April, pp. 25-34.
Singer, Milton (1984). Man's Glassy Essence: Explorations in Semiotic Anthropology. Bloomington: Indiana Univ. Press.

Sontag, Susan (1978). Illness as Metaphor. N.Y.: Farrar, Straus and Giroux.

Staiano, Kathryn Vance (1979a). A semiotic definition of illness. Semiotica 28(1-2): 107-125.

Staiano, Kathryn Vance (1979b). A semiotic approach to ritual drama. Semiotica 28 (3/4):225-246.

Staiano, Kathryn Vance. (1981). Alternative therapeutic systems in Belize: a semiotic framework. Social Science and Medicine, 15B (3): 317-332.

Staiano, Kathryn Vance (1982). Medical semiotics: Redefining an ancient craft. Semiotica 38(3/4): 319-346.

Sussman, Linda K. (1981). Unity in diversity in a polyethnic society; the maintenance of medical pluralism on Mauritius. Social Science and Medicine 15B(3): 247-260.

Szasz, Thomas (1970). Ideology and Insanity: Essays on the Psychiatric Dehumanization of Man. Garden City, N.Y.: Anchor Books.

Szasz, Thomas (1973). Mental illness as a metaphor. Nature 242: 305-307.

Szasz, Thomas (1974). The Myth of Mental Illness. New York: Harper and Row (Rev. Ed.).

Szasz, Thomas (1976). Schizophrenia, The Sacred Symbol of Psychiatry. New York: Basic Books.

Taylor, Douglas MacRae (1951). The Black Carib of British Honduras. New York: Viking Fund Publications in Anthropology, No. 17.

Thomas, Lewis (1974). The Lives of a Cell. N.Y.: Bantam Books.

Thomas, Lewis (1979). The Medusa and the Snail: More Notes of a Biology Watcher. N.Y.: Bantam Books.

Turner, Victor (1967). Forest of Symbols. Ithaca, N.Y.: Cornell Univ. Press.

Turner, Victor (1968). Drums of Affliction. Oxford: Clarendon Press.

Twumasi, Patrick (1979). A social history of the Ghanaian pluralistic medical system. Medical Anthropology, 13B (Special Issue) (4): 349

Unschuld, Paul (1975). Medico-cultural conflicts in Asian settings: an explanatory theory. Social Science and Medicine, 9: 303-312.

Von Uexküll, Thure (1982). Semiotics and medicine. Semiotica 38(3/4): 205-215.

Waitzkin, Howard B. and Barbara Waterman (1974). The Exploitation of Illness in Capitalist Society. N.Y.: The Bobbs-Merrill Co.

Watzlawick, Paul, J.H. Beavin, and D. D. Jackson (1967). Pragmatics of Human Communication. New York: W.W. Norton and Co.

Wells, Marilyn M. (1980). Circling with the ancestors: Hugulendii symbolism in ethnic group maintenance. Belizean Studies 8(6): 1-9.

Wells, Marilyn M. (1982a). *Dugu* visibility: the role of a religious ceremony in status politics. Tennessee Anthropologist 7: 75-88.

Wells, Marilyn M. (1982b). The symbolic use of *guseue* among the Garif (Black Carib) of Central America. Anthropological Quarterly 55(1): 44-55.

Whipple, Emory (1976). Pia Manadi. Belizean Studies, Vol. 4, No. 4: 1-18.

Winner, I.P. and T.G. Winner (1976). The semiotics of cultural texts. Semiotica, 18: 101-156.

Winner, Irene Portis (1979). Ethnicity, modernity and theory of culture texts. In: Semiotics of Culture (I.P. Winner and Jean Umiker-Sebeok, eds.) The Hague: Mouton Publ.: 103-148.

Woods, Clyde M. (1977). Alternative curing strategies in a changing medical situation. Medical Anthropology, 1(3) 25-54.

Young, Allan (1982). The Amhara medical system. In: African Health and Healing Systems: Proceedings of a Symposium. (P. Stanley Yoder, ed.) Los Angeles: Crossroads Press, pp. 21-41.

Appendix A

Additional Expressions Used in Discussions of Illness or Presentation of Signs

My head feels funny
I have an uncomfortable feeling in my stomach.
I felt cold on my stomach
I spit up mucus
I had a stomach infection
I had a kidney problem
I urine all the time
I am thirsty all the time
I felt my mouth twitch
I get a jerk on my toe and it turned bad
I feel weak on my knees
I have a strain on my leg
I have sickness inside privates from strain when I fell down.
I have a boil inside
I have a bad sickness
I feel hot in the night
I have sweet blood
He had arthritis pain in the joints from time he was small
I feel weak
She doesn't have passage for baby
My mind is not settled
This is an unexpected illness [uncommon]
I feel gripe inside my body
He has uncontrollable behavior
There is something wrong in the brain
The body is reducing
I can't swallow
I have eaten something against the body
Something acted on the nerves
Her illness was nerves
I suffer from lack of sleep
He isn't eating properly
I have backache

I have stoppage of water
She is talking foolish
I am unable to move about
He is out his senses
The outer part of the body broke out with little bumps
My body feels heavy
The mind is not contented
The heart is not functioning good
The blood looks waterish
I had a blood rash
The blood leaves the womb and clots down, gets solid
The heart pumps the blood too slow
I have hemorrhage from the nose
My heart is jumping
I don't feel like to do anything
I have a cold in the womb
My eyes are running water
I feel like my leg is sleeping
I think someone is tampering with me [*obeah, abiñariguile*]
My blood is low
My blood is poor
My blood is weak
I have high blood
I feel my brains are coming out of my head
The sight in my eye is dim
I have a bad feeling
Things get blurred
I have liver trouble
It hurts when I try to read
I can't see so far
The skin feel as if something walk over me
My whole body hurts
I am feeling feverish
The heart trembles
I feel my stomach open
My eyes are going bad
The fever flies in the head like crazy
I have pressing of the heart
The heart beats like bop, bop
Eyes straining like when looking at something
I have low blood pressure
He was stillborn from an eclipse of the moon
He had water head from an eclipse of the moon
Feels like my heart is beating fast at night
Talks funny and does unpredicatable things
There was a chafe on my neck like a rash, but deeper
I felt dizzy as though something around the ear was sick
I feel trembling in my body
I feel my heart beating hard
I feel discouraged
He is not so strong
He isn't so sound from inside
The navel swollen like a hernia
He has bumps on the lower eyelid
I have watering eyes
I have liver spots from dirty blood

I have tingling in my hands
I have numbness in my hands
I have cramps over my entire body
My joints hurt
I feel my head swinging
I don't feel strong
My tongue is swollen
The mouth is twitching
I feel my head heavy
My food won't digest
I have cramps inside from chills
I don't have no appetite
I have pain in all the joints
I am unrestful from the illness
He has choking from asthma
I feel like there are blunt needles in my foot

Appendix B

Patent Preparations and Biomedically Justified Preparations

Tonics

Mattelvol
3 S's - also tonic for children's blood
Phosferine Tablets
Agapodium
Codol
Multiple 12
Seven Seas - also to exercise veins, nerves, bones
Iron and Yeast Tablets - tonic for children
Geritol
Scott's Emulsion - tonic for children
Ruby Wine
Liquifruta - tonic for children
Beet Iron and Wine
Confrom 12
Ferrol
One-a-Day - vitamins, tonic
Polyvisol - for children
Glucodin - for weakness

External Use Only [Sores, Wounds, Pain, Sprains]

Cuticura powder
Benque
Bay Rum
Alcohol
Carbonegros soap
Detol
Penicillin ointment
Sulphur
Thermogene
Camphor

Internal and External Use [Multiple Uses]

Vicks Vapo-Rub
Dr. Castro's Balsalm
Benjamin's Healing Oil
Linament

Purge

P.L.
DeWitts
Castor Oil
Brooklet's Tablets
Magnesia
Epsom salts

Pain, generalized

Anacin
Aspro
APC
Aspirin
Phrensic
Chases

Upset Stomach, Pain in the Stomach

Alka-Seltzer
Andrews
Eno

Fever

Aspirin
Phrensic
Aspro
Anacin
APC

Worms

DeWitts
Tetrax

Pressure

Andrews
Aspirin

Cough

Formula 44

Heart

Red Lavinda

Women's Problems (?)

Dr. Rose's Pills

Loose Stools

Sulfaguidine

Undetermined

Clorodine

Appendix C

Medicines used in Bush Preparations

NOTE: This list includes items which are not, strictly speaking, "bush" medicines, that is, they are not all plants or plant products. Nevertheless, they are utilized as components in bush medicines or constitute a component of what is generally referred to as bush medicine. Not all uses have been listed. Many of these items are combined, though any may be used alone. No attempt was made to determine the scientific name for any of these items.

Piece-of-Eight - poor blood
Sink am Bible - diabetes
Mint - upset stomach
Mayflower (with bluing, coconut leaf, seawater, to cure child who couldn't walk)
Coconut leaf (see Mayflower)
Gangwao - belly ache, blood, causes an erection in men and said to stimulate sexual desire in women
Hammond's Leaf (also Almond's Leaf) - for high blood pressure
Jackass bitters - purge, remove inside cold, diabetes, fever, tonic, bathe with contrebo, jackass bitters to feel good; for giddiness
Contrebo - purge, remove inside cold, diabetes, tonic, to give appetite, fever, to build blood, malaria, senility
Billy Web bark - purge, remove inside cold, diabetes (also used with several other bush: jackass, contrebo, sorasee, palo de hombre) cleaning out, give appetite
Sorasee - pressure, purify blood, diabetes, rub on sores, purge, tonic, pain in belly, cleaning after baby, fever, clean stomach, with garlic for worms, with water for inflammation, with Marigold and Fresh Cut for asthma, with orange skin and garlic for pain in belly; with epsom salts for flame in belly, itch
Coconut water - from green coconuts, to cause someone to pass urine
Cow Foot leaf - rub to bring warmth to cold site; sprain, helps keep heart on a cool system, used for treatment of uncommon illnesses
Custard Apple leaf - bind on affected area for pain
Palo de Hombre - to cause an erection in men, for diabetes (with Billy Web)
Provision bark - builds blood
Fever grass - for fever, high blood pressure
Apasote - worms, relief of pain (external), fever, pain in stomach
Onion-like plant (unnamed) - mixed with coconut milk, garlic for sores (external application), drunk for asthma
Skagineal - for headaches

Tree-of-Life - for headache - applied externally
Marigold - with Fresh Cut and sorasee for asthma
Fresh Cut - see above
Corn - burned and dried with fresh cow's milk for weakness and for blood
Bokut leaf - pressure (with Hammond's leaf and garlic), for pressure (with Pia leaf and Matapalo)
China root - tonic, develops blood
Sour orange - for cooling in summer
Cashuneen - draws heat out of body
Grapefruit - for diabetes
Senna - purge
Scandinine - headache, to draw heat out, for hemorrhoids (external or ingested), stops blood in stool
Banana with skin, boiled - for vitamins
Matapalo (with pia leaf) for pain in back; (with bokut) for pressure
Pia leaf - with matapalo for pain in back
Tunna - for headache, applied externally
Ruda - with mint for vexation
Mountain cow hoof - with garlic, rum, nutmeg to cure "tongue strung up from vexation"
Piñon leaf - blisters inside mouth
Amansoza - for cold on the stomach
Hirusulu - for chest cold
Yababwano - loose stools and vomiting
Ganabis root - purge, cold stomach, dysentery, poor blood
Ganabis leaf - purge, itch, backache (with ganabis root, epsom salts, sorasee, and cream of tartar)
Caro - high blood pressure
Makakao leaf - for sores
Gahela leaf (with guava skin for vomiting [emetic])
Guava skin - see above
Trumpet leaf - cough (with garlic)
Ganapistola - for too much heat in the body
Christ's Cane - sores on body, dropsy, to wash the blood
Gombo limbo (*tura heurunai*) bark - for sore inside
Balsalm copayba -purge
Santa Maria leaf - clean insides (probably same as Cow Foot leaf)
Siwapat - pain in joints, insect bites, twisted veins and swelling
Cabbage bark - poor blood
Guava leaf - stops vomiting
Olivera - bitters
Vine-of-Life - for headache (probably same as Tree-of-Life)
Mesina - reduces swelling
Bongolingo gum - for purge (same as gombo limbo?)
Maliba - headache, applied esternally
Dunginau - coughs
Hibiscus - tonic
Worm plant - worms
Gumbolibo milk of breadfruit tree (?) - for pain in back
Roseapple leaf - for pressure
Mangrove (gurura) - to treat *idáhadu*
Crabu bark - to treat *obeah*
Two-cat-tails - to treat *idáhadu*
Garlic titie, garlic leaves - to keep spirits away, for blood
Flor de muerte - fever, mix with rum and rub body for fever, evil spirits, headache, causes sweating
Umiala - to get rid of evil spirits

Cashew bark - to get rid of evil spirits
Oudlice (hamuterie?) - protects against evil spirits
Essence root - protects against evil spirits, keeps spirits in check
Bue - tobacco smoked during *dugu*
Bisi nut - pain in belly; taken to avoid poisonings
Cedar bark - evil spirits, treatment of *idáhadu*, inside injuries
Copali - to keep evil spirits in check
Waiuri - *idáhadu*, evil spirits, treatment of miscellaneous illnesses
Lamuru - *idáhadu*, evil spirits, miscellaneous illnesses
Haliwalu - to get rid of evil spirits
Lime - rubbed on head for pressure; also used for asthma with cocount oil and linament; rubbed on head for headache; use with epsom salts for purge; used for relief of pain (external application), nausea
Aniseed (same as anise?) - used with Billy Web Bark, contrebo as a tonic in the morning, gives appetite
Asafetida - used with contrebo, aniseed, garlic
Nutmeg - applied to infant's navel after birth
Anise, baby oil - to be swallowed by babies after birth to clean them out
Black tea and Cod Liver Oil - for loose stools
Clavo, anise, romero - for change of life
Eggs and nutmeg - applied as plaster for mole drop
Spice seed (aniseed?) - for women after birth of child
Honey - liver trouble, sores in the mouth
Guinea pepper - pain in the belly
Cream of tartar - with epsom salts, ganabis leaf and root - for purge
Shark's oil - for tuberculosis
Tiger fat - for asthma
Olive oil - for nointing
Coconut oil, linament - for tonsils, external massage, asthma
Mint (peppermint?) - for stomach
Bluing - for salve
Ginger - pain in the stomach (with garlic)
Garlic - for evil spirits, pain in the stomach, wind, gas, with sorasee for worms
Honey, soft candle wax, and nutmeg - for cough
Turpentine, raw rum, alcohol, bitter ginger - used as massage following stroke
Pumble stone - burned in fire, put in well water, strained water drunk for palpitations
Quicksilver - prevention against enemies (inserted under skin)
Spanish medicine: mansinilla, ginger, nutmeg, garlic, aniseed, clavo, romero, alosema - to clean woman after baby; to pass wind; 'Recipes' for Spanish medicine differed across informants
Achote - used externally to heal sores
Seaweed - used as a tonic and to cause an erection in men
Pepper - appendicitis, cancer, purges nicotine
Corn water - chicken pox, measles, used as coolant for system
Pineapple - used to treat a cold in the penis
Sweet basil - earache
Soft candle wax - sprain
Alum - sores for body, plaster for heat in head, sores in the mouth
Eggshells - cataracts
Kerosene - asthma
Altamisa - used after birth
Sweet oil - takes old cold, earache
Boiled rat - asthma
Conch shell - gets rid of evil spirits
Licorice - cough

Index

Bei Fragen zur Produktsicherheit wenden Sie sich bitte an:
If you have any questions regarding product safety,
please contact:

Walter de Gruyter GmbH
Genthiner Straße 13
10785 Berlin
productsafety@degruyterbrill.com